ARCO

NURSING SCHOOL AND ALLIED HEALTH ENTRANCE EXAMINATIONS

15th Edition

ARCO

NURSING SCHOOL AND ALLIED HEALTH ENTRANCE EXAMINATIONS

15th Edition

Marion F. Gooding, RN, Ph.D.
Professor of Nursing
North Carolina Central University
Durham, North Carolina

CONTRIBUTING EDITORS

Mattie Moss, Ed.D.
Mathematics

Leslie Maduro-Davis, B.A.
Mathematics

Charles R. George, Ph.D.
Life Sciences

Sumana Banerjee, Ph.D.
Biology

Duana A. Dreyer, Ph.D.
Anatomy and Physiology

James M. Schooler, Ph.D.
Chemistry

Doris E. Wilson, B.A.
Language Arts

THOMSON ™
ARCO

Australia • Canada • Mexico • Singapore • Spain • United Kingdom • United States

THOMSON

ARCO

An ARCO Book

ARCO is a registered trademark of Thomson Learning, Inc., and is used herein under license by Peterson's.

About The Thomson Corporation and Peterson's

With revenues of US$7.2 billion, The Thomson Corporation (www.thomson.com) is a leading global provider of integrated information solutions for business, education, and professional customers. Its Learning businesses and brands (www.thomsonlearning.com) serve the needs of individuals, learning institutions, and corporations with products and services for both traditional and distributed learning.

Peterson's, part of The Thomson Corporation, is one of the nation's most respected providers of lifelong learning online resources, software, reference guides, and books. The Education Supersite℠ at www.petersons.com—the Internet's most heavily traveled education resource—has searchable databases and interactive tools for contacting U.S.-accredited institutions and programs. In addition, Peterson's serves more than 105 million education consumers annually.

For more information, contact Peterson's, 2000 Lenox Drive, Lawrenceville, NJ 08648; 800-338-3282; or find us on the World Wide Web at www.petersons.com/about.

Fifteenth Edition

Library of Congress Number: 9503-6421

ISBN: 0-02-863542-6

Printed in the United States of America

9 8 7 04 03

CONTENTS

Part I

INFORMATION ABOUT NURSING AND ALLIED HEALTH PROGRAMS AND ENTRANCE EXAMINATIONS

ABOUT THE NURSING PROFESSION

SELECTING A NURSING CAREER

Regardless of which kind of nursing program you choose to enter, you will have opportunities to provide an important service to humanity. You may enter nursing at one level and expand your skills through practice and additional education. Advancement within the nursing profession comes about in several ways. A practical nurse may decide to become a registered nurse, an upward move. A registered nurse may decide to move from the hospital setting into community-based care, a horizontal move that expands the types of services a nurse can provide. A registered nurse who does not have a baccalaureate degree may decide to earn one in order to step up to a management position.

There are four kinds of programs that prepare for entrance into nursing:

The practical-nurse programs are usually offered in vocational schools, hospitals, and community colleges. The program varies from 9 to 18 months. The courses include the basic sciences and medical-surgical, pediatric, and obstetrical nursing. Some mental-health concepts are included. The major focus is on technical skills. A practical nurse works under the supervision of a registered nurse (RN).

The associate-degree nurse is a graduate of a two-year college program that is designed with a balance between clinical nursing courses (medical, surgical, psychiatric, obstetrical, and pediatric nursing) and general-education courses (biological and physical sciences, behavioral sciences, humanities, and electives) to provide a background for making important judgments about patient care. The graduate is prepared for technical expertise in the assessment, planning, and delivery of direct patient care in the hospital setting.

The graduate of the hospital-based diploma program functions on the nursing team in the same manner as the associate-degree nurse. Most diploma programs are 24 to 30 months in length, and the non-nursing courses may be offered through a college.

The baccalaureate nursing program is four years in length and is offered in senior colleges and universities. The required courses in the biological, physical, and behavioral sciences are both basic and advanced. These general-education requirements, along with courses that provide a broad liberal-arts background, are taken during the first two years. The major clinical courses are offered in the third and fourth years and include the five clinical areas identified above, with an emphasis on community-health nursing and the role of the professional nurse as a manager. Most nursing programs offering the professional baccalaureate degree admit graduates from the diploma and associate degree programs with varying degrees of advanced standing.

The graduates of all four programs take a licensing examination. At the present time, there are two kinds of licenses: the practical-nurse license and the registered-nurse license for graduates of the diploma, associate degree, and baccalaureate degree programs.

A nurse may continue studies to receive a master's degree and a doctorate with a major in clinical specialties, teaching, administration, or research, depending on his or her career choice. There is a great demand for nurses in hospitals, schools, clinics, public-health agencies, and many other settings throughout the world. Nurses may become anesthetists, enter the military, or become writers, consultants, or private practitioners. Nursing provides a basis for many careers and, more importantly, a personally and financially satisfying experience.

SELECTING A NURSING PROGRAM

The first factor you should take into consideration is your career goal. Do you plan to work in hospitals as a member of the health team? Is your ultimate goal to function as a manager or an administrator? Are you primarily interested in teaching? Do you want to specialize in a specific clinical area? Are you planning to work in a community setting providing services to families? Is your ultimate goal to become an entrepreneur?

The rapidly moving trend in nursing today is to license two levels of nursing for entry into the professional services. The assistant level will be represented by graduates of the associate degree nursing programs; the professional level, by graduates of the baccalaureate nursing programs. Baccalaureate education in nursing forms the foundation for graduate education in nursing, where specialization as a clinical practitioner, administrator, and teacher occurs. Other types of graduates (practical nurse and diploma) will achieve these credentials through career mobility programs.

A second factor to consider is costs. The demands for full-time study and the length of the program may necessitate resigning from your job.

A third factor is whether you qualify for admission. As the levels of performance increase, so do the academic requirements. In some cases, a student may enter at the associate degree level and upon graduating and receiving a license (RN), enter the baccalaureate program because the requirements are different for the RNs.

Once you have matched your career with a program, you should use the guidelines listed below to make your final choice.

1. Is the program approved by the state regulating body (Board of Nursing)?
2. Is the program accredited by a voluntary agency (National League for Nursing)?
3. What is the program's reputation in terms of graduate performance?
4. How does the social and academic environment meet your needs?

SELECTING AN ALLIED HEALTH PROGRAM

Occupations related to allied health are rapidly expanding. The criteria for selecting a program are similar to those for nursing:

1. If a license is required to practice, be certain that the program is approved by the regulating body.
2. Check to see if the program is accredited by the appropriate voluntary agency.
3. Find out how well the graduates are performing on the licensing examination.
4. How well does the program meet your short- and long-term career goals?

The most popular allied health careers are described below.

Occupation	Work Description	Education Needed
Clinical and Medical Lab Technician	Perform tests in labs to get information for doctors to use. Use chemicals, microscopes, and other technical equipment.	OJT, Two-Year CC, Bachelor's, Master's
Emergency Medical Technician	Administer first aid treatment to sick or injured persons and transport them to medical facilities. Work as a member of an emergency medical team.	OJT, One-Year CC, Two-Year CC

Occupation	Work Description	Education Needed
Medical Lab Technician	Perform routine tests in medical laboratories for use in the treatment and diagnosis of diseases.	OJT, Two-Year CC, Bachelor's, Master's
Medical Record Technician	Compile and maintain medical records of hospital clinic patients.	OJp, Two-Year CC
Occupational Therapist	Plan, organize, and conduct programs to facilitate rehabilitation of mentally, physically, or emotionally handicapped people.	Bachelor's, Master's
Physical Therapist	Plan, organize, and administer treatment in order to restore mobility and prevent and relieve pain for those suffering from a disabling injury or disease.	Bachelor's, Master's
Radiologic Technologist	Take x-rays to help doctors diagnose illness. Also use radioactive materials to treat patients.	Two-Year CC
Respiratory Therapist	Specialize in the evaluation, treatment, and care of patients with breathing disorders.	Two-Year CC, Bachelor's

Key: OJT-On the Job Training, CC-Community College, HS-High School.

FINANCIAL AID SOURCES

With the increasing costs of education, and the decreasing federal sources for financial aid, the competition for funds is increasing. It is therefore important to know what the sources are, the eligibility requirements, and how to apply. It is also important to apply as early as possible to a variety of programs.

To initiate the application process, get a financial aid form from your local high school counseling office, or directly from the school to which you are seeking admission. This form must be completed and mailed to the *College Scholarship Service* (address is on the form). In approximately six weeks, a report is sent back that identifies whether you are eligible for financial aid. This report must be sent to the school of your selection so that the amount you are eligible for and amount you will have to pay can be determined.

The amount of money a recipient can receive is dependent on the need analysis derived from the financial aid form and the financial aid program in which the nursing school, college, or university is participating. The school usually prepares a financial aid package that is a combination of financial sources to make up for the difference between the amount the student is able to contribute and the total costs for the nursing program.

Some financial aid programs are loans, which must be paid back at a low interest rate over a prolonged period of time. Other sources are grants and scholarships, which do not have to be paid back. The obligation for debt payment requires serious thought on the part of the student since a default can affect his or her credit ranking.

When shopping for financial aid, check the accreditation status of the nursing program and the institution's eligibility for such aid. All nursing programs accredited by the National League for Nursing are eligible for federal funding, but some institutions have limited federal sources due to high default rates.

FEDERAL SOURCES OF FINANCIAL AID

Pell Grants are awarded to undergraduate students who have not previously earned a degree. The grant does not have to be repaid and may be supplemented by other funds. Eligibility is based on need which is calculated by a formula. The amount of the awards vary yearly and depend on program funding. The maximum award in 1997–98 was $2,700 per year. You do not have to be a full-time student.

Direct and FFEL Stafford Loans

These federal loans are of two kinds; subsidized awarded on the basis of need with no interest before you start repayment, and unsubsidized which is not based on need and you will be charged interest from the time the loan is disbursed. Dependent students may borrow $2,625 the first year, $3,500 the second year, and $5,500 the third and the fourth year. Independent students may receive $6,625 the first year, $7,500 the second year, and $10,500 a year for the remaining two years.

Plus Loans

Plus loans enable parents with good credit histories to borrow to pay the education expenses of each child who is a dependent undergraduate student enrolled at least half time. The yearly time is equal to your cost of attendance minus any other financial aid received.

Consolidation Loans

These loans are designed to help the students and parents simplify loan repayment by allowing the borrowers to consolidate several types of federal loans in one loan with one payment schedule.

Campus-Based Programs (Administered by Financial Aid Office)

- **Federal Supplemental Educational Opportunity Grants (SEOG)** are for undergraduates with exceptional financial need and give priority to students who received Federal Pell Grants. You can receive between $100 and $4,000 a year depending on need, the financial level of the school, and the financial aid policies.
- **Federal Work Study** provides a work-study program for undergraduates and graduate students in financial need. Students are allowed to earn money through community service and work related to your course of study.
- **Federal Perkins Loan** is a low-interest (5 percent) loan for both undergraduate and graduate students with exceptional financial need. Your school is the lender and the loan must be repaid to the school. Loans may be granted in the amount of $3,000 for each year of undergraduate study up to $15,000, and $5,000 each year of graduate/professional study up to $30,000.

For additional information on federal loans call 1-800-4-FED-AID or pick-up from your local campus financial aid office, *The Student Guide: Financial Aid*, from the U.S. Department of Education.

OTHER SOURCES OF FINANCIAL AID

Your public library is a good source for identifying foundations, religious organizations, fraternities and sororities, and civic groups that provide scholarships and/or loans for educational purposes. In addition, the military offers scholarships through the ROTC Program. You should also seek sources from the organizations related to your field of interest. Your program of choice can provide specific information and assistance.

SPECIAL FEATURES OF THIS BOOK

SIMULATED TESTS

By studying the more than 1,300 test questions in this book, which are similar to the items included in the entrance examinations, you will review material already learned, gain new knowledge, and become familiar with the format of timed tests. The sections for the registered-nurse and practical-nurse examinations are separated; however, the entire book may be used to prepare for all examinations.

TEST-TAKING SKILLS

By following the guidelines presented on test-taking skills, you will be able to increase your chances for success by using the "educated guess" technique.

PRESENTATION OF BASIC CONCEPTS

The verbal ability, mathematics, and science sections include a summary of basic facts, principles, and concepts related to the content area. This provides a study guide and helps you select correct answers.

EXPLANATORY ANSWERS

For selected tests, explanations of the correct answers are given. This provides another opportunity to reinforce principles which apply to the test items.

SPECIAL FEATURES OF THE FIFTEENTH EDITION

- New section for Allied Health exams
- Updated test material
- Expanded contributions from distinguished item writers
- New section on test taking skills and techniques
- Complete and updated information on financial aid
- Hundreds of new test question items

ABOUT THE EXAMINATIONS

Registered nursing programs, practical/vocational nursing programs, and allied health programs require different entrance examinations.

For registered nursing programs, you may be required to take either the Entrance Examination for Schools of Nursing (RNEE), the Pre-Admission Examination-RN, the PSB-Nursing School Aptitude Examination (RN), or the Nurse Entrance Test (NET). All exams evaluate the academic ability of applicants in key areas of the basic nursing curriculum. For information about the RNEE, write to:

The Psychological Corporation
555 Academic Court
San Antonio, Texas 78204-2498

For information about the Pre-Admission Examination-RN, write to:
National League for Nursing
350 Hudson Street
New York, New York 10014

For information about the PSB-Nursing School Aptitude Examination (RN), write to:
Psychological Services Bureau
P.O. Box 327
St. Thomas, Pennsylvania 17252

For information about the Nurse Entrance Test, write to:
Educational Resources, Inc.
10200 W. 75th Street
Shawnee Mission, Kansas 66204

The entrance examinations for practical/vocational nursing programs assess your knowledge of areas essential to the basic practical/vocational nursing curriculum. You may be required to take either the Entrance Examination for Schools of Practical/Vocational Nursing (PNEE), the Pre-Admission Examination-PN, or the PSB-Aptitude for Practical Nursing Examination. For information about the PNEE, write to the Psychological Corporation. For information about the Pre-Admission Examination-PN, write to the National League for Nursing. For information about the PSB-Aptitude for Practical Nursing Examination, write to the Psychological Services Bureau.

Allied health programs entrance examinations measure academic ability and scientific knowledge in order to identify qualified applicants. The Allied Health Admissions Test (AHPAT) is administered by the Psychological Corporation; the Psychological Services Bureau offers the PSB-Health Occupations Aptitude Examination.

CONTENT AND FORMAT OF THE EXAMINATIONS

Registered Nursing Entrance Exams

The Psychological Corporation's Entrance Examination for Schools of Nursing (RNEE) contains approximately 230 multiple-choice questions, and takes about three and one-half hours. The proctor arranges for a break midway through the test. The test format is as follows:

Test Section	Content	# of Questions
Verbal Ability	Uses synonym and antonym identification to measure vocabulary and verbal reasoning.	Approximately 50 questions
Numerical Ability	Emphasizes arithmetic operations including word problems, percentages and fractions, and fundamental algebra and geometry.	Approximately 40 questions
Life Sciences	Focuses on principles and concepts of the biological sciences specifically related to body structure and functions, heredity and development, microorganisms and health.	Approximately 40 questions

Test Section	Content	# of Questions
Physical Sciences	Measures understanding of principles and concepts of chemistry and physics, which includes the nature of matter, changes, and energy.	Approximately 40 questions
Reading Skill	Determines ability to draw inferences, interpret, and evaluate reading passages from natural and social sciences.	Approximately 45 questions

NOTE: Occasionally, there is an extra experimental section included on the exam. It will be based on one of the five content areas. This section has no effect on your score; however, you will not be told which section is the experimental one.

The National League for Nursing's Pre-Admission Examination-RN contains three multiple-choice tests and takes approximately three and one-half hours. The test format is as follows:

Section	Content	Time
Verbal Ability (2 Subtests)	1. Word knowledge: uses word identification to test vocabulary. 2. Reading comprehension: presents five reading passages of a scientific or general nature; tests ability to identify main idea and supporting details, and to analyze and interpret material.	Approximately one hour
Mathematics	Includes computation and word problems; emphasizes proportions, decimals, percentages, basic algebra and geometry.	Approximately one hour
Science	Measures understanding of general principles of biology, chemistry, physics, general science.	Approximately one hour

NOTE: Experimental items are included that do not affect your test score.

The Psychological Services Bureau's Nursing School Aptitude Examination (RN) contains five tests and three subtests, and takes about one hour and forty-five minutes. The test format is as follows:

Test Section	Content	# of Questions
Academic Aptitude (3 Subtests)	1. Verbal: emphasizes vocabulary-related questions. 2. Arithmetic: focuses on skill and computational speed with arithmetic. 3. Non-Verbal: deals with recognizing relationships and differences between objects; measures mental manipulation and reasoning.	Subtest 1: 30 questions Subtest 2: 30 questions Subtest 3: 30 questions

Test Section	Content	# of Questions
Spelling	Measures written expression or communication skills.	50 questions
Reading Comprehension	Determines ability to interpret passages, understand direct statements, infer ideas and purposes, and derive author's intent.	40 questions
Information in the Natural Sciences	Tests understanding of biology, chemistry, health, safety, etc., at an elementary level.	90 questions
Vocational Adjustment Index	Ascertains an individual's characteristic lifestyle by examining his or her educational and occupational adjustment.	90 questions

The Nurse Entrance Test (NET) given by Educational Resources is the newest type of entrance examination for registered nursing programs. It takes approximately two and one-half hours and is divided into seven subtests. Of these, three cover subjects considered to be *cognitive* (related to knowledge and achievement), and four cover subjects considered to be *noncognitive* (related to psychological-social factors). You do not have to study for the noncognitive tests. The test format is as follows:

Type	Subtest	Content
COGNITIVE	Essential Math Skills	Tests basic arithmetic operations including whole numbers, fractions, decimals, percentages, ratios, and basic algebra.
	Reading Comprehension Skills	Evaluates inferential reading level for science-related material; reading passages have a tenth-grade level of vocabulary and sentence syntax.
	Reading Rate	Estimates the number of words per minute that the student is able to read in a test or study situation.
NONCOGNITIVE	Test-Taking Skills	Measures student abilities to write objective, essay, and standardized examinations.
	Stress Level Profile	Judges student's ability to cope with five personal stressors: family life, social life, the work place, academics, and time/money.
	Social Interaction Profile	Assesses passive and aggressive social interaction attitudes of the student within a group.
	Learning Style Inventory	Determines auditory, visual, group, solitary, oral and writing dependent learner styles.

Practical Nursing Entrance Exams

The Entrance Examination for Schools of Practical/Vocational Nursing (PNEE) given by the Psychological Corporation contains approximately 300 multiple-choice questions, and takes about three and one-half hours, including a break period. The test format is as follows:

Test Section	Content	# of Questions
Verbal Ability	Uses synonym and antonym identification to measure vocabulary and verbal reasoning.	Approximately 75 questions
Numerical Ability	Emphasizes arithmetic operations including word problems, percentages and ratios, and fundamental algebra. Focuses on understanding and applying quantitative concepts and relationships.	Approximately 60 questions
Science	Measures understanding of principles and concepts of biology, chemistry, health, and the physical sciences.	Approximately 75 questions
Reading Skill	Determines ability to read and understand passages from natural and social sciences.	Approximately 45 questions

NOTE: Occasionally, there is an extra experimental section included on the exam. It will be based on one of the five content areas. This section has no effect on your score; however, you will not be told which section is the experimental one.

The National League for Nursing's Pre-Admission Examination-PN has the same test format as their registered nursing exam; however, its contents are at a level appropriate for applicants to practical/vocational programs. The test format is as follows:

Test Section	Content	Time
Verbal Ability (2 Subtests)	1. Word knowledge: uses word identification to test vocabulary. 2. Reading comprehension: presents five reading passages of a scientific or general nature: tests ability to identify main idea and supporting details, and to analyze and interpret material.	Approximately one hour
Mathematics	Includes computation and word problems; emphasizes proportions, decimals, percentages, basic algebra and geometry.	Approximately one hour
Science	Measures understanding of general principles of biology, chemistry, physics, general science.	Approximately one hour

NOTE: Experimental items are included that do not affect your test score.

The Psychological Services Bureau's Aptitude for Practical Nursing Examination contains five tests and three subtests, and takes about two hours and fifteen minutes. The test format is as follows:

Test Section	Content	# of Questions
Academic Aptitude (3 Subtests)	1. Verbal: emphasizes vocabulary-related questions. 2. Arithmetic: focuses on skill and computational speed with arithmetic. 3. Non-Verbal: deals with recognizing relationships and differences between objects; measures mental manipulation and reasoning.	Subtest 1: 30 questions Subtest 2: 30 questions Subtest 3: 30 questions
Spelling	Measures written expression or communication skills.	50 questions
Information in the Natural Sciences	Determines understanding of biology, chemistry, health, safety, hygiene, etc., at an elementary level.	90 questions
Judgment and Comprehension in Practical Nursing Situations	Evaluates how a nurse—both as a student and as a practitioner—exercises judgment in his/her working relationships.	50 questions
Vocational Adjustment Index	Ascertains an individual's characteristic lifestyle by examining his or her educational and occupational adjustment.	90 questions

Allied Health Programs Entrance Exams

The Psychological Corporation's Allied Health Professions Admissions Test (AHPAT) contains about 300 multiple-choice questions and lasts approximately three and one-half hours, including a short break period. The test format is as follows:

Test Section	Content	# of Questions
Verbal Ability	Uses synonym and antonym identification to measure vocabulary and verbal reasoning.	Approximately 75 questions
Quantitative Ability	Emphasizes nonverbal arithmetic exercises, problem solving, and applications in algebra, geometry, and basic trigonometry to interpret ability to reason through and understand quantitative concepts.	Approximately 50 questions
Biology	Focuses on the principles and concepts of basic biology, especially human biology, including cell biology, heredity, human structure and function, bacteria and viruses, evolution, and plants.	Approximately 50 questions

Test Section	Content	# of Questions
Chemistry	Focuses on the principles and concepts of basic chemistry, including atoms and molecules, formulas, equations, bonding, element and periodic relationships, states of matter, solutions, chemical equilibrium, acids, bases, electro-chemistry, kinetics, and nuclear and organic chemistry.	Approximately 50 questions
Reading Comprehension	Determines ability to comprehend, analyze, and interpret reading passages on science-oriented topics.	Approximately 45 questions

The Psychological Services Bureau's Health Occupations Aptitude Examination contains five tests and three subtests, and takes about two hour and fifteen minutes. The test format is as follows:

Test Section	Content	# of Questions
Academic Aptitude (3 Subtests)	1. Verbal: emphasizes vocabulary-related questions. 2. Arithmetic: focuses on skill and computational speed with arithmetic. 3. Non-Verbal: deals with recognizing relationships and differences between objects; measures mental manipulation and reasoning.	Subtest 1: 30 questions Subtest 2: 30 questions Subtest 3: 30 questions
Spelling	Measures written expression or communication skills.	60 questions
Reading Comprehension	Determines ability to interpret passages, understand direct statements, infer ideas and purposes, and derive author's intent.	50 questions
Information in the Natural Sciences	Tests understanding of biology, chemistry, health, safety, hygiene, etc., at an elementary level.	90 questions
Vocational Adjustment Index	Ascertains an individual's characteristic lifestyle by examining his or her educational and occupational adjustment.	90 questions

HOW TO APPLY FOR AN ENTRANCE EXAMINATION

The procedures for applying for an entrance examination for nursing school or for an allied health program will be provided by the specific school that you have selected. The school will notify you which examination it requires, where the local testing centers are located, and the specific time you are scheduled to take the examination. An application card must be completed and submitted with a test fee. You must follow all instructions given by the specific program for which you are applying. All applications and test results are handled through the specific schools.

ADMINISTRATION OF THE EXAMINATIONS

The examinations are administered by qualified persons, usually in a testing center. You will be scheduled to take the tests along with other candidates. Specific directions for taking the examinations will be given by the person proctoring the examination. All tests are timed. The proctor will tell you when to begin and when to stop.

All answers are placed on a separate answer sheet so that your results can be analyzed by computer. The computerized answer sheets are similar to the answer sheets in this book.

Answer sheets are sent to the respective testing centers for analysis. A computerized report is sent to the program from which the application was obtained, and the person taking the examination can also receive a report. The average time for receiving the test results is three weeks.

The tests are developed from a blueprint that identifies the number and type of items. There are several forms for each examination. If the blueprint calls for ten items related to understanding electrolytes, each form will have ten such items, but the specific test items may differ. That is why this book provides a variety of test items along with basic guidelines for answering similar questions.

HOW TO INTERPRET TEST SCORES

SIMULATED REPORT OF PERFORMANCE

NLN Pre-Admission Examination

Applicant	**Identification No.**	**Test Date**
Mary Brown, 100 Oaks Road Clearview, OK 74835	6-5081-599	04/11/97

		Percentile Norms*		
TEST	**SCORE**	**DI**	**AD**	**ALL**
Verbal Ability	026	22	20	21
Mathematics	013	20	29	24
Science	024	20	18	18
Composite	082	17	20	19

**Percentile Norms Are Based on Performance of:*

	Indiv.	**Prog.**	**States**	**Period**
Applicants to Diploma Programs	995	61	20	1997
Applicants to Associate Degree Programs	1449	43	20	1997
All Applicants to Basic Nursing Programs	2756	114	27	1997

Norms not available for applicants to baccalaureate degree programs.

Report Date	**Program Code**	**Head**
05/13/97	99-999	Department of Nursing, Centerville State Community College, P.O. Box 341, Centerville, OK 74830

The sample above represents a test score report. Notice that it is an individual report with the examinee name and identification number. This sample is for the NLN Pre-admission Examination. The scores represent the candidate's achievement on each one of the subtests on the examination.

The score for each test represents the number of correct items. The composite score (a standard score) reflects the score achieved in relation to the group average, with a composite of 100 being the mean or midpoint. The candidate in this sample scored well below the group mean. The scores are then compared with all of the examinees who took the test in 1997. See the lower portion of sample, which gives an indication of how the candidate's achievement on this examination compares with other examinees on a nationwide basis. The information is reported in percentiles, that is, the percentage of individuals who took the test and scored lower than this candidate did. Therefore, the 50th percentile represents a midpoint. Percentiles above 50 are considered above average and percentiles below 50 are considered below average. A percentile of 74 would be interpreted as the examinee did as well as or better than 74 percent of the group.

There are two groups (norms): those who apply to diploma programs (DI) and those applying to associate-degree programs (AD). The third percentile, ALL, describes performance in relation to both groups. In the example on page 15, the individual scored below the 50th percentile in all subtests. This level of performance is reflected in the composite scores for DI, AD, and ALL.

The Psychological Corporation's methods of reporting and interpreting test results on the registered and practical nursing entrance examinations and the Allied Health Professions Admissions Test are similar to those of the National League for Nursing. The RNEE scores are given as scaled scores and percentile ranks for each test section and for the entire test. The PNEE scores are given as raw scores and percentile ranks for the test by section and as a whole. The AHPAT score report is broken down as raw scores and percentile ranks for each test section.

The Psychological Services Bureau provides a student test record and profile chart for the registered nursing, practical nursing, and health occupations examinations. Test results are given as raw scores and percentile ranks for each test and subtest; a graph depicts the student's performance in comparison to the average grades.

Educational Resources distributes two types of score reports for the NET. The individual student summary, which contains a profile of 31 computer-generated diagnostic scores, is sent to each examinee. The composite group report, which contains a class profile and a student report for each examinee, is sent to each registered nursing program.

Each program determines how these scores will be used in the admission process. It is, therefore, advisable to seek this information directly from the program to which you are applying.

PREPARING FOR THE EXAMINATIONS

REDUCING TEST ANXIETY

Anxiety results from a threat to our well-being that might be real or perceived to be real. This threat affects our feelings of self-esteem, makes us uncomfortable in that it presents us with stress, and our behavior changes in an attempt to seek relief.

Many people become anxious or "uptight" about taking a test because someone is going to make a judgement about them, based on their test performance. Consequently, this leads to a test of their self-esteem. Is your self-esteem strong enough for you to think positively?. . . "I can pass this test!" Or, do you lack confidence in yourself, and assume . . . "I am going to fail." What can you do to prevent this situation?

First, you must realize that anxiety can be productive as well as destructive. Anxiety is an energizer and you want to direct this energy towards the goals you have set. You must remove the imagined threats. For example, you may have the idea that the admission test will determine your entire future in that if you don't pass the test, you won't be admitted to the program of your choice. The fact of the matter is that admission tests are used along with many other kinds of information to determine your eligibility for entering a program. So this is not a real threat. On the other hand, if you are not prepared to take this test and have made no effort to get ready, then you do have a real threat.

The secret to success is being confident and that goes hand in hand with your level of self-esteem. If you believe that you can pass a test then you will feel good about yourself. You can gain that confidence by completing the practice tests in this book with an 80% or above score in all areas. That would be proof that you can perform well on the admission test.

There are several things that you can do to relieve the stress that results from anxiety. You can set up a time-framed plan for studying from this book. Schedule a few pages per day and avoid last minute cramming.

Ventilation is good for the soul and reduces anxiety. Talk to a friend about why you're taking the test and why you would need to know the subject matter included in the admission test. Explore the "what if" situation and the related options for achieving your career goals.

Provide yourself with an outlet, something physical that you enjoy. Blow off your steam to alleviate your tension.

Think back to how you have handled stress and anxiety in your past experiences. It's alright to use defense mechanisms. Tell your significant other he/she is making you nervous. Eat a whole quart of ice cream, just this once, if it makes you feel good.

Positive thinking is a must. Imagine yourself receiving the results of your test enclosed in a letter of congratulations which you share with your family and friends. Make plans for the next step towards achieving your career goals. Imagine the pleasurable feeling and comfort that comes from peace of mind. You'll do just fine!

ANSWERING TEST ITEMS

After completing the overview of a section, answer the sample tests. Please note that many items are multiple-choice. This type of item requires knowing the answer or making an educated guess. (You are not penalized for guessing wrong on these examinations.) Therefore, you should go through the entire test, answering all the questions that you know, and then go back to the items you are not sure about to make an educated guess. This is how it's done.

1. *Carefully* read the question (the *stem*). Look for clues or the main ideas in the stem that will lead you to the correct answer.
2. Go through the entire examination, answering all questions that you feel sure about. This will give you an overall idea of what the test is about and lessen the time pressure, and you may run across related items that will help you to answer those you aren't sure about.
3. Now go back to those items you didn't answer and use the test-taking techniques. First, look for the key word(s) or clue(s) in the stem. Keeping that in mind, try to eliminate those options that do not relate to the clue. Look at the remaining options to identify similarities and differences. Compare the difference with the clue to see if you can eliminate another option. Select the remaining option.

Example: Which of the following observations may be an indication of high blood pressure?

(A) flushed skin
(B) pale skin
(C) cold skin
(D) weak pulse

What is the *clue*?

Answer: high pressure

Can I eliminate any options?

Answer: Yes. There is a direct relationship between pressure and force; therefore, (D) cannot be the correct answer.

What are the similarities and differences among options (A), (B), and (C)?

Answer: They all relate to changes in skin characteristics. However, items (B) and (C) are alike. As a matter of fact, if (B) were correct, (C) would also be correct.

The selected answer, then, is (A).

Now, let's assume that the following question is also on the test.

Why do some people with high blood pressure have flushed skin?

(A) The pulse weakens, and blood pools in the skin.
(B) The skin temperature lowers, and the skin blood vessels dilate.
(C) The increased pressure increases the volume of blood to the arteries.
(D) The increased pressure forces the arteries to dilate.

Based on your experience with the previous item, you would immediately eliminate options (A) and (B). Looking at (C) and (D), you might think that both would cause reddened skin. However, you would either eliminate (D) because it contradicts the relationship between pressure and volume, or you would select (C) because it supports the relationship between pressure and volume.

PLEASE PRACTICE THIS TECHNIQUE WITH THE SAMPLE ITEMS!

A summary of the steps for preparing to take a nursing-school entrance examination is presented below:

1. Study the concepts and principles presented in each section so that you will have a good base of knowledge.
2. Study one section at a time over a period of time—whatever is reasonable for your learning style. Do not cram!
3. Take the tests related to each section immediately after studying the explanatory materials.
4. Follow all directions for each test carefully.
5. Utilize the guidelines for test-taking as presented in this section.
6. Check your answers in order to diagnose your strengths and weaknesses.
7. Seek additional information from reliable resources in the areas in which you are weak.

Part II

PRACTICE FOR REGISTERED NURSING SCHOOL ENTRANCE EXAMINATIONS

UNIT I: VERBAL ABILITY

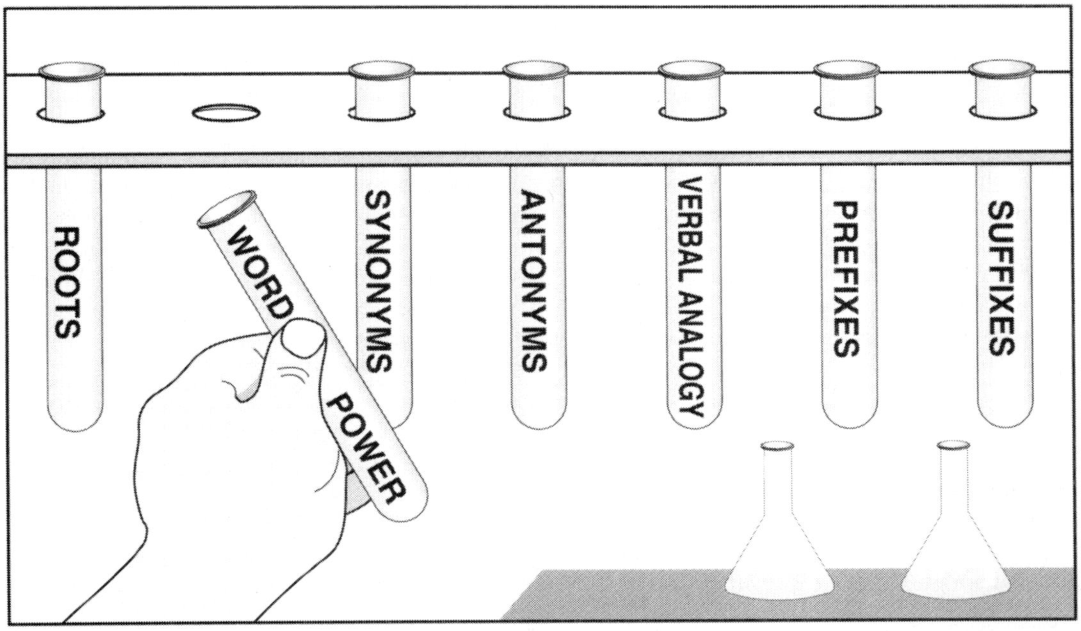

WHAT VERBAL ABILITY IS AND HOW IT IS MEASURED

Verbal ability may be defined as skill with word usage and comprehension. It is often evaluated in the form of written vocabulary tests. These vocabulary tests measure the test taker's ability to recall and produce *lexical units.* A lexical unit is a word or group of words possessing a specific meaning. A single word can have a variety of meanings in different contexts (that is, phrases or sentences). For this reason, a single word may represent several lexical units. Consider the following example:

Her answer to the question was *right.*

She handed the paper to the person on her *right.*

She has a *right* to know the results of the test.

She felt compelled to help *right* the wrong that was done.

The vocabulary test usually includes words from your *active* vocabulary—those words that you see, hear, and use frequently—and words from your *passive* vocabulary—words that you have heard and seen, and might comprehend, but that you rarely if ever use. It also includes words that may be common in written language but are not often used in spoken expression, and vice versa.

Measurement of verbal skill encompasses many elements. Although vocabulary test items may or may not appear on your test, it is advisable to study and practice with the kind of material presented in this verbal ability section. Words and their meanings are vital for good scores on tests of reading comprehension, effective writing, and current usage. Expanding your vocabulary will result in a marked improvement in your scores in these and similar subjects.

EXTENDING YOUR VOCABULARY

A good command of words is essential to most aspects of your life. Words can broaden your vistas and reveal new interests in your daily environment and activities. Such discoveries may never be accessible to you if your vocabulary remains restricted or too specialized.

Effective expression is essential to making and maintaining meaningful social relationships. An extensive vocabulary will help you to convey ideas, desires, and information. If you are enrolled in school, regardless of the level, you will learn faster and enjoy the process more if you are "fortified" with a large, effective vocabulary. Your comprehension of a broad range of words will help you to determine what you do *not* understand and will help you remedy the situation by posing intelligent questions.

Your word power directly affects your work. If you are seeking to improve your occupational status through a job change or a promotion from your present position, a better command of words will undoubtedly help you to succeed. This fact has been proven time and again through scientific studies conducted by educators, psychologists, sociologists, and personnel specialists. Many employers require a battery of tests, the results of which are used in determining which applicants are best suited to an available position. Frequently these tests incorporate a number of items designed to measure verbal ability.

Attaining a leadership role depends on, among other things, the extent of your vocabulary. Leadership tasks demand that you get your ideas across, that you speak and are heard. You will need to use all your expressive powers to voice your opinion with conviction. Articulation can furnish you with an astonishing amount of persuasive power.

A larger vocabulary will help you feel secure and competent in every undertaking. Let's explore the means by which this vocabulary may be acquired.

The following strategies are designed to increase your vocabulary and help you achieve word mastery. Word mastery implies reaching a level of verbal ability at which you can both recognize and comprehend words—and use them frequently and properly.

1. Read as much as you can, taking care not to confine yourself to one kind of reading material. Seek variety in what you read—periodicals, newspapers, nonfiction, novels and other fiction, poetry, prose, essays, etc. Reading from a broad range of material will accelerate your vocabulary growth. You will learn the meaning of words by context. This means that at times you will not know the definition of an isolated word, but the words or phrase with which this word appears will be familiar and therefore provide a clue to its meaning.

2. Take vocabulary tests. There are many practice books containing word tests; we recommend *Webster's New World™ Power Vocabulary.* These tests are challenging and make an enjoyable leisure-time activity. More important, they are fast vocabulary builders.

3. Listen to lectures, discussion, and talks given by people who speak well. TV and radio are excellent means of learning new terminology coming into common usage in the English language. A word of caution: You cannot always rely on a speaker's pronunciation. Always check your dictionary for proper pronunciation.

4. Use a dictionary when you are not certain of a word's meaning. If you do not have access to a dictionary when you encounter the word, make a note of it (and its context) and research it at your earliest convenience. Find out how it is pronounced, what words are related to it, and its finer shades of meaning and correct usage. A good dictionary is a must! Any one of the following is highly recommended:

   Funk and Wagnall's Standard College Dictionary

   Webster's New World™ Dictionary

   Random House College Dictionary

Also, use of the following is encouraged: *Roget's International Thesaurus*; *Webster's New World Dictionary™ of Synonyms*; and *Harper Dictionary of Contemporary Usage*.

5. Word games, such as Scrabble® and Boggle®, are an effective and pleasurable means of encountering new words. Crossword puzzles, anagrams, and similar word games provide a relaxing method of acquiring new vocabulary. Most of these puzzles are published in varying degrees of difficulty. Start with the easy level and progress to the expert. You will find it a challenging learning experience.
6. Review the etymological charts and diagrams in this book, which explain word derivations. A knowledge of roots, or stems, of words will enable you to infer the meaning of new words having roots similar to words you already know.
7. Study words by central ideas. It is difficult to study and retain isolated words. Even context clues sometimes are not enough to help you remember a word, its meaning, or its appropriate use. Studying vocabulary by central idea encourages you to consider groups of related words. As you learn each term, you associate it with some other word. For example: The words *ingest, devour, consume, voracious, edible, delectable*, and *palatable* are all tied to the principle idea of eating. The central idea strategy of studying words will not only provide you with a basis for remembering the word but will also motivate you to use the word in your everyday oral and written expression. Frequent use of the word will in turn ensure your ability to recall its meaning in a testing situation. This word study method also fosters comprehension of jargon or word usage peculiar to specific fields. A number of workbooks and study materials present words according to a central idea and feature exercises formatted to this method. Such books may be found in the "study aids" section of most bookstores.

Be sure to record all new words in a notebook dedicated to that purpose. Make notes alongside each entry that include a simple definition or synonym, finer shades of meaning, related forms, and sample sentences of the word in context. Finally, make these words your own. Use them in your writing and speaking. Remember—verbal ability is a skill you can improve at any age.

The purpose of this section is to provide you with practice exercises representative of the three most common kinds of verbal-ability test items: synonyms, antonyms, and verbal analogies. This section covers these question types in three separate subsections.

An explanation of each kind of test item, helpful study hints, and test-taking strategies precede each subsection. Subsections also include a 75-question, multiple-choice test. An answer key follows each sample test to help you evaluate your performance immediately and to help you determine areas of weakness. You may wish to use these answer keys to compile a word study list.

ETYMOLOGY—KEY TO WORD RECOGNITION

Etymology is the study of the history and origin of words. It explains how a word came into being, the place of its beginning, and how it has been used through the ages. The etymology of a word also outlines alterations in its meaning, usage, and spelling through the years.

Although the term "etymology" sounds somewhat complex and weighty, the science itself is not difficult to understand. Etymologies may be simple and concise or lengthy and intricate. To find them, you should use your dictionary. Etymologies are usually found at the beginning of a definition of a principal entry (the word you are looking up, usually printed in heavy type), enclosed in brackets and placed directly before the definition.

arris\'ar ə s*n,pl* **arris** or **arrises** [probably modif. of MF *areste*, lit., fishbone, fr LL *arista*, ear of grain]: the sharp edge or salient angle formed by the meeting of two surfaces, esp. in moldings.

You probably should familiarize yourself with the abbreviations used to denote the origin of words. Consult the front pages of your dictionary where you will find a guide to the use of that particular publication. Look for a heading that refers to etymologies or abbreviations and symbols used in etymologies. These keys will help you interpret a word's entry. For instance, the entry printed above uses the abbreviations MF and LL indicating that the entry *arris* is derived from Middle French or Late Latin.

Many English words have their origin in Greek and Roman myths and legends. If you are well-read, you may already have an edge in using the etymological method of determining word meaning. For instance, if you have read the story of the mythical king Tantalus, you would understand the derivation of the verb *tantalize.* King Tantalus, after his death, was punished for his wickedness by being placed in water up to his chin. When he stooped to drink, the water would recede. Above his head, branches laden with fruit bobbed out of his reach. So from the name Tantalus came the word *tantalize*, meaning "to tease."

A great many of the words we use daily came into our language from the Latin and Greek. Approximately half the words in the dictionary are derived from Latin. Many Latin words and phrases have been borrowed and adopted by other languages. European languages such as French and Spanish came directly from Latin and are known as Romance languages. Consequently, if you are or have been a student of Latin, you will find it easier to build your vocabulary.

Many foreign terms were absorbed into English as parts of several different words related in meaning to each other. These parts of words fall into three groups.

Roots (or stems)—These carry the basic meaning and are combined with each other and with prefixes and suffixes to create other words with related meanings.

Prefixes—Letter combinations with their own particular meaning that appear at the beginning of a word.

Suffixes—Letter combinations with their own particular meaning that appear at the end of a word.

The lists of roots, prefixes, and suffixes in this section are accompanied by words in which the letter combinations appear. Use the dictionary to look up any words that are not clear in your mind.

Remember that this section is not meant for easy reading. It is a guide to a program of study that will prove invaluable if you do your part. Do not try to absorb too much at one time. If you can put in a half-hour every day, your study will yield better results.

After you have done your preliminary work and have formed a better idea of how words are formed in English, schedule the various vocabulary tests we have provided. They cover a wide variety of the vocabulary questions commonly encountered on examinations. These lengthy tests are not meant to be taken all at one time. Space them out. Adhere closely to the directions, which differ for the different kinds of tests. Keep an honest record of your scores. Study your corrected mistakes and look them up in your dictionary. Concentrate closely on each sample test . . . and watch your scores improve.

KNOW YOUR ROOTS

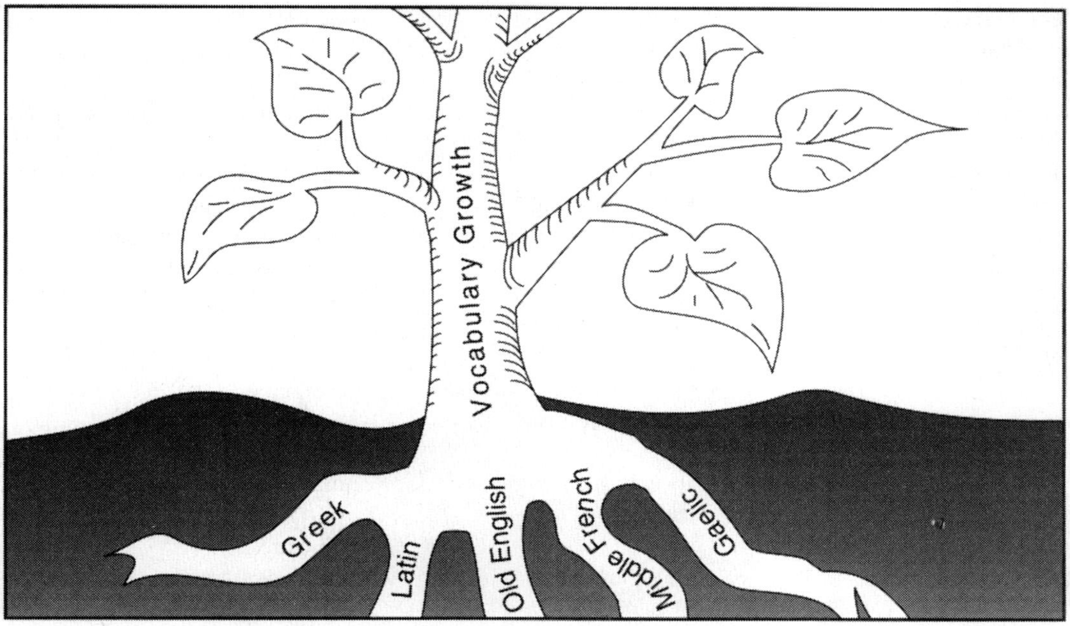

ROOTS OR STEMS

The root or stem is that part of the word that conveys the basic meaning of the word. For example, in the word *introduction, duct* is the root. It means "lead." *Intro-* means *within, into,* and *-tion* is a noun ending. Hence, the meaning of introduction—a "leading into."

Below is a chart of common stems. See how well you "know your roots."

STEMS

Stem	Meaning	Example
ag, ac	do	agenda, action
agri	farm	agriculture
aqua	water	aquatic
auto	self	automatic
biblio	book	bibliography
bio	life	biography
cad, cas	fall	cadence, casual
cap, cep, cept	take	captive, accept
capit	head	capital, decapitate
ced, cede, ceed, cess	go	intercede
celer	speed	accelerate
chrom	color	monochromatic
chron	time	chronological
cide, cis	cut	incision
clude, clud, clus	close, close in	include, cluster
cog, cogn	knowledge of	recognize
cur, curs	run	recur, cursive

Stem	Meaning	Example
ded	give	dedicate
dent, dont	tooth	dental
duce, duct	lead	induce, deduct
fact, fect, fict	make, do	perfect, fiction, factory
fer, late	carry	refer, dilate, transfer, translate
flect, flex	bend, turn	reflect
fring, fract	break	infringe, refract
graph, gram	picture, writing	graphic, telegram
greg	group, gather	gregarious, congregation
gress, grad	step, walk	progress, degrade
hydr	water	hydrate
ject	throw	inject
jud	right	judicial
junct	join	conjunction
juris	law, justice	jurist
lect, leg	read, choose	collect, legible
logue	speech, speaking	dialogue
logy	study of	psychology
loq, loc	speak	elocution
lude, lus	play, perform	elude, ludicrous
manu	by hand	manuscript
mand	order	remand
mar	sea	maritime
med	middle	intermediate
ment, mem	mind, memory	mention
meter	measure	thermometer
micro	small	microscope
min	lessen	miniature
mis, miss, mit	send	remit, dismiss
mot, mov	move	remote, remove
mute	change	commute, mutation
naut	sailor, sail	nautical
nounce, nunci	declare, state	announce, enunciate
ped, pod	foot	pedal
pel, pulse	drive, push	dispel, impulse
pend, pense	hang	depend, dispenser
plac	please	placate
plic	fold	implicate
port	carry	portable
pose, pone	put, place	depose, component
reg, rect	rule	regulate, direct
rupt	break	disruption
sec, sect	cut	bisect
sed	remain	sedentary
sert	weave, bind	insert
serve	keep, save	preserve
scend, scent	climb	ascent
scribe, script	write	describe, transcript
sist	stand, set	insist
spect	look	inspect
spire, spirat	breath, breathe	perspire

Stem	**Meaning**	**Example**
strict	tighten	restrict
tain	hold	detain
term	end	terminate
tract	draw, drag	detract
tort	twist	distort
vene, vent	come	intervene, invent
vict	overcome, conquer	evict
volve, volu	roll, turn	evolve, evolution

PREFIXES AND SUFFIXES

DOWN TO THE LETTER

Prefixes and suffixes are the "beginning and end!" We will begin by reviewing the term *prefix.* A prefix is a letter-combination attached to the beginning of a word; it usually carries a meaning independent of the word to which it is attached. For example, the prefix *semi* means "half." It can be added to many words—*semicircle, semilunar, semiprofessional, semiformal.* Attaching a prefix sometimes requires the placement of a hyphen between the prefix and the root word. A hyphen is used when the prefix is attached to a proper noun: *all-American, pro-British, anti-Fascist, un-Christian.*

A suffix is a combination of letters attached to the end of a word and usually possessing a meaning separate from the word to which it is affixed, for example: *-less* (without)—*careless, hopeless, meaningless.* Usually, affixing a suffix to a word changes its part of speech, for example: *Assert* (verb)—*assertion* (noun); *beautiful* (adjective)—*beautifully* (adverb).

Study the following prefix and suffix charts to increase your understanding of related words and inflected (changed) forms.

PREFIXES

Prefix	**Meaning**	**Example**
a	not	amoral
ab, a	away from	absent
ad, ac, ag, at	to	advent, accrue, attract, aggressive
an	without	anarchy
ante	before	antedate
anti	against	antipathy
aud, audit	hear	auditor
bene	well	beneficent
bi	two	bicameral
cap, capt, cept	take, seize, hold	capture
ced, cess	go, yield	rescind, recess
circum	around	circumspect
com, con, col	together	commit, confound, collate
contra	against	contraband
cred, credit	believe	credible
de	from, down	descend
dic, dict	say	dictionary

dis, di	apart	distract, divert
dom	home, rule	domicile, dominate
duc, duct	lead	induce
ex, e	out	exit, emit
extra	beyond	extracurricular
fac, fact	make	facsimile
in, im, ir, il, un	not	inept, irregular, illegal
in, im	in, into	interest, imbibe
inter	between	interscholastic
intra, intro	within	intramural
mal	bad	malcontent
mis	wrong	misnomer
non	not	nonentity
ob	against	obstacle
omni	all	omnivorous
per	through	permeate
peri	around	periscope
poly	many	polytheism
post	after	postmortem
pre	before	premonition
pro	forward	propose
re	again	review
se	apart	seduce
semi	half	semicircle
sub	under	subvert
sui	self	suicide
super	above	superimpose
sur	on, upon	surcharge
trans	across	transpose
un	not	unwelcome
vice	instead of	vice-president

SUFFIXES

Suffix	Meaning	Example
able, ible	capable of being	capable, reversible
age	state of	storage
al	pertaining to	instructional
ance	relating to	reliance
ary	relating to	dictionary
ate	act	confiscate
ation	action	radiation
cy	quality	democracy
ed	past action	subsided
ence	relating to	confidence
er, or	one who	adviser, actor
ic	pertaining to	democratic
ing	present action	surmising
ious	full of	rebellious

ish	like, as	childish
ive	having the quality of	creative
ize	to make like	harmonize
less	without	hopeless
ly	the quality of	carefully
ment	result	amusement
ness	the quality of being	selfishness
ty	condition	sanity

INCREASED WORD POWER FROM BEGINNING TO END

Using the etymological approach can simplify the process by which you attack the monumental feat of learning medical terminology. By knowing that the suffix *itis* implies inflammation and *ectomy* means "the cutting out or removal of," you can easily deduce that the term *appendicitis* means "inflammation of the appendix" and *appendectomy* means "the cutting out or removal of the appendix."

Now that you have studied the various letter combinations or word components, see if you can make an educated guess at the meanings of the terms listed below. Start with the root or stem. Next, add the suffix and/or prefix to the interpretation in the order that provides a clear definition. The result will be increased word power from "beginning to end!" It's as challenging as a jigsaw puzzle! Be sure to compare your definitions with those in the dictionary.

decapitate	colloquy
emissary	aggregation
incursion	retractable
involuted	implacable
convocation	celerity

SYNONYMS

THE NAME'S THE SAME

Synonyms are words that share meanings. The English language abounds in synonyms. In your effort to acquire word mastery, you must learn to express your ideas without redundancy and constant use of overworked words. Effective writing and speaking may be achieved through the precise use of synonyms.

Words such as *brave* and *courageous*, which may allude to an identical quality, can be used interchangeably. Some synonyms, however, differ in definition or usage. For example, *fewer* refers to number, while *less* refers to quantity: John has *fewer* books and *less* money than his brother. These words are indeed similar in meaning, but one cannot be substituted for the other.

The adjectives *beautiful* and *handsome* both describe someone or something attractive or pleasing to the eye. Nevertheless, you would not usually speak of a "beautiful man" or a "handsome young lady." In our society, common usage would cause one to reverse these expressions to "beautiful young lady" and "handsome man."

A study of the finer shades of meaning of synonyms will help you be more precise when you convey your exact feelings or mental picture of an object or scene. For instance, if you were to say, "The *bottom* of the lamp is made of Indian brass and features intricate carvings," one might simply envision the underside of the lamp. However, if you were to substitute *base* for the word *bottom*, one would instead get a visual image of something highly decorative that supports the upper structure of the lamp. So even though the "name" appears to be the same, an investigation into various shades of definition will assist you in distinguishing variations in usage.

If you wish to expand your vocabulary of synonyms and familiarize yourself with their correct use, you will find the following reference books helpful:

Webster's New World™ Dictionary of Synonyms

Crabb's English Synonyms

Roget's International Thesaurus

Harper Dictionary of Contemporary Usage

FAMILIAR SURROUNDINGS?

The most common way of testing vocabulary on a standardized test is in context, that is, to present the items in a sentence or phrase so that you can see how a word is used. You can then determine whether the word is used as a noun, a verb, an adjective, etc. The test, therefore, is designed to encourage the extraction of word meaning from context; however the context will not be so explicit that you can easily infer the meaning of a word.

More specifically, the synonym test item is usually a multiple-choice item that appears in one of three formats:

Type A—Given an underlined or italicized word in a complete sentence, the test-taker is required to identify which of the four other words is a synonym for the underlined or italicized word.

Example: The disinterested witness was able to give a *candid* account of the incident.

(A) complete
(B) impartial
(C) biased
(D) candescent

Type B—Given an underlined or italicized word in a phrase, the test-taker is required to identify which of the four other words is a synonym for the underlined or italicized word.

Example: The *emaciated* patient

(A) discharged
(B) emancipated
(C) emotional
(D) shriveled

Type C—Given a sentence with a missing word, the test-taker is required to identify which of the four other words best completes the sentence.

Example: An *apology* is appropriate when a person feels

(A) sorry
(B) apathetic
(C) rejected
(D) elated

OR

Example: He is a *staunch* supporter of the presidential candidate. Staunch means

(A) stubborn
(B) faithful
(C) inflexible
(D) hopeful

Especially Special: Scientific Terms

When preparing for an entrance exam for programs leading to science-related careers, it is beneficial to familiarize yourself with the specialized vocabulary of this discipline. Remember, even though the general public considers scientific jargon confusing, technical terms are imperative for scientific communication. If you plan to study science, your ability to comprehend the terminology of the field could indicate how well you will do in the related course work. Your entrance exam may measure your scientific vocabulary skills.

Mastery of specialized vocabulary—or any vocabulary for that matter—can best be achieved by learning words as you encounter them in your reading. However, when preparing for an entrance exam, you may want to employ the following strategies:

1. Review "Know Your Roots" and "Prefixes and Suffixes" on pages 25–29 of this publication.
2. Read a variety of scientific articles, science textbook chapters, etc.
3. Try to understand the unfamiliar words that you encounter in these readings as they are used in context.
4. If you cannot grasp the meaning from context, then put your knowledge of roots and affixes to work. Take the word apart and see if you can determine a meaning that fits the context (or if you are in the testing situation, a meaning that comes close to one of the multiple-choice items).
5. If Step 4 does not yield a reasonable definition, then check the footnotes, glossary, or index of the text you are reading. If you find the word in the index, skim the pages listed for that word, checking for either its definition or its contextual usage.
6. If you cannot find a definition of the word in the material that you are reading, look it up in a dictionary. It would be best to use a scientific dictionary or encyclopedia. There are dictionaries that are for specific areas of study, such as geography, modern history, politics, and biology.
7. Once you have come up with a definition for the word, you may want to write it on an index card (word on one side, definition on the other). After accumulating a number of these vocabulary cards, carry them in your pocket or book bag. Flip through them when you have a spare moment (commuting by train or bus, sitting in the waiting room of the dentist or doctor, etc.).
8. Become accustomed to recognizing words that stand for concepts rather than facts. To a scientist, a concept is a generalization or an idea based on information or knowledge that explains a phenomenon. Read the following paragraph and underline those words which you feel represent scientific concepts.

   Karotyping is a process that enables scientists to study the chromosomes of human beings. Sometimes the study can be made even before birth. Chromosomes can best be observed during metaphase in mitosis. At this point they are coiled. Skin cells are good to use in making a Karyotype because they divide frequently. Some genetic disorders can be identified just by looking at the Karyotype of a person.

   If you underlined Karyotype process, metaphase, mitosis, and genetic disorders, you would be correct. These words represent ideas. They cannot be touched and they have no exact physical form or boundaries, yet they are real because they represent scientific facts.
9. Finally, learn to connect symbols to words. A scientific symbol is an abbreviation that stands for a word or concept.

Example: $C_6H_{12}O_6$ represents glucose, a chemical compound.

You will have the opportunity to practice your use of these vocabulary expansion strategies as you encounter scientific terms on the verbal ability practice test and final verbal ability examination in this book. The answers to several of the questions in the reading comprehension test involve scientific terms. These questions are indicated by asterisks.

In completing a synonym test item, remember to look for a word which means the same, or almost the same, as the target word in the item (the underlined or italicized word). Do not be distracted by a word that is a look-alike, that is, one that looks similar or begins with the same three or four letters but is unrelated in meaning. When possible, apply the etymological approach of interpreting roots, prefixes, and suffixes. Now try completing the sample synonym test. There is a total of 75 items. An answer key appears on page 40.

SYNONYMS TEST ANSWER SHEET

1. Ⓐ Ⓑ Ⓒ Ⓓ	20. Ⓐ Ⓑ Ⓒ Ⓓ	39. Ⓐ Ⓑ Ⓒ Ⓓ	58. Ⓐ Ⓑ Ⓒ Ⓓ
2. Ⓐ Ⓑ Ⓒ Ⓓ	21. Ⓐ Ⓑ Ⓒ Ⓓ	40. Ⓐ Ⓑ Ⓒ Ⓓ	59. Ⓐ Ⓑ Ⓒ Ⓓ
3. Ⓐ Ⓑ Ⓒ Ⓓ	22. Ⓐ Ⓑ Ⓒ Ⓓ	41. Ⓐ Ⓑ Ⓒ Ⓓ	60. Ⓐ Ⓑ Ⓒ Ⓓ
4. Ⓐ Ⓑ Ⓒ Ⓓ	23. Ⓐ Ⓑ Ⓒ Ⓓ	42. Ⓐ Ⓑ Ⓒ Ⓓ	61. Ⓐ Ⓑ Ⓒ Ⓓ
5. Ⓐ Ⓑ Ⓒ Ⓓ	24. Ⓐ Ⓑ Ⓒ Ⓓ	43. Ⓐ Ⓑ Ⓒ Ⓓ	62. Ⓐ Ⓑ Ⓒ Ⓓ
6. Ⓐ Ⓑ Ⓒ Ⓓ	25. Ⓐ Ⓑ Ⓒ Ⓓ	44. Ⓐ Ⓑ Ⓒ Ⓓ	63. Ⓐ Ⓑ Ⓒ Ⓓ
7. Ⓐ Ⓑ Ⓒ Ⓓ	26. Ⓐ Ⓑ Ⓒ Ⓓ	45. Ⓐ Ⓑ Ⓒ Ⓓ	64. Ⓐ Ⓑ Ⓒ Ⓓ
8. Ⓐ Ⓑ Ⓒ Ⓓ	27. Ⓐ Ⓑ Ⓒ Ⓓ	46. Ⓐ Ⓑ Ⓒ Ⓓ	65. Ⓐ Ⓑ Ⓒ Ⓓ
9. Ⓐ Ⓑ Ⓒ Ⓓ	28. Ⓐ Ⓑ Ⓒ Ⓓ	47. Ⓐ Ⓑ Ⓒ Ⓓ	66. Ⓐ Ⓑ Ⓒ Ⓓ
10. Ⓐ Ⓑ Ⓒ Ⓓ	29. Ⓐ Ⓑ Ⓒ Ⓓ	48. Ⓐ Ⓑ Ⓒ Ⓓ	67. Ⓐ Ⓑ Ⓒ Ⓓ
11. Ⓐ Ⓑ Ⓒ Ⓓ	30. Ⓐ Ⓑ Ⓒ Ⓓ	49. Ⓐ Ⓑ Ⓒ Ⓓ	68. Ⓐ Ⓑ Ⓒ Ⓓ
12. Ⓐ Ⓑ Ⓒ Ⓓ	31. Ⓐ Ⓑ Ⓒ Ⓓ	50. Ⓐ Ⓑ Ⓒ Ⓓ	69. Ⓐ Ⓑ Ⓒ Ⓓ
13. Ⓐ Ⓑ Ⓒ Ⓓ	32. Ⓐ Ⓑ Ⓒ Ⓓ	51. Ⓐ Ⓑ Ⓒ Ⓓ	70. Ⓐ Ⓑ Ⓒ Ⓓ
14. Ⓐ Ⓑ Ⓒ Ⓓ	33. Ⓐ Ⓑ Ⓒ Ⓓ	52. Ⓐ Ⓑ Ⓒ Ⓓ	71. Ⓐ Ⓑ Ⓒ Ⓓ
15. Ⓐ Ⓑ Ⓒ Ⓓ	34. Ⓐ Ⓑ Ⓒ Ⓓ	53. Ⓐ Ⓑ Ⓒ Ⓓ	72. Ⓐ Ⓑ Ⓒ Ⓓ
16. Ⓐ Ⓑ Ⓒ Ⓓ	35. Ⓐ Ⓑ Ⓒ Ⓓ	54. Ⓐ Ⓑ Ⓒ Ⓓ	73. Ⓐ Ⓑ Ⓒ Ⓓ
17. Ⓐ Ⓑ Ⓒ Ⓓ	36. Ⓐ Ⓑ Ⓒ Ⓓ	55. Ⓐ Ⓑ Ⓒ Ⓓ	74. Ⓐ Ⓑ Ⓒ Ⓓ
18. Ⓐ Ⓑ Ⓒ Ⓓ	37. Ⓐ Ⓑ Ⓒ Ⓓ	56. Ⓐ Ⓑ Ⓒ Ⓓ	75. Ⓐ Ⓑ Ⓒ Ⓓ
19. Ⓐ Ⓑ Ⓒ Ⓓ	38. Ⓐ Ⓑ Ⓒ Ⓓ	57. Ⓐ Ⓑ Ⓒ Ⓓ	

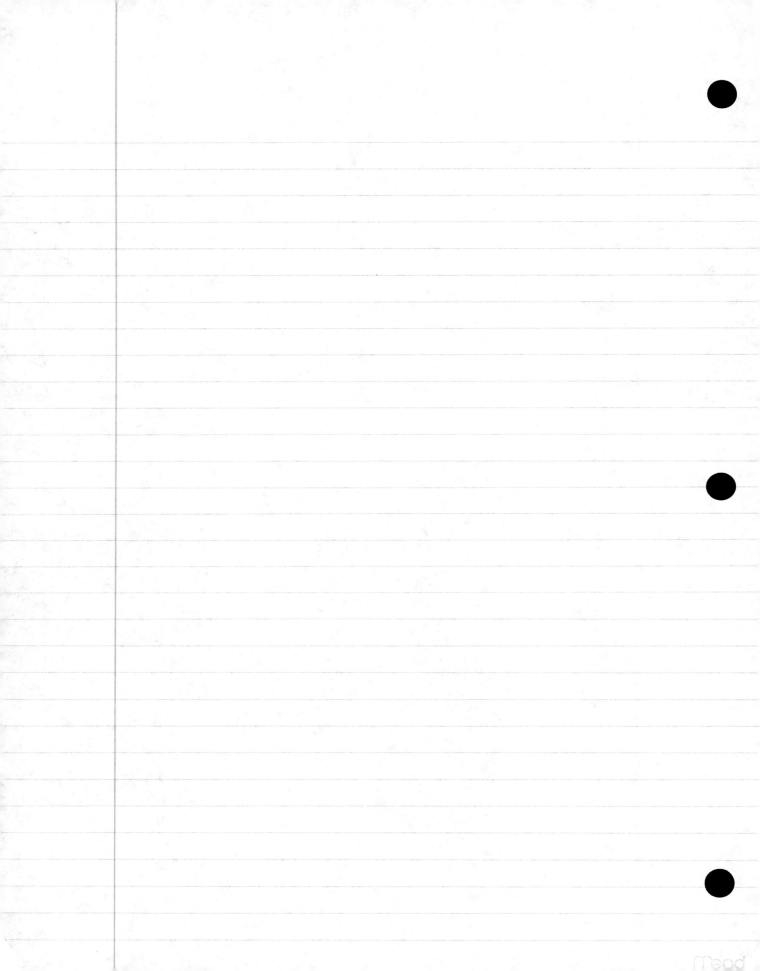

SYNONYMS TEST

75 QUESTIONS • TIME—30 MINUTES

Directions: In each of the sentences below, one word is italicized. Following each sentence are four words or phrases. For each sentence, choose the word or phrase that most nearly corresponds in meaning with the italicized word.

1. The *diction* acceptable in speech is usually more informal than that required in writing.

   (A) conviction
   (B) language
   (C) discourse
   (D) decrement

2. It is apparent that Mr. Smith is the most *sedulous* and active member of the group.

   (A) hideous
   (B) generous
   (C) infirm
   (D) industrious

3. During the hockey game several *altercations* took place.

   (A) fracases
   (B) substitutions
   (C) alterations
   (D) plays

4. The carrot is a perfect illustration of a *biennial.*

   (A) occurring quarterly
   (B) occurring once in two years
   (C) perennial
   (D) bisection

5. She has run the *gamut* of clerical jobs in this office.

   (A) periphery
   (B) margin
   (C) range
   (D) imperception

6. His deeds amounted to nothing more than those of a *sanctimonious* hypocrite.

   (A) parsimonious
   (B) perpetual
   (C) intrinsic
   (D) affectedly pious

7. He displayed the manners of an *urbane* gentleman.

   (A) suave
   (B) poignant
   (C) spasmodic
   (D) pensive

8. The *slogan* is appropriate for both the product and its service.

   (A) catchword
   (B) sample
   (C) design
   (D) passage

9. The *chloroplasts* in plant cells is where photosynthesis takes place.

   (A) organelles
   (B) mitochondria
   (C) ribosomes
   (D) vacuoles

10. He was determined to *foil* the scheme of his opponent.

    (A) heighten
    (B) secure
    (C) disencumber
    (D) thwart

11. The examiner *purported* to be an official representative.

    (A) addressed
    (B) claimed
    (C) propitiated
    (D) conciliated

12. The ship carried refugees of every *persuasion.*

    (A) mediocrity
    (B) sort
    (C) prospectus
    (D) compendium

13. The child could not *recollect* the incident.

(A) remember
(B) dubitate
(C) interrogate
(D) illumine

14. The Supreme Court *rescinded* the law.

(A) complicated
(B) inveigled
(C) revoked
(D) accepted

15. The implementation of the plan was given *scant* consideration.

(A) audacious
(B) fervid
(C) little
(D) clothed

16. The key speaker in his lengthy presentation *scoffed* at religion.

(A) exonerated
(B) amplified
(C) confuted
(D) mocked

17. She completed the *sprint* with a sudden surge of energy.

(A) relaxation
(B) adventure
(C) run
(D) convergence

18. The content of the message was *urgent.*

(A) privileged
(B) amendable
(C) pressing
(D) absolved

19. A *simulated* rescue mission was conducted by the forest rangers.

(A) pretended
(B) superficial
(C) stimulated
(D) simultaneous

20. A *histamine* is released from the tissues when the cells are injured.

(A) A histone
(B) An amine
(C) A stimulant
(D) An isoenzyme

21. Her quickening gait seemed regulated by the *pulse* of the big city.

(A) utility
(B) pace
(C) reverence
(D) solace

22. The language of the publication is *unsophisticated* but informative.

(A) ponderous
(B) elaborate
(C) simple
(D) superficial

23. All the evidence presented pointed to *willful* execution of a crime.

(A) deliberate
(B) eminent
(C) amicable
(D) remorseful

24. There is no *provision* for deadlines in the contract.

(A) improvement
(B) convenience
(C) aggregation
(D) stipulation

25. The furnishings *impart* an air of elegance to the room.

(A) communicate
(B) indemnify
(C) reinforce
(D) disguise

26. She exhibited great *valor* in handling the emergency.

(A) ingeniousness
(B) courage
(C) discretion
(D) optimism

27. Various courses were *fused* in the revision of the curriculum.

(A) required
(B) implicated
(C) combined
(D) involved

28. Production of complex molecules is accomplished by *replication.*

(A) duplication
(B) synthesis
(C) fixation
(D) reproduction

29. The task of choosing one from so many qualified applicants *bewildered* the employer.

    (A) perplexed
    (B) aggravated
    (C) subdued
    (D) infuriated

30. The revision of the city plan incorporated adjustments in the projected *modes* of transportation.

    (A) increments
    (B) expenditures
    (C) means
    (D) modifications

31. The politician sought to *aggrandize* himself at the expense of the people.

    (A) exhaust
    (B) subjugate
    (C) sacrifice
    (D) exalt

32. The newcomer made an effort to *mingle* with the crowd.

    (A) argue
    (B) mix
    (C) disrupt
    (D) flout

33. If an organization's programs were described as *philanthropic,* the programs would be

    (A) primitive
    (B) deleterious
    (C) extraneous
    (D) benevolent

34. If the traits of a nation's leader were *covetous,* they were

    (A) greedy
    (B) exemplary
    (C) disparate
    (D) adventitious

35. Rabbits *breed* offspring rapidly.

    (A) raise
    (B) gather
    (C) propagate
    (D) destroy

36. It was necessary to *iterate* one procedure of the experiment.

    (A) adjust
    (B) defend
    (C) ferment
    (D) repeat

37. A shadow of a man *loomed* ominously in the dimly lit corridor.

    (A) asserted
    (B) yielded
    (C) appeared
    (D) rebuffed

38. Alcohol consumption often exerts a *malign* influence on an individual.

    (A) ecstatic
    (B) injurious
    (C) luminous
    (D) gloomy

39. The girl is reported to have left of her own *volition.*

    (A) flight
    (B) will
    (C) repudiation
    (D) recognizance

40. The most important *mutation* is one occurring in the gametes.

    (A) fertilization
    (B) meoisis
    (C) deamination
    (D) change

41. The *similitude* between the original painting and the reproduction is remarkable.

    (A) incongruity
    (B) connection
    (C) resemblance
    (D) relationship

42. A *prudent* individual will save some portion of his or her wage.

    (A) judicious
    (B) terse
    (C) audacious
    (D) laconic

43. His decision to return home was *instinctive.*

(A) spontaneous
(B) turbid
(C) premeditated
(D) irrelevant

44. The mountain *torrent* flowed over the rocks.

(A) slide
(B) avalanche
(C) deluge
(D) air

45. The book was written to embody all aspects of life science.

(A) combat
(B) eliminate
(C) abjure
(D) incorporate

46. Her sudden decision is typical of her *impetuous* behavior.

(A) contemptible
(B) sophisticated
(C) impulsive
(D) fallacious

47. It is fitting that we *eulogize* one who has contributed so greatly to our society.

(A) promulgate
(B) praise
(C) denigrate
(D) append

48. The convention hall swelled with the *vociferation* of various campaign groups.

(A) clamor
(B) taciturnity
(C) oblivion
(D) discernment

49. The blackmailer has placed her in a *precarious* position.

(A) mellifluous
(B) intrusive
(C) unusual
(D) unstable

50. Her display of so much fine china was too *ostentatious.*

(A) pretentious
(B) inconspicuous
(C) ascribable
(D) candid

51. To *manifest* interest

(A) conceal
(B) diminish
(C) augment
(D) display

52. *Banter* and laughter

(A) discourse
(B) singing
(C) toasting
(D) raillery

53. *Aesthetic* value

(A) practical
(B) artistic
(C) monetary
(D) intrinsic

54. Confirmed his *apostasy*

(A) defiance
(B) defection
(C) belief
(D) inference

55. The *cryptic* message

(A) cynical
(B) mysterious
(C) critical
(D) censorious

56. New witnesses *emerged*

(A) deviated
(B) divested
(C) declined
(D) appeared

57. The *contumacious* youngster

(A) exuberant
(B) rebellious
(C) awkward
(D) mischievous

58. *Cognizant* of the ill will

(A) ignorant
(B) aware
(C) insensitive
(D) remorseful

59. *Glacial* region

(A) glass-like
(B) illiberal
(C) frigid
(D) reticent

60. *Instigated* the rebellion

(A) quelled
(B) incited
(C) assisted
(D) depressed

61. A fight *ensued*

(A) followed
(B) terminated
(C) was avoided
(D) culminated

62. *Retrospect* of events

(A) review
(B) concept
(C) knowledge
(D) awareness

63. *Malice* toward my friend

(A) adoration
(B) sympathy
(C) ill will
(D) apathy

64. *Saturated* with moisture

(A) void of
(B) mixed with
(C) full of
(D) replaced with

65. *Debilitating* to people

(A) invigorating
(B) stimulating
(C) tolerable
(D) weakening

66. Ten years' *servitude*

(A) freedom
(B) lethargy
(C) vicissitude
(D) bondage

67. *Relish* the thought

(A) enjoy
(B) dread
(C) spread
(D) implant

68. A *lackadaisical* attitude

(A) enthusiastic
(B) complacent
(C) profound
(D) indifferent

69. To *hoist* the sails

(A) cast
(B) raise
(C) prepare
(D) repair

70. *Asperse* the family's good name

(A) slander
(B) fathom
(C) extol
(D) palliate

71. *Sordid* details

(A) bizarre
(B) wretched
(C) primordial
(D) exaggerated

72. Sudden *alienation*

(A) agitation
(B) inception
(C) subsidence
(D) isolation

73. *Biotin* is widely distributed in organisms.

(A) Vitamin H
(B) Vitamin D
(C) Chyme
(D) Plasmodia

74. *Accede* to the request

(A) attend
(B) refer
(C) adjust
(D) agree

75. The *proximity* of the lake

(A) worthlessness
(B) nearness
(C) level
(D) ebullition

SYNONYMS TEST ANSWER KEY

1. **B**
2. **D**
3. **A**
4. **B**
5. **C**
6. **D**
7. **A**
8. **A**
9. **A**
10. **D**
11. **B**
12. **B**
13. **A**
14. **C**
15. **C**
16. **D**
17. **C**
18. **C**
19. **A**
20. **B**
21. **B**
22. **C**
23. **A**
24. **D**
25. **A**
26. **B**
27. **C**
28. **A**
29. **A**
30. **C**
31. **D**
32. **B**
33. **D**
34. **A**
35. **C**
36. **D**
37. **C**
38. **B**
39. **B**
40. **D**
41. **C**
42. **A**
43. **A**
44. **C**
45. **D**
46. **C**
47. **B**
48. **A**
49. **D**
50. **A**
51. **D**
52. **D**
53. **B**
54. **B**
55. **B**
56. **D**
57. **B**
58. **B**
59. **C**
60. **B**
61. **A**
62. **A**
63. **C**
64. **C**
65. **D**
66. **D**
67. **A**
68. **D**
69. **B**
70. **A**
71. **B**
72. **D**
73. **A**
74. **D**
75. **B**

ANTONYMS

THE TURNABOUTS

In the preceding part of this section, emphasis was placed on synonyms or words with similar or identical meanings. You are now ready to make a "turnabout" and embark upon increasing your word power from a contrasting point of view. Antonyms are words that are opposite in meaning. Some very explicit and simple samples are: *hot/cold, strong/weak, sit/stand, night/day, and lazy/industrious.*

Antonyms are extremely useful to express contrast. The use of certain antonyms can result in the verbal creation of a universal portrait or concept. For instance, everyone associates the name "Scrooge" with *penny-pinching* or *miserly* traits. The Dickens character was anything but philanthropic, a term that characterizes people or agencies who devote themselves to helping and giving to humanity. Therefore, if you read that "a former Scrooge has transformed himself into a philanthropist" you would surmise that the person being described has had a complete change of heart. The term *philanthropist* has been contrasted with a symbol of *miserly* and *penny-pinching* traits.

In taking a test measuring your comprehension of verbal contrasts, be certain to select a response that is the same part of speech as the term in question. Although *discourtesy* and *insolent* share the same shade of meaning, one could not be substituted for the other—the former is a noun and the latter an adjective. Therefore, they could not play identical roles in a sentence.

If you are stumped by any one test item, move on quickly to the next. When you have completed the test, and if time permits, return to any test item(s) you have skipped. Mentally put the various word choices, including the test item, in a sentence. Then remove the test item again.

Example: Polite

(A) desperate
(B) discourtesy
(C) insolent
(D) discriminate

For the above example, make up a sentence using the word *polite* and then substitute the options in its place, such as "The boy is *discourtesy*" and "The boy is *insolent*." Obviously, *insolent* is the correct response, as it is the word opposite in meaning to *polite* and best fits the sentence pattern "The boy is . . ."

USING PREFIXES

Another helpful technique in taking antonym tests is the close examination of prefixes. Review the etymological information before attempting the sample antonym test, and pay special attention to prefixes. Prefixes can often be the key to contrast in meaning. For example, the prefixes *un*, *im*, and *in* frequently denote the opposite meaning of the word to which they are affixed: *happy/unhappy; adequate/ inadequate; polite/impolite*. These examples make it apparent that the actual meaning of the prefixes is "not." The prefixes *in* and *ex* are opposite in meaning. *In* means, "in," "into," "inside;" and *ex* means "out," "outside of."

If the target word is internal, which of the following words would you select as its antonym?

(A) interior
(B) ephermeral
(C) illegal
(D) external

Of course, *external* is the correct response. Study the list of contrasting prefixes below. Then try your hand at making the "turnabout!"

CONTRASTING PREFIXES

ad, ac, ag, at (to)	*ab, a* (away from)
ante (before)	*post* (after)
anti, contra (against)	*pro* (for)
bene (well, good)	*mal* (bad)
corn, con, col (together)	*dis, di* (apart)
con, com (with)	*an* (without)
eu (good)	*dys* (bad)
in, im (in)	*e, ex* (out)
hypo (under)	*hyper* (over)
pro (forward)	*retro* (backward)
sub (under)	*super, sur* (above)

ANTONYMS TEST ANSWER SHEET

1. Ⓐ Ⓑ Ⓒ Ⓓ	20. Ⓐ Ⓑ Ⓒ Ⓓ	39. Ⓐ Ⓑ Ⓒ Ⓓ	58. Ⓐ Ⓑ Ⓒ Ⓓ
2. Ⓐ Ⓑ Ⓒ Ⓓ	21. Ⓐ Ⓑ Ⓒ Ⓓ	40. Ⓐ Ⓑ Ⓒ Ⓓ	59. Ⓐ Ⓑ Ⓒ Ⓓ
3. Ⓐ Ⓑ Ⓒ Ⓓ	22. Ⓐ Ⓑ Ⓒ Ⓓ	41. Ⓐ Ⓑ Ⓒ Ⓓ	60. Ⓐ Ⓑ Ⓒ Ⓓ
4. Ⓐ Ⓑ Ⓒ Ⓓ	23. Ⓐ Ⓑ Ⓒ Ⓓ	42. Ⓐ Ⓑ Ⓒ Ⓓ	61. Ⓐ Ⓑ Ⓒ Ⓓ
5. Ⓐ Ⓑ Ⓒ Ⓓ	24. Ⓐ Ⓑ Ⓒ Ⓓ	43. Ⓐ Ⓑ Ⓒ Ⓓ	62. Ⓐ Ⓑ Ⓒ Ⓓ
6. Ⓐ Ⓑ Ⓒ Ⓓ	25. Ⓐ Ⓑ Ⓒ Ⓓ	44. Ⓐ Ⓑ Ⓒ Ⓓ	63. Ⓐ Ⓑ Ⓒ Ⓓ
7. Ⓐ Ⓑ Ⓒ Ⓓ	26. Ⓐ Ⓑ Ⓒ Ⓓ	45. Ⓐ Ⓑ Ⓒ Ⓓ	64. Ⓐ Ⓑ Ⓒ Ⓓ
8. Ⓐ Ⓑ Ⓒ Ⓓ	27. Ⓐ Ⓑ Ⓒ Ⓓ	46. Ⓐ Ⓑ Ⓒ Ⓓ	65. Ⓐ Ⓑ Ⓒ Ⓓ
9. Ⓐ Ⓑ Ⓒ Ⓓ	28. Ⓐ Ⓑ Ⓒ Ⓓ	47. Ⓐ Ⓑ Ⓒ Ⓓ	66. Ⓐ Ⓑ Ⓒ Ⓓ
10. Ⓐ Ⓑ Ⓒ Ⓓ	29. Ⓐ Ⓑ Ⓒ Ⓓ	48. Ⓐ Ⓑ Ⓒ Ⓓ	67. Ⓐ Ⓑ Ⓒ Ⓓ
11. Ⓐ Ⓑ Ⓒ Ⓓ	30. Ⓐ Ⓑ Ⓒ Ⓓ	49. Ⓐ Ⓑ Ⓒ Ⓓ	68. Ⓐ Ⓑ Ⓒ Ⓓ
12. Ⓐ Ⓑ Ⓒ Ⓓ	31. Ⓐ Ⓑ Ⓒ Ⓓ	50. Ⓐ Ⓑ Ⓒ Ⓓ	69. Ⓐ Ⓑ Ⓒ Ⓓ
13. Ⓐ Ⓑ Ⓒ Ⓓ	32. Ⓐ Ⓑ Ⓒ Ⓓ	51. Ⓐ Ⓑ Ⓒ Ⓓ	70. Ⓐ Ⓑ Ⓒ Ⓓ
14. Ⓐ Ⓑ Ⓒ Ⓓ	33. Ⓐ Ⓑ Ⓒ Ⓓ	52. Ⓐ Ⓑ Ⓒ Ⓓ	71. Ⓐ Ⓑ Ⓒ Ⓓ
15. Ⓐ Ⓑ Ⓒ Ⓓ	34. Ⓐ Ⓑ Ⓒ Ⓓ	53. Ⓐ Ⓑ Ⓒ Ⓓ	72. Ⓐ Ⓑ Ⓒ Ⓓ
16. Ⓐ Ⓑ Ⓒ Ⓓ	35. Ⓐ Ⓑ Ⓒ Ⓓ	54. Ⓐ Ⓑ Ⓒ Ⓓ	73. Ⓐ Ⓑ Ⓒ Ⓓ
17. Ⓐ Ⓑ Ⓒ Ⓓ	36. Ⓐ Ⓑ Ⓒ Ⓓ	55. Ⓐ Ⓑ Ⓒ Ⓓ	74. Ⓐ Ⓑ Ⓒ Ⓓ
18. Ⓐ Ⓑ Ⓒ Ⓓ	37. Ⓐ Ⓑ Ⓒ Ⓓ	56. Ⓐ Ⓑ Ⓒ Ⓓ	75. Ⓐ Ⓑ Ⓒ Ⓓ
19. Ⓐ Ⓑ Ⓒ Ⓓ	38. Ⓐ Ⓑ Ⓒ Ⓓ	57. Ⓐ Ⓑ Ⓒ Ⓓ	

ANTONYMS TEST

75 QUESTIONS • TIME—30 MINUTES

Directions: For each of the following questions, select the word opposite in meaning to the word printed in capital letters.

1. DEFACE
   (A) defame
   (B) embellish
   (C) vilify
   (D) disfigure
2. SUPERFLUOUS
   (A) coarse
   (B) transient
   (C) insufficient
   (D) abundant
3. ASSUAGE
   (A) presume
   (B) agitate
   (C) alleviate
   (D) absorb
4. AUGURY
   (A) gentility
   (B) relentlessness
   (C) supremacy
   (D) science
5. TERMINATE
   (A) withhold
   (B) construe
   (C) repel
   (D) initiate
6. VITIATE
   (A) liquidate
   (B) revive
   (C) validate
   (D) slander
7. JUBILANT
   (A) lugubrious
   (B) irrepressible
   (C) discernible
   (D) jocular
8. HOSTILE
   (A) affable
   (B) awkward
   (C) judicious
   (D) coxcombical
9. TACITURN
   (A) tactful
   (B) talkative
   (C) crucial
   (D) impetuous
10. LAGGARDLY
   (A) laboriously
   (B) languidly
   (C) briskly
   (D) cowardly
11. PHLEGMATIC
   (A) vital
   (B) apparent
   (C) conversant
   (D) apprehensive
12. LOATHSOME
   (A) alluring
   (B) mournful
   (C) indifferent
   (D) preposterous
13. EXALT
   (A) degrade
   (B) gratify
   (C) expose
   (D) desiderate
14. PACIFY
   (A) conciliate
   (B) palliate
   (C) quell
   (D) exasperate

15. SUBSEQUENT
   (A) worthless
   (B) inactive
   (C) preceding
   (D) demeaning

16. ULTIMATE
   (A) initial
   (B) equitable
   (C) irrefutable
   (D) turbid

17. LEEWAY
   (A) relevance
   (B) restriction
   (C) protection
   (D) satisfaction

18. PRETENTIOUS
   (A) flagrant
   (B) diabolical
   (C) officious
   (D) modest

19. QUANDARY
   (A) certainty
   (B) mediocrity
   (C) ruthlessness
   (D) criterion

20. SAGACIOUS
   (A) obtuse
   (B) scurrilous
   (C) indulgent
   (D) impertinent

21. SAVANT
   (A) savage
   (B) master
   (C) neophyte
   (D) constituent

22. SQUALID
   (A) staunch
   (B) stately
   (C) avaricious
   (D) equivocal

23. EXQUISITE
   (A) exorbitant
   (B) inobscure
   (C) extraneous
   (D) ordinary

24. FACILITATE
   (A) falsify
   (B) delude
   (C) hinder
   (D) assimilate

25. FLAWLESS
   (A) pertinent
   (B) conventional
   (C) defective
   (D) complacent

26. RECOMPENSE
   (A) renovate
   (B) misrequite
   (C) miscompute
   (D) sanction

27. FERVENT
   (A) nonchalant
   (B) lenient
   (C) meager
   (D) liable

28. AVERT
   (A) pursue
   (B) forestall
   (C) reject
   (D) relinquish

29. ARID
   (A) fragrant
   (B) moist
   (C) parched
   (D) odoriferous

30. IMPERATIVE
   (A) conceptive
   (B) illustrative
   (C) speculative
   (D) optional

31. SUCCINCT
   (A) corporeal
   (B) graphic
   (C) princely
   (D) loquacious

32. JEOPARDY
   (A) security
   (B) discernment
   (C) curiosity
   (D) tedium

33. SOMBER
    (A) insipid
    (B) congruous
    (C) festive
    (D) voluminous

34. EXOTIC
    (A) diachronic
    (B) erotic
    (C) common
    (D) harmonious

35. AFFILIATE
    (A) annihilate
    (B) disassociate
    (C) proffer
    (D) disparage

36. SINISTER
    (A) auspicious
    (B) immaculate
    (C) fanatical
    (D) transitory

37. INEXTRICABLE
    (A) intricate
    (B) judicious
    (C) disentangled
    (D) desperate

38. PROFLIGATE
    (A) insolvent
    (B) virtuous
    (C) redundant
    (D) incessant

39. TURBULENT
    (A) diaphanous
    (B) tranquil
    (C) formidable
    (D) diffident

40. UNWARRANTED
    (A) justifiable
    (B) baneful
    (C) depleted
    (D) contemplated

41. PLAINTIVE
    (A) embellished
    (B) peccant
    (C) rational
    (D) gleeful

42. ORNATE
    (A) unadorned
    (B) deft
    (C) subtle
    (D) conspicuous

43. ABROGATE
    (A) ratify
    (B) reconcile
    (C) abridge
    (D) alleviate

44. ABASE
    (A) cede
    (B) dignify
    (C) repudiate
    (D) engulf

45. RENOUNCE
    (A) claim
    (B) deride
    (C) conceive
    (D) alienate

46. SABOTAGE
    (A) compensate
    (B) reinforce
    (C) restrain
    (D) release

47. OBLIVIOUS
    (A) latent
    (B) integrant
    (C) repugnant
    (D) cognizant

48. SUBMISSIVE
    (A) offensive
    (B) tactless
    (C) incompliant
    (D) manifest

49. NURTURE
    (A) distinguish
    (B) impart
    (C) neglect
    (D) disclose

50. PRUDENCE
    (A) compunction
    (B) dilemma
    (C) anticipation
    (D) recklessness

51. LAMENT

(A) rejoice
(B) acclaim
(C) surmise
(D) deceive

52. GRUELING

(A) relaxing
(B) satisfying
(C) taming
(D) suppressing

53. TRIVIAL

(A) nugatory
(B) ungainly
(C) critical
(D) solicitous

54. ZENITH

(A) vitality
(B) rage
(C) reverence
(D) nadir

55. UNOBTRUSIVE

(A) resonant
(B) interfering
(C) controlled
(D) subjective

56. REFRACTIVE

(A) cryptic
(B) interruptive
(C) applicable
(D) direct

57. REBUFF

(A) exclusion
(B) disturbance
(C) recall
(D) encouragement

58. ADVERSARY

(A) opponent
(B) administrator
(C) accomplice
(D) enemy

59. ANTAGONIST

(A) rival
(B) protagonist
(C) analyst
(D) pessimist

60. ALIEN

(A) native
(B) anonymous
(C) verified
(D) copious

61. ERUDITE

(A) contagious
(B) inadvertent
(C) benevolent
(D) ignorant

62. PARAMOUNT

(A) admissible
(B) inconsequential
(C) tolerable
(D) supreme

63. SURREPTITIOUS

(A) authoritative
(B) candid
(C) vulnerable
(D) subjugated

64. MENDACIOUS

(A) meddlesome
(B) incomparable
(C) malicious
(D) creditable

65. UNCTUOUS

(A) awkward
(B) dubious
(C) furtive
(D) disputable

66. IMPETUOUS

(A) subdued
(B) unmitigated
(C) substantial
(D) egregious

67. PENURIOUS

(A) frugal
(B) extravagant
(C) plausible
(D) absurd

68. ODIOUS

(A) attentive
(B) considerate
(C) acceptable
(D) unascertained

69. OSTENSIBLE
    - (A) hidden
    - (B) preliminary
    - (C) authentic
    - (D) unsuitable

70. DELETERIOUS
    - (A) distressing
    - (B) beneficial
    - (C) grievous
    - (D) delirious

71. IGNOMINY
    - (A) honor
    - (B) aversion
    - (C) perplexity
    - (D) remoteness

72. COMPATIBLE
    - (A) dexterous
    - (B) repugnant
    - (C) incongruous
    - (D) captivating

73. PREMEDITATED
    - (A) devoted
    - (B) condescending
    - (C) improvised
    - (D) supposed

74. PERNICIOUS
    - (A) restorative
    - (B) conclusive
    - (C) tractable
    - (D) capricious

75. UMBRAGE
    - (A) pique
    - (B) monstrous
    - (C) reliance
    - (D) amity

ANTONYMS TEST ANSWER KEY

1. **B**
2. **C**
3. **B**
4. **D**
5. **D**
6. **C**
7. **A**
8. **A**
9. **B**
10. **C**
11. **A**
12. **A**
13. **A**
14. **D**
15. **C**
16. **A**
17. **B**
18. **D**
19. **A**
20. **A**
21. **C**
22. **B**
23. **D**
24. **C**
25. **C**
26. **B**
27. **A**
28. **A**
29. **B**
30. **D**
31. **D**
32. **A**
33. **C**
34. **C**
35. **B**
36. **A**
37. **C**
38. **B**
39. **B**
40. **A**
41. **D**
42. **A**
43. **A**
44. **B**
45. **A**
46. **B**
47. **D**
48. **C**
49. **C**
50. **D**
51. **A**
52. **A**
53. **C**
54. **D**
55. **B**
56. **D**
57. **D**
58. **C**
59. **B**
60. **A**
61. **D**
62. **B**
63. **B**
64. **D**
65. **A**
66. **A**
67. **B**
68. **C**
69. **A**
70. **B**
71. **A**
72. **C**
73. **C**
74. **A**
75. **D**

SKILL WITH VERBAL ANALOGIES

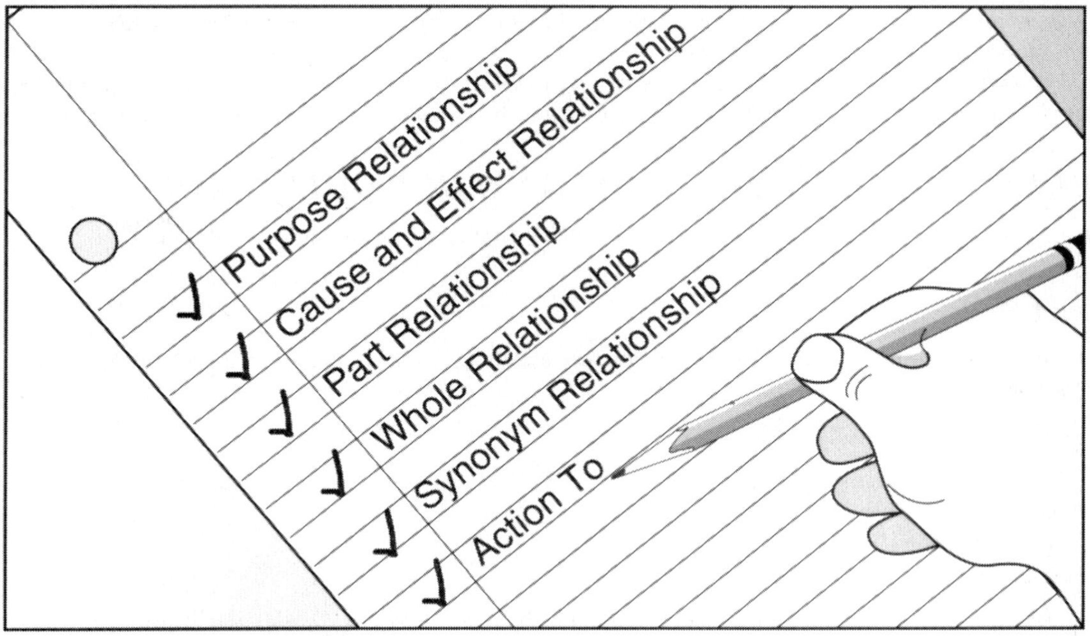

The verbal analogy is one variation of the vocabulary question often encountered on nursing school tests. It tests your understanding of word meanings and your ability to grasp relationships between words and ideas. This practice in mental agility will help you do better with all the other questions on the test.

In addition to their simple meanings, words carry subtle shades of implication that depend in some degree upon the relationship they bear to other words. There are various classifications of relationship, such as similarity (synonyms) and opposition (antonyms). Careful students will try to examine each shade of meaning they encounter.

The ability to detect the exact nature of the relationship between words is a function of your intelligence. In a sense, the verbal analogy test is a vocabulary test. But it is also a test of your ability to analyze meanings, think things out, and see the relationships between ideas and words. In mathematics, this kind of situation is expressed as a proportion problem: 3:5::6:*X*. Sometimes, verbal analogies are written in this mathematical form:

CLOCK : TIME :: THERMOMETER:

(A) hour
(B) degrees
(C) climate
(D) temperature

Or the question may be put:

CLOCK is to TIME as THERMOMETER is to

(A) hour
(B) degrees
(C) climate
(D) temperature

The problem is to determine which of the lettered words has the same relationship to *thermometer* as *time* has to *clock*. The best way of determining the correct answer is to provide a word or phrase that shows the relationship between these words. In the above example, "measures" is a word expressing the relationship. However, this may not be enough. The analogy must be exact. *Climate* or *weather* would not be exact enough. *Temperature*, of course, is the correct answer.

You will find that many of the choices you have to select from have some relationship to the third word. Select the one with a relationship that *best* approximates the relationship between the first two words.

THREE FORMATS FOR VERBAL ANALOGY QUESTIONS

Some standardized tests provide four answer choices (A,B,C,D) and some five (A,B,C,D,E).

Type 1

From the four pairs of words that follow, you are to select the pair related in the same way as are the words of the first pair.

SPELLING : PUNCTUATION ::

(A) pajamas : fatigue
(B) powder : shaving
(C) bandage : cut
(D) biology : physics

Spelling and *Punctuation* are elements of the mechanics of English; *Biology* and *Physics* are two of the subjects that make up the field of science. The other choices do not possess this part: part relationship. Therefore, (D) is the correct choice.

Type 2

Another popular format gives two words followed by a third word. The latter is related to one word in a group of choices in the same way that the first two words are related.

WINTER : SUMMER :: COLD

(A) wet
(B) future
(C) hot
(D) freezing

Winter and *Summer* bear an opposite relationship. *Cold* and *hot* have the same kind of opposite relationship. Therefore, (C) is the correct answer.

Type 3

Still another analogy format has a variable construction. Any four relationship elements may not be specified. From choices offered—regardless of position—you are to select the one choice that completes the relationship with the other three items. In this example the third element is not specified.

SUBMARINE : FISH ::___: BIRD

(A) kite
(B) limousine
(C) feather
(D) chirp

Both a *submarine* and a *fish* are usually found in the water; both a *kite* and a *bird* are customarily seen in the air. (A), consequently, is the correct answer.

This third type is used in the Miller Analogy Test, considered one of the most reliable and valid tests for selection of graduate students for universities and high-level personnel for government, industry, and business.

CATEGORIZING THE KINDS OF ANALOGY RELATIONSHIPS

1. Purpose Relationship

   GLOVE : BALL ::

   (A) hook : fish
   (B) winter : weather
   (C) game : pennant
   (D) stadium : seats

   (Answer: A)

2. Cause-and-Effect Relationship

   RACE : FATIGUE ::

   (A) track : athlete
   (B) ant : bug
   (C) fast : hunger
   (D) walking : running

   (Answer: C)

3. Part : Whole Relationship

   SNAKE : REPTILE ::

   (A) patch : thread
   (B) removal : snow
   (C) struggle : wrestle
   (D) hand : clock

   (Answer: D)

4. Part : Part Relationship

   GILL : FIN ::

   (A) tube : antenna
   (B) instrument : violin
   (C) sea : fish
   (D) salad : supper

   (Answer: A)

5. Action : Object Relationship

   KICK : FOOTBALL ::

   (A) kill : bomb
   (B) break : pieces
   (C) question : team
   (D) smoke : pipe

   (Answer: D)

6. Object : Action Relationship

   STEAK : BROIL ::

   (A) bread : bake
   (B) food : eat
   (C) wine : pour
   (D) sugar : spill

   (Answer: A)

7. Synonym Relationship

   ENORMOUS : HUGE ::

   (A) rogue : rock
   (B) muddy : unclear
   (C) purse : kitchen
   (D) black : white

   (Answer: B)

8. Antonym Relationship

   PURITY : EVIL ::

   (A) suavity : bluntness
   (B) north : climate
   (C) angel : horns
   (D) boldness : victory

   (Answer: A)

9. Place Relationship

   MIAMI : FLORIDA ::

   (A) Chicago : United States
   (B) New York : Albany
   (C) United States : Chicago
   (D) Albany : New York

   (Answer: D)

10. Degree Relationship

    WARM : HOT ::

    (A) glue : paste
    (B) climate : weather
    (C) fried egg : boiled egg
    (D) bright : genius

    (Answer: D)

11. Characteristic Relationship

    IGNORANCE : POVERTY ::

    (A) blood : wound
    (B) money : dollar
    (C) schools : elevators
    (D) education : stupidity

    (Answer: A)

12. Sequence Relationship

    SPRING : SUMMER ::

    (A) Thursday : Wednesday
    (B) Wednesday : Monday
    (C) Monday : Sunday
    (D) Wednesday : Thursday

    (Answer: D)

13. Grammatical Relationship

    RESTORE : CLIMB ::

    (A) segregation : seem
    (B) into : nymph
    (C) tearoom : although
    (D) overpower : seethe

    (Answer: D)

14. Association Relationship

    DEVIL : WRONG ::

    (A) color : sidewalk
    (B) slipper : state
    (C) ink : writing
    (D) picture : bed

    (Answer: C)

15. Numerical Relationship

    4 : 12 ::

    (A) 10 :16
    (B) 9 : 27
    (C) 3 : 4
    (D) 12 : 6

    (Answer: B)

POINTS TO REMEMBER

In many analogy questions, the incorrect choices may be related in some way to the first two words. Don't let this association mislead you. For example, in number 4 (part : part relationship), the correct answer is (A), *tube : antenna*. Choice (C), *sea : fish*, is incorrect, although these two latter words are associated in a general sense with the first two words (*gill : fin*).

Often, the relationship of the first two words may apply to *more than one* of the choices given. In such a case, you must narrow down the initial relationship in order to get the correct choice. For example, in number 6 (object: action relationship), a *steak* is something that you *broil*. Now let us consider the choices: *bread* is something that you *bake*; food is something that you *eat*; wine is something that you *pour* and *sugar* is something that you (can) *spill*. Thus far, each choice seems correct. Let us now narrow down the relationship: a *steak* is something that you *broil* with *heat*. The only choice that fulfills this *complete* relationship is (A), *bread*—something that you *bake* with *heat*. It follows that (A) is the correct choice.

Remember that the keys to analogy success are:

Step One: Determine the relationship between the first two words.

Step Two: Find the same relationship among the choices that follow the first two words.

VERBAL ANALOGIES TEST ANSWER SHEET

PART A

1. Ⓐ Ⓑ Ⓒ Ⓓ	8. Ⓐ Ⓑ Ⓒ Ⓓ	15. Ⓐ Ⓑ Ⓒ Ⓓ	22. Ⓐ Ⓑ Ⓒ Ⓓ
2. Ⓐ Ⓑ Ⓒ Ⓓ	9. Ⓐ Ⓑ Ⓒ Ⓓ	16. Ⓐ Ⓑ Ⓒ Ⓓ	23. Ⓐ Ⓑ Ⓒ Ⓓ
3. Ⓐ Ⓑ Ⓒ Ⓓ	10. Ⓐ Ⓑ Ⓒ Ⓓ	17. Ⓐ Ⓑ Ⓒ Ⓓ	24. Ⓐ Ⓑ Ⓒ Ⓓ
4. Ⓐ Ⓑ Ⓒ Ⓓ	11. Ⓐ Ⓑ Ⓒ Ⓓ	18. Ⓐ Ⓑ Ⓒ Ⓓ	25. Ⓐ Ⓑ Ⓒ Ⓓ
5. Ⓐ Ⓑ Ⓒ Ⓓ	12. Ⓐ Ⓑ Ⓒ Ⓓ	19. Ⓐ Ⓑ Ⓒ Ⓓ	
6. Ⓐ Ⓑ Ⓒ Ⓓ	13. Ⓐ Ⓑ Ⓒ Ⓓ	20. Ⓐ Ⓑ Ⓒ Ⓓ	
7. Ⓐ Ⓑ Ⓒ Ⓓ	14. Ⓐ Ⓑ Ⓒ Ⓓ	21. Ⓐ Ⓑ Ⓒ Ⓓ	

PART B

1. Ⓐ Ⓑ Ⓒ Ⓓ Ⓔ	8. Ⓐ Ⓑ Ⓒ Ⓓ Ⓔ	15. Ⓐ Ⓑ Ⓒ Ⓓ Ⓔ	22. Ⓐ Ⓑ Ⓒ Ⓓ Ⓔ
2. Ⓐ Ⓑ Ⓒ Ⓓ Ⓔ	9. Ⓐ Ⓑ Ⓒ Ⓓ Ⓔ	16. Ⓐ Ⓑ Ⓒ Ⓓ Ⓔ	23. Ⓐ Ⓑ Ⓒ Ⓓ Ⓔ
3. Ⓐ Ⓑ Ⓒ Ⓓ Ⓔ	10. Ⓐ Ⓑ Ⓒ Ⓓ Ⓔ	17. Ⓐ Ⓑ Ⓒ Ⓓ Ⓔ	24. Ⓐ Ⓑ Ⓒ Ⓓ Ⓔ
4. Ⓐ Ⓑ Ⓒ Ⓓ Ⓔ	11. Ⓐ Ⓑ Ⓒ Ⓓ Ⓔ	18. Ⓐ Ⓑ Ⓒ Ⓓ Ⓔ	25. Ⓐ Ⓑ Ⓒ Ⓓ Ⓔ
5. Ⓐ Ⓑ Ⓒ Ⓓ Ⓔ	12. Ⓐ Ⓑ Ⓒ Ⓓ Ⓔ	19. Ⓐ Ⓑ Ⓒ Ⓓ Ⓔ	
6. Ⓐ Ⓑ Ⓒ Ⓓ Ⓔ	13. Ⓐ Ⓑ Ⓒ Ⓓ Ⓔ	20. Ⓐ Ⓑ Ⓒ Ⓓ Ⓔ	
7. Ⓐ Ⓑ Ⓒ Ⓓ Ⓔ	14. Ⓐ Ⓑ Ⓒ Ⓓ Ⓔ	21. Ⓐ Ⓑ Ⓒ Ⓓ Ⓔ	

PART C

1. Ⓐ Ⓑ Ⓒ Ⓓ Ⓔ	8. Ⓐ Ⓑ Ⓒ Ⓓ Ⓔ	15. Ⓐ Ⓑ Ⓒ Ⓓ Ⓔ	22. Ⓐ Ⓑ Ⓒ Ⓓ Ⓔ
2. Ⓐ Ⓑ Ⓒ Ⓓ Ⓔ	9. Ⓐ Ⓑ Ⓒ Ⓓ Ⓔ	16. Ⓐ Ⓑ Ⓒ Ⓓ Ⓔ	23. Ⓐ Ⓑ Ⓒ Ⓓ Ⓔ
3. Ⓐ Ⓑ Ⓒ Ⓓ Ⓔ	10. Ⓐ Ⓑ Ⓒ Ⓓ Ⓔ	17. Ⓐ Ⓑ Ⓒ Ⓓ Ⓔ	24. Ⓐ Ⓑ Ⓒ Ⓓ Ⓔ
4. Ⓐ Ⓑ Ⓒ Ⓓ Ⓔ	11. Ⓐ Ⓑ Ⓒ Ⓓ Ⓔ	18. Ⓐ Ⓑ Ⓒ Ⓓ Ⓔ	25. Ⓐ Ⓑ Ⓒ Ⓓ Ⓔ
5. Ⓐ Ⓑ Ⓒ Ⓓ Ⓔ	12. Ⓐ Ⓑ Ⓒ Ⓓ Ⓔ	19. Ⓐ Ⓑ Ⓒ Ⓓ Ⓔ	
6. Ⓐ Ⓑ Ⓒ Ⓓ Ⓔ	13. Ⓐ Ⓑ Ⓒ Ⓓ Ⓔ	20. Ⓐ Ⓑ Ⓒ Ⓓ Ⓔ	
7. Ⓐ Ⓑ Ⓒ Ⓓ Ⓔ	14. Ⓐ Ⓑ Ⓒ Ⓓ Ⓔ	21. Ⓐ Ⓑ Ⓒ Ⓓ Ⓔ	

VERBAL ANALOGIES TEST

75 QUESTIONS • TIME—75 MINUTES

Directions: In the following questions, you are to determine the relationship between the first pair of capitalized words and then decide which of the answer choices shares a similar relationship with the third capitalized word. Parts A and B of this test are written in mathematical form (expressed as proportion problems). Part A's questions have four answer choices, Part B's questions have five. Part C is written so that relationships are expressed with "is to" and "as."

PART A

25 QUESTIONS • TIME—10 MINUTES

1. GUN : SHOTS :: KNIFE :
   (A) run
   (B) cuts
   (C) hat
   (D) bird
2. EAR : HEAR :: EYE :
   (A) table
   (B) hand
   (C) see
   (D) foot
3. FUR : MAMMAL :: FEATHERS :
   (A) bird
   (B) neck
   (C) feet
   (D) bill
4. HANDLE : HAMMER :: KNOB :
   (A) key
   (B) room
   (C) shut
   (D) door
5. SHOE : FOOT :: HAT :
   (A) coat
   (B) nose
   (C) head
   (D) collar
6. WATER : DRINK :: BREAD :
   (A) cake
   (B) coffee
   (C) eat
   (D) pie
7. FOOD : MAN :: GASOLINE:
   (A) gas
   (B) oil
   (C) automobile
   (D) spark
8. EAT : FAT :: STARVE :
   (A) thin
   (B) food
   (C) bread
   (D) thirsty
9. MAN : HOUSE :: BIRD :
   (A) fly
   (B) insect
   (C) worm
   (D) nest
10. GO : COME :: SELL :
    (A) leave
    (B) buy
    (C) money
    (D) papers

11. PENINSULA : LAND :: BAY :
    - (A) boats
    - (B) pay
    - (C) ocean
    - (D) colony
12. HOUR : MINUTE :: MINUTE :
    - (A) hour
    - (B) week
    - (C) second
    - (D) short
13. ABIDE : DEPART :: STAY :
    - (A) over
    - (B) home
    - (C) play
    - (D) leave
14. JANUARY : FEBRUARY :: JUNE :
    - (A) July
    - (B) May
    - (C) month
    - (D) year
15. BOLD : TIMID :: ADVANCE :
    - (A) proceed
    - (B) retreat
    - (C) campaign
    - (D) soldiers
16. ABOVE : BELOW :: TOP :
    - (A) spin
    - (B) bottom
    - (C) surface
    - (D) side
17. LION : ANIMAL :: ROSE :
    - (A) smell
    - (B) leaf
    - (C) plant
    - (D) thorn
18. TIGER : CARNIVOROUS :: HORSE :
    - (A) cow
    - (B) nervous
    - (C) omnivorous
    - (D) herbivorous
19. SAILOR : NAVY :: SOLDIER :
    - (A) gun
    - (B) cap
    - (C) hill
    - (D) army
20. PICTURE : SEE :: SOUND :
    - (A) noise
    - (B) music
    - (C) hear
    - (D) bark
21. SUCCESS : JOY :: FAILURE :
    - (A) sadness
    - (B) success
    - (C) fail
    - (D) work
22. HOPE : DESPAIR :: HAPPINESS :
    - (A) frolic
    - (B) fun
    - (C) joy
    - (D) sadness
23. PRETTY : UGLY :: ATTRACT :
    - (A) fine
    - (B) repel
    - (C) nice
    - (D) draw
24. PUPIL : TEACHER :: CHILD :
    - (A) parent
    - (B) dolly
    - (C) youngster
    - (D) obey
25. CITY : MAYOR :: ARMY :
    - (A) navy
    - (B) soldier
    - (C) general
    - (D) private

PART B

25 QUESTIONS • TIME—10 MINUTES

1. REMUNERATIVE : PROFITABLE :: FRAUDULENT:

(A) lying
(B) slander
(C) fallacious
(D) plausible
(E) reward

2. AX : WOODSMAN :: AWL :

(A) cut
(B) hew
(C) plumber
(D) pierce
(E) cobbler

3. SURGEON : SCALPEL :: BUTCHER :

(A) mallet
(B) cleaver
(C) chisel
(D) wrench
(E) medicine

4. CAT : FELINE :: HORSE :

(A) equine
(B) tiger
(C) quadruped
(D) carnivore
(E) vulpine

5. ADVERSITY : HAPPINESS :: VEHEMENCE :

(A) misfortune
(B) gaiety
(C) troublesome
(D) petulance
(E) serenity

6. NECKLACE : ADORNMENT :: MEDAL :

(A) jewel
(B) metal
(C) bravery
(D) bronze
(E) decoration

7. GUN : HOLSTER :: SWORD :

(A) pistol
(B) scabbard
(C) warrior
(D) slay
(E) plunder

8. ARCHEOLOGIST : ANTIQUITY :: ICHTHYOLOGIST :

(A) theology
(B) ruins
(C) horticulture
(D) marine life
(E) mystic

9. SHOE : LEATHER :: HIGHWAY :

(A) passage
(B) road
(C) asphalt
(D) trail
(E) journey

10. SERFDOM : FEUDALISM :: ENTREPRENEUR :

(A) laissez faire
(B) captain
(C) radical
(D) agriculture
(E) capitalism

11. FIN : FISH :: PROPELLER :

(A) automobile
(B) airplane
(C) grain elevator
(D) water
(E) canoe

12. PULP : PAPER :: HEMP :

(A) rope
(B) baskets
(C) yarn
(D) cotton
(E) wood

13. SKIN : MAN :: HIDE :

(A) scales
(B) fur
(C) animal
(D) hair
(E) fish

14. RAIN : DROP :: SNOW :

(A) ice
(B) cold
(C) zero
(D) flake
(E) sleet

15. WING : BIRD :: HOOF :

(A) dog
(B) foot
(C) horse
(D) girl
(E) horseshoe

16. CONSTELLATION : STAR :: ARCHIPELAGO :

(A) continent
(B) peninsula
(C) country
(D) island
(E) river

17. ACCOUNTANCY : BOOKKEEPING :: COURT REPORTING :

(A) law
(B) judgment
(C) stenography
(D) lawyer
(E) judge

18. ABSENCE : PRESENCE :: STABLE :

(A) steady
(B) secure
(C) safe
(D) changeable
(E) influential

19. RUBBER : FLEXIBILITY :: PIPE :

(A) iron
(B) copper
(C) pliability
(D) elasticity
(E) rigidity

20. SAFETY VALVE : BOILER :: FUSE :

(A) motor
(B) house
(C) wire
(D) city
(E) factory

21. SCHOLARLY : UNSCHOLARLY :: LEARNED :

(A) ignorant
(B) wise
(C) skilled
(D) scholarly
(E) literary

22. IMMIGRANT : ARRIVAL :: EMIGRATION :

(A) leaving
(B) alienation
(C) native
(D) welcoming
(E) emigrant

23. GOVERNOR : STATE :: GENERAL :

(A) lieutenant
(B) navy
(C) army
(D) captain
(E) admiral

24. LETTER CARRIER : MAIL :: MESSENGER :

(A) value
(B) dispatches
(C) easy
(D) complicated
(E) fast

25. CLOTH : COAT :: GINGHAM :

(A) doll
(B) cover
(C) washable
(D) dress
(E) dressmaker

PART C

25 QUESTIONS • TIME—10 MINUTES

1. BOAT is to DOCK as AIRPLANE is to
   (A) wing
   (B) strut
   (C) engine
   (D) wind
   (E) hangar
2. OAT is to BUSHEL as DIAMOND is to
   (A) gram
   (B) hardness
   (C) usefulness
   (D) carat
   (E) ornament
3. MEDICINE is to EXAMINATION as LAW is to
   (A) jurist
   (B) court
   (C) interrogation
   (D) contract
   (E) suit
4. PARENT is to COMMAND as CHILD is to
   (A) obey
   (B) will
   (C) women
   (D) love
   (E) achieve
5. CAPTAIN is to VESSEL as DIRECTOR is to
   (A) touring party
   (B) board
   (C) travel
   (D) orchestra
   (E) musician
6. FATHER is to DAUGHTER as UNCLE is to
   (A) son
   (B) daughter
   (C) son-in-law
   (D) niece
   (E) aunt
7. PISTOL is to TRIGGER as MOTOR is to
   (A) wire
   (B) dynamo
   (C) amperes
   (D) barrel
   (E) switch
8. CUBE is to PYRAMID as SQUARE is to
   (A) box
   (B) solid
   (C) pentagon
   (D) triangle
   (E) cylinder
9. PROFIT is to SELLING as FAME is to
   (A) buying
   (B) cheating
   (C) bravery
   (D) praying
   (E) loving
10. BINDING is to BOOK as WELDING is to
    (A) box
    (B) tank
    (C) chair
    (D) wire
    (E) pencil
11. GYMNASIUM is to HEALTH as SCHOOL is to
    (A) sick
    (B) study
    (C) books
    (D) knowledge
    (E) library
12. RIGHT is to WRONG as SUCCEED is to
    (A) aid
    (B) profit
    (C) fail
    (D) error
    (E) gain
13. INDIAN is to AMERICA as ABORIGINE is to
    (A) Hindustan
    (B) Mexico
    (C) soil
    (D) magic
    (E) Australia
14. WEALTH is to MERCENARY as GOLD is to
    (A) lucre
    (B) miner
    (C) fame
    (D) eleemosynary
    (E) South Africa

15. BOTTLE is to BRITTLE as TIRE is to

(A) elastic
(B) scarce
(C) rubber
(D) spheroid
(E) automobile

16. SOPRANO is to HIGH as BASS is to

(A) violin
(B) good
(C) low
(D) fish
(E) soft

17. OLFACTORY is to NOSE as TACTILE is to

(A) tacit
(B) bloody
(C) finger
(D) handkerchief
(E) stomach

18. STREET is to HORIZONTAL as BUILDING is to

(A) tall
(B) brick
(C) broad
(D) vertical
(E) large

19. ALLEGIANCE is to LOYALTY as TREASON is to

(A) obedience
(B) rebellion
(C) murder
(D) felony
(E) homage

20. CANVAS is to PAINT as MOLD is to

(A) clay
(B) cloth
(C) statue
(D) art
(E) aesthetic

21. FISH is to FIN as BIRD is to

(A) wing
(B) five
(C) feet
(D) beak
(E) feathers

22. CONQUEST is to ASCENDANCY as DEFEAT is to

(A) omission
(B) frustration
(C) censure
(D) subjugation
(E) mastery

23. SOLUTION is to MYSTERY as COMPLETION is to

(A) puzzle
(B) books
(C) college
(D) school
(E) detective

24. ALUMNUS is to ALUMNA as PRINCE is to

(A) castle
(B) king
(C) knight
(D) country
(E) princess

25. OCCULT is to OVERT as SECRET is to

(A) abstract
(B) outward
(C) science
(D) tarry
(E) concealed

VERBAL ANALOGIES TEST ANSWER KEY

Part A	*Part B*	*Part C*
1. **B**	1. **C**	1. **E**
2. **C**	2. **E**	2. **D**
3. **A**	3. **B**	3. **C**
4. **D**	4. **A**	4. **A**
5. **C**	5. **E**	5. **B**
6. **C**	6. **E**	6. **D**
7. **C**	7. **B**	7. **E**
8. **A**	8. **D**	8. **D**
9. **D**	9. **C**	9. **C**
10. **B**	10. **E**	10. **B**
11. **C**	11. **B**	11. **D**
12. **C**	12. **A**	12. **C**
13. **D**	13. **C**	13. **E**
14. **A**	14. **D**	14. **A**
15. **B**	15. **C**	15. **A**
16. **B**	16. **D**	16. **C**
17. **C**	17. **C**	17. **C**
18. **D**	18. **D**	18. **D**
19. **D**	19. **E**	19. **B**
20. **C**	20. **A**	20. **A**
21. **A**	21. **A**	21. **A**
22. **D**	22. **A**	22. **D**
23. **B**	23. **C**	23. **A**
24. **A**	24. **B**	24. **E**
25. **C**	25. **D**	25. **B**

LET'S PUT YOU TO THE TEST

Now that you have thoroughly reviewed the various kinds of verbal-ability items and are familiar with the test-taking strategies associated with them, let's put you to the test.

Pay strict attention to the time allotted for each section of the test and do your best to adhere to the time limits. Read the directions for each part of the test before attempting to answer any of the items.

This test has three parts: A—Synonyms; B—Antonyms; C—Verbal Analogies. The total time allotted for this test is 50 minutes. Have extra pencils available in case of point breakage, so as not to lose testing time.

An answer key is provided at the end of the test so that you can evaluate your performance. Remember, this is a simulation of the "real thing," so be honest with yourself and save the glance at the answer key until after you have completed the test.

FINAL VERBAL ABILITY EXAMINATION ANSWER SHEET

PART A: SYNONYMS

1. Ⓐ Ⓑ Ⓒ Ⓓ	10. Ⓐ Ⓑ Ⓒ Ⓓ	19. Ⓐ Ⓑ Ⓒ Ⓓ	28. Ⓐ Ⓑ Ⓒ Ⓓ
2. Ⓐ Ⓑ Ⓒ Ⓓ	11. Ⓐ Ⓑ Ⓒ Ⓓ	20. Ⓐ Ⓑ Ⓒ Ⓓ	29. Ⓐ Ⓑ Ⓒ Ⓓ
3. Ⓐ Ⓑ Ⓒ Ⓓ	12. Ⓐ Ⓑ Ⓒ Ⓓ	21. Ⓐ Ⓑ Ⓒ Ⓓ	30. Ⓐ Ⓑ Ⓒ Ⓓ
4. Ⓐ Ⓑ Ⓒ Ⓓ	13. Ⓐ Ⓑ Ⓒ Ⓓ	22. Ⓐ Ⓑ Ⓒ Ⓓ	31. Ⓐ Ⓑ Ⓒ Ⓓ
5. Ⓐ Ⓑ Ⓒ Ⓓ	14. Ⓐ Ⓑ Ⓒ Ⓓ	23. Ⓐ Ⓑ Ⓒ Ⓓ	32. Ⓐ Ⓑ Ⓒ Ⓓ
6. Ⓐ Ⓑ Ⓒ Ⓓ	15. Ⓐ Ⓑ Ⓒ Ⓓ	24. Ⓐ Ⓑ Ⓒ Ⓓ	33. Ⓐ Ⓑ Ⓒ Ⓓ
7. Ⓐ Ⓑ Ⓒ Ⓓ	16. Ⓐ Ⓑ Ⓒ Ⓓ	25. Ⓐ Ⓑ Ⓒ Ⓓ	34. Ⓐ Ⓑ Ⓒ Ⓓ
8. Ⓐ Ⓑ Ⓒ Ⓓ	17. Ⓐ Ⓑ Ⓒ Ⓓ	26. Ⓐ Ⓑ Ⓒ Ⓓ	35. Ⓐ Ⓑ Ⓒ Ⓓ
9. Ⓐ Ⓑ Ⓒ Ⓓ	18. Ⓐ Ⓑ Ⓒ Ⓓ	27. Ⓐ Ⓑ Ⓒ Ⓓ	

PART B: ANTONYMS

1. Ⓐ Ⓑ Ⓒ Ⓓ	11. Ⓐ Ⓑ Ⓒ Ⓓ	21. Ⓐ Ⓑ Ⓒ Ⓓ	31. Ⓐ Ⓑ Ⓒ Ⓓ
2. Ⓐ Ⓑ Ⓒ Ⓓ	12. Ⓐ Ⓑ Ⓒ Ⓓ	22. Ⓐ Ⓑ Ⓒ Ⓓ	32. Ⓐ Ⓑ Ⓒ Ⓓ
3. Ⓐ Ⓑ Ⓒ Ⓓ	13. Ⓐ Ⓑ Ⓒ Ⓓ	23. Ⓐ Ⓑ Ⓒ Ⓓ	33. Ⓐ Ⓑ Ⓒ Ⓓ
4. Ⓐ Ⓑ Ⓒ Ⓓ	14. Ⓐ Ⓑ Ⓒ Ⓓ	24. Ⓐ Ⓑ Ⓒ Ⓓ	34. Ⓐ Ⓑ Ⓒ Ⓓ
5. Ⓐ Ⓑ Ⓒ Ⓓ	15. Ⓐ Ⓑ Ⓒ Ⓓ	25. Ⓐ Ⓑ Ⓒ Ⓓ	35. Ⓐ Ⓑ Ⓒ Ⓓ
6. Ⓐ Ⓑ Ⓒ Ⓓ	16. Ⓐ Ⓑ Ⓒ Ⓓ	26. Ⓐ Ⓑ Ⓒ Ⓓ	36. Ⓐ Ⓑ Ⓒ Ⓓ
7. Ⓐ Ⓑ Ⓒ Ⓓ	17. Ⓐ Ⓑ Ⓒ Ⓓ	27. Ⓐ Ⓑ Ⓒ Ⓓ	37. Ⓐ Ⓑ Ⓒ Ⓓ
8. Ⓐ Ⓑ Ⓒ Ⓓ	18. Ⓐ Ⓑ Ⓒ Ⓓ	28. Ⓐ Ⓑ Ⓒ Ⓓ	38. Ⓐ Ⓑ Ⓒ Ⓓ
9. Ⓐ Ⓑ Ⓒ Ⓓ	19. Ⓐ Ⓑ Ⓒ Ⓓ	29. Ⓐ Ⓑ Ⓒ Ⓓ	39. Ⓐ Ⓑ Ⓒ Ⓓ
10. Ⓐ Ⓑ Ⓒ Ⓓ	20. Ⓐ Ⓑ Ⓒ Ⓓ	30. Ⓐ Ⓑ Ⓒ Ⓓ	40. Ⓐ Ⓑ Ⓒ Ⓓ

PART C: VERBAL ANALOGIES

1. Ⓐ Ⓑ Ⓒ Ⓓ	8. Ⓐ Ⓑ Ⓒ Ⓓ	15. Ⓐ Ⓑ Ⓒ Ⓓ	22. Ⓐ Ⓑ Ⓒ Ⓓ
2. Ⓐ Ⓑ Ⓒ Ⓓ	9. Ⓐ Ⓑ Ⓒ Ⓓ	16. Ⓐ Ⓑ Ⓒ Ⓓ	23. Ⓐ Ⓑ Ⓒ Ⓓ
3. Ⓐ Ⓑ Ⓒ Ⓓ	10. Ⓐ Ⓑ Ⓒ Ⓓ	17. Ⓐ Ⓑ Ⓒ Ⓓ	24. Ⓐ Ⓑ Ⓒ Ⓓ
4. Ⓐ Ⓑ Ⓒ Ⓓ	11. Ⓐ Ⓑ Ⓒ Ⓓ	18. Ⓐ Ⓑ Ⓒ Ⓓ	25. Ⓐ Ⓑ Ⓒ Ⓓ
5. Ⓐ Ⓑ Ⓒ Ⓓ	12. Ⓐ Ⓑ Ⓒ Ⓓ	19. Ⓐ Ⓑ Ⓒ Ⓓ	
6. Ⓐ Ⓑ Ⓒ Ⓓ	13. Ⓐ Ⓑ Ⓒ Ⓓ	20. Ⓐ Ⓑ Ⓒ Ⓓ	
7. Ⓐ Ⓑ Ⓒ Ⓓ	14. Ⓐ Ⓑ Ⓒ Ⓓ	21. Ⓐ Ⓑ Ⓒ Ⓓ	

FINAL VERBAL ABILITY EXAMINATION

100 QUESTIONS • TIME—50 MINUTES

PART A: SYNONYMS

35 QUESTIONS • TIME—35 MINUTES

Directions: In each of the sentences below, one word is in italics. Following each sentence are four words or phrases. For each sentence, select the word or phrase that best corresponds in meaning to the italicized word.

1. The chart *classifies* these organisms.

   (A) fuses
   (B) categorizes
   (C) controls
   (D) camouflages

2. On many teams, a player may face a *penalty* for irresponsible or unruly behavior.

   (A) arrangement
   (B) gratification
   (C) punishment
   (D) precaution

3. He used the *allotted* study time to complete his assignments.

   (A) authorized
   (B) designated
   (C) agreed
   (D) alerted

4. When examining the *notochord,* you will find it to be a flexible, rodlike structure.

   (A) backbone
   (B) muscle
   (C) tissue
   (D) pharynx

5. It was apparent that he had attempted to *concoct* an alibi.

   (A) inculcate
   (B) conceal
   (C) reveal
   (D) fabricate

6. The City Council could have avoided this *sanction* by passing the ordinance.

   (A) preliminary plan
   (B) obliteration
   (C) veneration
   (D) penalty

7. *Lipids* are organic compounds that store and release large amounts of energy.

   (A) Enzymes
   (B) Diatoms
   (C) Proteins
   (D) Fats

8. The soldiers retreated to a position of *comparative* safety.

   (A) objective
   (B) relative
   (C) subjective
   (D) scientific

9. Geologists *assure* us that our earth is a few billion years old.

   (A) guarantee
   (B) instruct
   (C) deny
   (D) assail

10. It has been said that he is a *connoisseur* of fine wines.

    (A) expert on
    (B) taster of
    (C) procurer of
    (D) vendor of

11. He *spurned* the name that had won him this dishonor.

    (A) lauded
    (B) extolled
    (C) acclaimed
    (D) repudiated

12. The well-dressed gentleman bowed *ceremoniously.*

    (A) without ritual
    (B) disrespectfully
    (C) serenely
    (D) formally

13. Food is moved through the digestive system by *peristalsis.*

    (A) periosteum
    (B) contractions
    (C) metabolism
    (D) protists

14. The annual parade *traversed* this magnificent city from the east to the west side.

    (A) was patronized
    (B) extended
    (C) crossed
    (D) augmented

15. *Enraptured* by the beauty of the mountains, they had not spoken for twenty minutes.

    (A) summoned
    (B) impeded
    (C) exonerated
    (D) entranced

16. The results of the experiment upheld the *contention* of those who supported the hypothesis.

    (A) realization
    (B) contiguity
    (C) argument
    (D) exhilaration

17. The *consensus* of the group

    (A) stipulation
    (B) regulation
    (C) conviction
    (D) collective opinion

18. Arthritis is a *chronic* disease that results from a faulty immune system.

    (A) long-lasting
    (B) serious
    (C) contagious
    (D) infectious

19. Mayan magnificence *abounds* in the small resort village of Kailuum.

    (A) is remote
    (B) is abundant
    (C) is significant
    (D) is inadequate

20. If enthusiasm for the project *waxed* under the direction of a newly appointed administrator, the level of excitement

    (A) stirred
    (B) waned
    (C) vanished
    (D) increased

21. *Void* of intellectual stimuli

    (A) composed
    (B) in excess
    (C) empty
    (D) full

22. The injuries sustained resulted in paralysis in two of the four *appendages.*

    (A) chambers
    (B) muscles
    (C) limbs
    (D) tubes

23. Security was *risked* to attain maximum career satisfaction.

    (A) ventured
    (B) squandered
    (C) exhausted
    (D) wasted

24. The fruit was *pared* and sliced for the salad.

    (A) divided
    (B) rinsed
    (C) peeled
    (D) sectioned

25. Biogenesis is *a theory* which supports that living things can be produced only from other living things.

    (A) a principle
    (B) an opinion
    (C) a rationale
    (D) an experimentation

26. The introduction *delineates* the book's content and format.

    (A) discredits
    (B) describes
    (C) sanctions
    (D) endorses

27. The x-ray clearly showed the torn *cartilage* in the knee.

    (A) tissue
    (B) ligament
    (C) tendon
    (D) membrane

28. The receptionist *confirmed* the appointment.

    (A) canceled
    (B) rescheduled
    (C) verified
    (D) recorded

29. Arthropod is the *phylum* which includes insects, spiders, centipedes, and surprisingly, shrimp.

    (A) the fifth highest taxonomical category of the animal kingdom
    (B) second highest taxonomical category of the animal kingdom
    (C) the fourth highest taxonomical category of the animal kingdom
    (D) the third highest taxonomical category of the animal kingdom

30. If the engine was *malfunctioning* at the time, it was

    (A) operative
    (B) operating incorrectly
    (C) firing
    (D) igniting

31. The clients were shocked at the *fraudulent* practices of the contractors.

    (A) thorough
    (B) extensive
    (C) legal
    (D) deceitful

32. The employer questioned the *competence* of his staff. The employer was not sure about their

    (A) honesty
    (B) punctuality
    (C) credibility
    (D) ability

33. The reading list included an *anthology* by a famous author.

    (A) collection of literary selections
    (B) annotated bibliography
    (C) archaeological study
    (D) autobiography

34. Some bacteria are mobile because of their *flagellum*.

    (A) cili
    (B) bacilli
    (C) cytoplasm
    (D) tails

35. He smiled *wryly*.

    (A) deceptively
    (B) nastily
    (C) ironically
    (D) delightedly

PART B: ANTONYMS

40 QUESTIONS • TIME—15 MINUTES

Directions: For each of the following test items, select the word that is opposite in meaning to the term printed in capital letters.

1. IMPERIOUS

(A) submissive
(B) valuable
(C) pointed
(D) positive

2. CAPRICIOUS

(A) whimsical
(B) judicious
(C) steadfast
(D) tranquil

3. CANTANKEROUS

(A) pleasant
(B) dubious
(C) effective
(D) awkward

4. FORBEARANCE

(A) indulgence
(B) pliancy
(C) politeness
(D) impatience

5. HAPHAZARD

(A) inefficient
(B) premeditated
(C) unsatisfactory
(D) blundering

6. INEFFABLE

(A) forgettable
(B) exquisite
(C) unorganized
(D) race

7. CHIMERICAL

(A) philosophical
(B) elite
(C) factual
(D) unimpressive

8. REPRESS

(A) reserve
(B) liberate
(C) thrust
(D) precipitate

9. ABOMINABLE

(A) agreeable
(B) loathsome
(C) sufficient
(D) degrading

10. UNETHICAL

(A) vulgar
(B) feasible
(C) pompous
(D) scrupulous

11. ANTECEDENT

(A) previous
(B) subsequent
(C) foregoing
(D) propitious

12. PONDEROUS

(A) delicate
(B) potent
(C) supportive
(D) massive

13. SUPPLICATION

(A) worship
(B) compassion
(C) entreaty
(D) disdain

14. POSITIVE

(A) negative
(B) sensitive
(C) diplomatic
(D) popular

15. RENEGADE
    (A) constant
    (B) extricate
    (C) obedient
    (D) heretical

16. DISREGARD
    (A) disown
    (B) respond
    (C) revoke
    (D) recover

17. WRATH
    (A) delight
    (B) travail
    (C) frivolity
    (D) detriment

18. TEDIOUS
    (A) ungainly
    (B) imperative
    (C) stimulating
    (D) suitable

19. EMBODY
    (A) impel
    (B) fuse
    (C) dissociate
    (D) collect

20. DEFERRABLE
    (A) urgent
    (B) furtive
    (C) inclined
    (D) deniable

21. HOMOGENOUS
    (A) invariable
    (B) homosexual
    (C) importunate
    (D) heterogenous

22. ADHERENT
    (A) disciple
    (B) repudiator
    (C) soothsayer
    (D) hypocrite

23. CRUDE
    (A) barbarous
    (B) refined
    (C) obscure
    (D) covetous

24. DAFT
    (A) cynical
    (B) sharp
    (C) prevalent
    (D) sensible

25. GRAPHIC
    (A) vague
    (B) illustrative
    (C) forcible
    (D) glacial

26. DEVASTATE
    (A) tolerate
    (B) obstruct
    (C) renovate
    (D) promote

27. STRINGENT
    (A) exacting
    (B) tough
    (C) influential
    (D) flexible

28. ACQUIESCE
    (A) contest
    (B) invest
    (C) dismiss
    (D) supply

29. BREVITY
    (A) abbreviation
    (B) length
    (C) ramification
    (D) delusion

30. FLAUNT
    (A) disavow
    (B) conserve
    (C) blight
    (D) astonish

31. CULTIVATE
    (A) restore
    (B) stifle
    (C) reinstate
    (D) nurture

32. DILATE
    (A) negate
    (B) abet
    (C) constrict
    (D) suspend

33. BEFITTING

(A) enhancing
(B) conciliatory
(C) inappropriate
(D) elegant

34. COHERENT

(A) illogical
(B) consecutive
(C) cognizant
(D) courtly

35. PALTRY

(A) political
(B) complaisant
(C) clever
(D) impressive

36. BUCOLIC

(A) urbane
(B) gallant
(C) valiant
(D) functional

37. EXTRAVAGANT

(A) coarse
(B) superior
(C) frugal
(D) typical

38. LENIENCY

(A) indulgence
(B) severity
(C) embroilment
(D) inequality

39. MANIFEST

(A) latent
(B) oblivious
(C) terminal
(D) languid

40. PLEBEIAN

(A) congenial
(B) ignoble
(C) scientific
(D) patrician

PART C: VERBAL ANALOGIES

25 QUESTIONS • TIME—10 MINUTES

Directions: In the following questions you are to determine the relationship between the first pair of capitalized words and then decide which of the answer choices shares a similar relationship with the third capitalized word.

1. CAT is to DOG as TIGER is to

(A) wild
(B) fur
(C) wolf
(D) bovine

2. SALINE is to SALT as SWEET is to

(A) sugar
(B) stale
(C) bread
(D) insipid

3. FLANNEL is to WOOL as LINEN is to

(A) cotton
(B) flax
(C) silk
(D) rayon

4. CONTEMPORARY is to PRESENT as POSTERITY is to

(A) past
(B) present
(C) future
(D) ancient

5. MOON is to EARTH as EARTH is to

(A) space
(B) moon
(C) sky
(D) sun

6. ACUTE is to CHRONIC as INTENSE is to

(A) sardonic
(B) tonic
(C) persistent
(D) pretty

7. VALLEY is to GORGE as MOUNTAIN is to
   - (A) freshet
   - (B) cliff
   - (C) steep
   - (D) high

8. EAST is to WEST as NORTHWEST is to
   - (A) southeast
   - (B) southwest
   - (C) north
   - (D) northeast

9. GASOLINE is to PETROLEUM as SUGAR is to
   - (A) oil
   - (B) cane
   - (C) plant
   - (D) sweet

10. AGGRAVATE is to TEASE as FONDLE is to
    - (A) vex
    - (B) wound
    - (C) embrace
    - (D) pursuit

11. LATITUDE is to LONGITUDE as WARP is to
    - (A) weave
    - (B) woof
    - (C) thread
    - (D) line

12. EDGE is to CENTER as EFFUSIVE is to
    - (A) unemotional
    - (B) exuberant
    - (C) eclectic
    - (D) eccentricity

13. DISCIPLE is to MENTOR as PROSELYTE is to
    - (A) opinion
    - (B) expedition
    - (C) leader
    - (D) football

14. SOPHISTICATION is to FINESSE as INEPTITUDE is to
    - (A) inefficiency
    - (B) artistry
    - (C) trickiness
    - (D) insatiability

15. CAPTAIN is to STEAMSHIP as PRINCIPAL is to
    - (A) interest
    - (B) school
    - (C) agent
    - (D) concern

16. DIME is to SILVER as PENNY is to
    - (A) mint
    - (B) copper
    - (C) currency
    - (D) value

17. REVERT is to REVERSION as SYMPATHIZE is to
    - (A) sympathetic
    - (B) symposium
    - (C) sympathy
    - (D) sympathizer

18. REGRESSIVE is to REGRESS as STERILE is to
    - (A) sterilization
    - (B) sterilize
    - (C) sterility
    - (D) sterilizer

19. DOWN is to UP as AGE is to
    - (A) year
    - (B) youth
    - (C) snow
    - (D) date

20. I is to MINE as MAN is to
    - (A) men
    - (B) his
    - (C) man's
    - (D) mine

21. DISLOYAL is to FAITHLESS as IMPERFECTION is to
    - (A) faithful
    - (B) depression
    - (C) foible
    - (D) decrepitude

22. NECKLACE is to PEARLS as CHAIN is to
    - (A) locket
    - (B) prisoner
    - (C) links
    - (D) clasp

23. DRIFT is to SNOW as DUNE is to

(A) hill
(B) rain
(C) sand
(D) hail

24. DILIGENT is to UNREMITTING as COMPLETE is to

(A) pretentious
(B) diametric
(C) adamant
(D) dietetic

25. SCHOONER is to VESSEL as PERSIMMON is to

(A) machine
(B) fruit
(C) engine
(D) vehicle

FINAL VERBAL ABILITY EXAMINATION ANSWER KEY

PART A: SYNONYMS

1. **B**	8. **B**	15. **D**	22. **C**	29. **B**
2. **C**	9. **A**	16. **C**	23. **A**	30. **B**
3. **B**	10. **A**	17. **D**	24. **C**	31. **D**
4. **A**	11. **D**	18. **A**	25. **A**	32. **D**
5. **D**	12. **D**	19. **B**	26. **B**	33. **A**
6. **D**	13. **B**	20. **D**	27. **A**	34. **D**
7. **D**	14. **C**	21. **C**	28. **C**	35. **C**

PART B: ANTONYMS

1. **A**	9. **A**	17. **A**	25. **A**	33. **C**
2. **C**	10. **D**	18. **C**	26. **C**	34. **A**
3. **A**	11. **B**	19. **C**	27. **D**	35. **D**
4. **D**	12. **A**	20. **A**	28. **A**	36. **A**
5. **B**	13. **D**	21. **D**	29. **B**	37. **C**
6. **A**	14. **A**	22. **B**	30. **A**	38. **B**
7. **C**	15. **C**	23. **B**	31. **B**	39. **A**
8. **B**	16. **B**	24. **D**	32. **C**	40. **D**

PART C: VERBAL ANALOGIES

1. **C**	6. **C**	11. **B**	16. **B**	21. **C**
2. **A**	7. **B**	12. **A**	17. **C**	22. **C**
3. **B**	8. **A**	13. **C**	18. **B**	23. **C**
4. **C**	9. **B**	14. **A**	19. **B**	24. **B**
5. **D**	10. **C**	15. **B**	20. **C**	25. **B**

UNIT II: MATHEMATICS

MATHEMATICS REVIEW

The review of mathematics in this section and the numerical ability tests include the following: basic quantitative problems involving addition, subtraction, multiplication, and division; calculations including decimals, fractions, percentages, and measurements; basic operations in algebra and geometry; and quantitative comparison question-types. Throughout the exercises, emphasis is placed on verbal problems in order to prepare you for the interpretations and methods required for problem-solving. The explanatory answers and problem solutions provide a variety of opportunities to review or to learn the numerical processes included on the prenursing examinations.

Study the guidelines listed below; they provide the major mathematics concepts needed for successful performance on your examination.

TIPS FOR STUDYING MATHEMATICS

In order to perform well on mathematics tests, it is important to be well prepared. In order to prepare well, you must know what material will be covered on the test. The mathematics guidelines and practice exercises in this book provide a review of materials that are covered on the mathematics section of the nursing school entrance examination. You can maximize your performance on the test by following the steps below.

1. Choose a place to study where you won't be distracted.
2. Set aside adequate time to study. Try to set aside at least one hour for each study session. Study and practice each day if possible. Make a study schedule and stick to it.
3. Give your full focus and attention to your studies.
4. Read the explanatory material in your book before doing any practice tests. Make sure that you understand what you're reading. Review information that you don't understand, and use other references when necessary.
5. Take the practice tests under test conditions. Read the instructions carefully. Complete tests in the amount of time suggested. Use the problem solving strategies below to help you solve problems.
6. Compare your answers with those provided in the book. Carefully review answers to questions that you missed.
7. Seek help if you don't understand a problem after several tries.
8. Review regularly and practice, practice, practice.

TEST-TAKING TIPS

There are four basic steps involved in solving mathematics problems. They are: Read the problem; plan how to solve the problem; solve the problem; and check your solution. These steps are explained in more detail in the tips given below.

- Read test instructions carefully. Note the amount of time allotted for completion of the test and pace yourself accordingly.
- Read each problem carefully for clarity and understanding. Make sure that you understand the concepts and terms being used. Try to restate the problem in your own words.
- Simplify the problem by breaking the problem down into smaller parts.
- Determine what information is given and what is to be found.
- Determine whether there is sufficient information given to solve the problem.
- Eliminate extraneous information.
- Choose a strategy for solving the problem.
- Express your answer in the number of units requested. You may be asked to express your answer in terms of minutes, feet, or hours or you may be asked to write your answer as a decimal or fraction.
- Check your solution to determine if it is reasonable. Does your answer appear to be unreasonably large or small?
- Don't spend too much time on a question that you find difficult. Move on to the next question and return to the problem after you complete the other test questions.
- Try an alternative strategy if the one you used didn't work.
- Review your answers if you finish before time is up. Check your computations very carefully.

GUIDELINES FOR MATHEMATICAL CALCULATIONS

I. WHOLE NUMBERS AND FRACTIONS

A. **Whole Numbers**

1. Whole numbers have **place-value** based on units of ten (decimal system). Therefore, it is extremely important that all whole numbers, including zeros, are lined up correctly in columns when adding and subtracting.

Example: a) Place values for the whole number 5264 are illustrated below.

$$5{,}264 = (5 \times 1000) + (2 \times 100) + (6 \times 10) + (4 \times 1)$$

b) Numbers are lined up according to place values in the following **addition** and **subtraction** examples.

$$\begin{array}{r} 5264 \\ +\ 478 \\ \hline 5742 \end{array} \qquad \begin{array}{r} 5264 \\ -\ 478 \\ \hline 4786 \end{array}$$

2. Use **multiplication** to determine the value of several quantities with the same value if the value of one quantity is given.

Example: If one loaf of bread costs 80 cents, how much will three loaves of bread cost? Multiply 3 times 80 cents: The answer is $2.40.

When multiplying be certain to include all zeros and keep the columns in line.

Example:

$$\begin{array}{r} 3600 \\ \times\underline{\ \ 507} \\ 25200 \\ 0000 \\ \underline{18000} \\ 1{,}825{,}200 \end{array}$$

3. Use **division** to determine the value of one quantity when the value of several quantities is given.

Example: Three loaves of bread cost \$2.40. How much will one loaf cost? Divide 3 into \$2.40. The answer is 80 cents. (3 is the divisor, \$2.40 is the dividend, and the quotient is .80)

DIVISIBILITY RULES:

a) If the last digit of a number is 0, 2, 4, 6, or 8, the number is divisible by 2.

b) If the last digit of a number ends in 0 or 5, the number is divisible by 5.

c) If the sum of the digits of a number is divisible by 3, the number is divisible by 3.

Example: The sum of the digits of 234 is 2 + 3 + 4 = 9. Since 9 is divisible by 3, 234 it is also divisible by 3 (234 ÷ 3 = 78).

d) If the sum of the digits of a number is divisible by 9, the number is divisible by 9. In the example above, it was shown that the sum of the digits of 234 is 9. By the above rule, we know that 234 is divisible by 9.

e) If the number represented by the last two digits of a number is divisible by 4, the number is divisible by 4.

32 is the number represented by the last two digits of 232. Since 32 is divisible by 4, the number 232 is divisible by 4.

f) Note that it is not possible to divide by zero.

4. A **prime number** is any whole number other than 0 or 1 that is only divisible by itself and 1.

Example: 17 is a prime number since it is only divisible by 1 and 17. The whole numbers 2, 3, 5, 7, and 11 are the first five prime numbers.

Divisibility rules can be used to find the prime factors of whole numbers.

Example: 24 is divisible by 2 (last digit is 4) and is divisible by 3 (sum of digits is 6)

a) $24 = 2 \times 2 \times 2 \times 3$
$ = 2^3 \times 3$

b)
$$\begin{array}{l} 2\underline{|24} \\ \ \ 2\underline{|12} \\ \ \ \ \ 2\underline{|6} \\ \ \ \ \ \ \ \ 3 \end{array}$$

c)

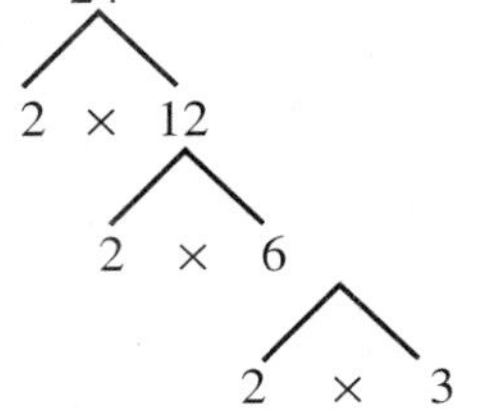

Two methods for determining the prime factors of a number are illustrated in examples b and c. In each method, keep dividing until your quotient is a prime number.

5. The **average** of a set of numbers is the sum of the numbers divided by the number of numbers added.

Example: The average of the numbers 10, 14, 17, and 23 is $\frac{10+14+17+23}{4} = \frac{64}{4} = 16$

6. The **square** of a number is the product obtained when a number is multiplied by itself.

Example: $4^2 = 4 \times 4 = 16$

7. The **square root** ($\sqrt{\ }$) of a given number is the number that yields the given number when multiplied by itself.

Example: $\sqrt{16} = 4$, since $4 \times 4 = 16$

8. The square of any whole number is called a **perfect square.** Conversely, the square root of a perfect square is a whole number.

Example: $4^2 = 16$ (a perfect square); thus $\sqrt{16} = 4$.

9. If a number is not a perfect square, you can **approximate the square root** of the number when a calculator is not available. One method of approximating the square root of a number is given below.

Example: Approximate the square root of 90 ($\sqrt{90}$).

a) Estimate the square root of the given number. Since 90 is between 81 and 100, the square root of 90 will be between 9 and 10. A possible estimate is 9.30.

b) Divide the given number by the estimated square root.

$90 \div 9.30 = 9.68$

c) Find the average of the resulting quotient and the estimated square root.

$\frac{9.68 + 9.30}{2} = 9.49$ (9.49 is the first approximation for $\sqrt{90}$)

d) Divide the given number by the average (first approximation) found above.

$90 \div 9.49 = 9.48$

e) Find the **average of the divisor** (first approximation) and the **quotient** found in step 4.

$\frac{9.49 + 9.48}{2} = 9.485$

The approximate square root of 90 is 9.485.

This process may be repeated to get a more accurate estimate of the square root of a number.

10. To add or subtract **radicals** (numbers expressed as square roots), the **radicands** (numbers under the radical) must be the same.

Example: $4\sqrt{12} + 3\sqrt{12} = 7\sqrt{12}$

Example: If the radicands are *not* the same, simplify the radicals and then see if they can be combined.

$3\sqrt{12} - 8\sqrt{3}$

$= 3(\sqrt{4} \times \sqrt{3}) - 8\sqrt{3}$ (12 can be factored as 4×3)

$= 3 \times 2\sqrt{3} - 8\sqrt{3}$ (Take $\sqrt{4}$, which equals 2)

$= 6\sqrt{3} - 8\sqrt{3}$

$= -2\sqrt{3}$

B. **Fractions**

A fraction is a part of something. A fraction is expressed using two terms: a **numerator**, which is the number above the fraction line, and a **denominator**, which is the number below the fraction line.

In the fraction $\frac{3}{4}$, the numerator is 3 and the denominator is 4.

A **proper fraction** is one whose numerator is less than its denominator. An **improper fraction** has a numerator that is equal to or greater than its denominator.

$\frac{4}{5}$ is a proper fraction and $\frac{7}{3}$ is an improper fraction.

An improper fraction can be expressed as a **mixed number,** which has both a whole and a fractional part. (Divide the denominator into the numerator to get the whole part, and the remainder will be the numerator and the divisor will be the denominator of the fractional part.)

Example: $\frac{7}{3} = 2\frac{1}{3}$

7 divided by 3 gives a quotient of 2 and a remainder of 1.

1. **Reducing Fractions**

Factor the numerator and denominator into prime factors and divide the numerator and denominator by the common factors. (The value of a fraction is unchanged when the numerator and denominator are multiplied or divided by the same number.)

Example: $\frac{35}{55} = \frac{7 \times 5}{11 \times 5} = \frac{7}{11}$

2. **Multiplying Fractions**

To multiply two fractions, multiply the two numerators to get the numerator of the product of the two fractions and multiply the two denominators to get the denominator of the product of the fractions. Then simplify the resulting fraction by reducing it to lowest terms and/or by changing it to a mixed number.

Example: $\frac{6}{9} \times \frac{3}{8} = \frac{18}{72} = \frac{2 \times 3 \times 3}{2 \times 2 \times 2 \times 3 \times 3} = \frac{1}{4}$

3. **Dividing Fractions**

To divide two fractions, invert the divisor then multiply the two fractions and simplify.

Examples: $\frac{9}{20} \div \frac{3}{4} = \frac{9}{20} \times \frac{4}{3} = \frac{36}{60} = \frac{2 \times 2 \times 3 \times 3}{2 \times 2 \times 3 \times 5} = \frac{3}{5}$

$2\frac{2}{3} \div 4 = \frac{8}{3} \times \frac{1}{4} = \frac{8}{12} = \frac{2 \times 2 \times 2}{2 \times 2 \times 3} = \frac{2}{3}$

Note that the mixed number $2\frac{2}{3}$ was changed to the improper fraction $\frac{8}{3}$, and the inversion of the whole number 4, which equals $\frac{4}{1}$, is $\frac{1}{4}$.

4. **Adding and Subtracting Fractions**

a) To add or subtract fractions with the **same**, or common, denominator, keep the common denominator and add or subtract the numerators of the fractions.

Examples: $\frac{7}{9} + \frac{4}{9} = \frac{11}{9}$

$\frac{15}{32} - \frac{5}{32} = \frac{10}{32} = \frac{5}{16}$

b) To add or subtract fractions with **different** denominators, express the fractions as equivalent fractions with a common denominator. The lowest common denominator is the smallest number that can be divided evenly by the denominators of the given fractions. To find the **lowest common denominator (LCD)** of two fractions, first express each denominator as a product of its prime factors. The lowest common denominator will be the number formed by multiplying each prime factor the largest number of times it occurs in the factorization of the denominators.

Examples: (1) $\frac{5}{9} + \frac{7}{12} = \frac{20}{36} + \frac{21}{36} = \frac{41}{36}$

Since $9 = 3 \times 3$ and $12 = 3 \times 4$, the lowest common denominator of 9 and 12 is $3 \times 3 \times 4 = 36$

(2) $\frac{7}{24} - \frac{9}{150}$

$150 = 2 \times 3 \times 5 \times 5$

$24 = 2 \times 2 \times 2 \times 3$

The largest number of times that 2 appears as a factor is 3 and the largest number of times that 5 appears as a factor is 2.3 appears as a factor only once in each of the factorizations.

Thus, the lowest common denominator of the two fractions is 600.

$2 \times 2 \times 2 \times 3 \times 5 \times 5 = 600$

$\frac{7}{24} - \frac{9}{150} = \frac{7}{24} \times \frac{25}{25} - \frac{9}{150} \times \frac{4}{4}$

$= \frac{175}{600} - \frac{36}{600} = \frac{139}{600}$

(3) $4\frac{2}{3} - 1\frac{3}{4} = 4\frac{8}{12} - 1\frac{9}{12}$

Since $\frac{9}{12}$ is greater than $\frac{8}{12}$, $4\frac{8}{12}$ is changed to $3 + 1 + \frac{8}{12}$

$= 3 + \frac{12}{12} + \frac{8}{12}$

$= 3 + \frac{20}{12}$ or $3\frac{20}{12}$

then $4\frac{8}{12} - 1\frac{9}{12} = 3\frac{20}{12} - 1\frac{9}{12}$

$= 2\frac{11}{12}$

5. **Comparison of Fractions**

To determine which of two fractions is larger, change the two fractions to equivalent fractions by expressing them as fractions with a common denominator and then comparing the numerators of the fractions. The fraction with the larger numerator is the larger fraction.

Example: Which is larger, $\frac{5}{6}$ or $\frac{7}{8}$?

24 is a common denominator for the two fractions, hence $\frac{5}{6} = \frac{20}{24}$ and $\frac{7}{8} = \frac{21}{24}$. Since $\frac{21}{24}$ is larger than $\frac{20}{24}$, $\frac{7}{8}$ is larger than $\frac{5}{6}$.

II. DECIMALS AND PERCENTS

A. **Decimals**

A common fraction can be expressed as a decimal. For example: $\frac{1}{2} = \frac{5}{10} = .5$ Each common fraction has an equivalent decimal form.

1. To change a common fraction to a decimal, divide the denominator of the fraction into the numerator.

Example: $\frac{3}{8} = .375$

2. When a decimal is changed to a fraction, the digits after the decimal point become the numerator. The denominator is 1 followed by as many zeros as there are decimal places. (The denominator can also be determined by raising 10 to a power. The power is the number of decimal places in the number.)

   An alternate method for changing a decimal to a common fraction is to count the number of decimal places in the decimal. One decimal place represents tenths, two decimal places hundredths, three decimal places thousandths, and so on. The numerical part of the decimal indicates how many tenths, hundredths, thousandths, etc., there are.

Examples: a) $0.540 = \frac{540}{1000}$ (Note that $1{,}000 = 10^3$. There are 3 decimal places in the number so the power is 3.)

b) $.48 = \frac{48}{100}$ (There are 48 hundredths)

3. **Adding and Subtracting Decimals**

Arrange the decimals vertically with the decimal points aligned under each other. (Express whole numbers as decimals by appending a decimal point at the end of the number and adding as many zeros as desired, i.e., 23 = 23.0)

Examples: a) Subtract 2.715 from 4

$$\begin{array}{r} 4.000 \\ \underline{-\,2.715} \\ 1.285 \end{array}$$

b) Add 11.3 + .968 + .24 + 3

$$\begin{array}{r} 11.300 \\ .968 \\ .240 \\ \underline{3.000} \\ 15.508 \end{array}$$

4. **Multiplying Decimals**

To multiply decimals, multiply as you would with whole numbers. The number of decimal places in the product is the sum of the number of decimal places in the two numbers being multiplied.

Example: Multiply 2.47 times .315, that is,

$$\begin{array}{r} 2.47 \\ \underline{\times\,.315} \\ .77805 \end{array}$$

$$\begin{array}{r} 247 \\ \underline{315} \\ 1\underline{235} \\ 247 \\ \underline{741} \\ 77805 \end{array}$$

There are 2 decimal places in 2.47 and 3 in .315; therefore; there are 5 decimal places in the product of the two numbers. The product is .77805.

5. **Dividing Decimals**

a) When a decimal is divided by a whole number, the decimal point in the quotient should be aligned with the decimal point in the dividend. Divide as you would with whole numbers.

Example: .264 divided by 12

```
     .022
12 ).264
     24
      24
      24
       0
```

b) To divide by a decimal, multiply the divisor by the multiple of 10 that will make the divisor a whole number and multiply the dividend by the same multiple of ten. Divide as you would with whole numbers.

Example: 2.752 divided by .16

```
.16 )2.752
```

Multiply the divisor and dividend by 100 to get a new divisor of 16 and dividend of 275.2

```
     17.2
16 )275.2
    16
     115
     112
       32
       32
        0
```

B. **Percents**

Percent means "by the hundredths." The symbol "%" denotes a percent. A percent can be expressed as a fraction with a denominator of 100.

$63\% = \frac{63}{100}$

1. Converting decimals and fractions to percents and vice-versa.

Examples: a) To convert a decimal to a percent, multiply the decimal by 100.

$.134 = .134 \times 100 = 13.4\%$

b) To convert a percent to a decimal, divide the percent by 100.

$47\% = \frac{47}{100} = .47$

2. To find a percent of a given number (the base), change the percent to a decimal and multiply the decimal times the base.

Examples: a) 35% of 80 = $.35 \times 80 = 28$

b) The number of patients admitted to GET WELL Hospital for drug overdoses was 24% higher in 1994 than in 1993. If 325 patients were admitted for drug overdoses in 1993, how many were admitted in 1994?

24% of 325 = $.24 \times 325 = 78$

$325 + 78 = 403$

There were 78 more patients in 1994 than 1993, making a total of 403 admitted for drug overdoses in 1994.

3. To determine the base when the percent and percentage are known, change the percent to a decimal and divide the percentage by the result. (Note that "is" can be interpreted as = and "of " as multiplication.)

Example: 32 is 20% of what number?

$32 = .20 \times B$ (B represents the base, which is the unknown number, and 32 is the percentage)

$\frac{32}{.20} = B$

$160 = B$

32 is 20% of 160.

4. To determine what percent a given percentage is of a base, divide the percentage by the base and change the resulting decimal to a percent.

Examples: a) What percent of 60 is 15?

$15 = P \times 60$ (60 is the base and 15 is the percentage)

$\frac{15}{60} = \frac{1}{4} = .25 = 25\%$

b) If a nurse with a salary of $40,000 receives a $2,000 bonus. What percent of his salary is his bonus? (That is, what percent of 40,000 is 2,000?)

$2000 = P \times 40000$

$P = \frac{2000}{40000} = \frac{1}{20} = .05$ or 5%

5. To find a percentage increase or percentage decrease in a verbal problem, write a fraction with the amount of increase or decrease as the numerator and the original amount as the denominator. Then change fraction to percentage.

Examples: A patient's prescription was decreased from 2 grams to 1.5 grams What is the percent of decrease of the new prescription?

The amount of decrease was .5 grams. What percent of 2 grams is .5 grams?

$.5 = \underline{?}\ \%$ of 2

$\frac{.5}{2} = .25 = 25\%$

The dosage was decreased by 25%.

6. To determine discount in verbal problems, change the percentage to a fraction or decimal, multiply by the original cost, and deduct this amount from the original cost.
7. For verbal problems dealing with **commission and taxes,** multiply the total value of the goods or services by the percentage of tax or commission.

III. RATIOS AND PROPORTIONS

A. **Ratios**

A ratio is the comparison of two numerical quantities by division.

Example: A box contains 3 red balls and 2 blue balls. The ratio of blue to red balls in the box is 2 to 3 or $\frac{2}{3}$.

B. **Proportions**

A proportion is a statement that two ratios are equivalent.

Example: The ratio of 4 to x is equivalent to the ratio of 5 to 10.

$$\frac{4}{x} = \frac{5}{10}$$

C. **Direct Proportions**

In a direct proportion, one quantity increases (↑) or decreases (↓) as the other increases or decreases. In other words, the direction of the changes is the same for both factors. (x increases as y increases or x decreases as y decreases.)

Example: One orange sells for 15 cents. How much will six oranges cost?

$$\frac{1 \text{ orange}}{15¢} = \frac{6 \text{ oranges}}{y\,¢}$$

Cross multiply: $1y = 6 \times 15$ $\quad y = 90¢$

The total cost increases as the number of oranges sold increases.

Example: Six oranges cost 90 cents. How much would one orange cost?

$$\frac{6 \text{ oranges}}{90¢} = \frac{1 \text{ orange}}{y\,¢}$$

Cross multiply: $6y = 90¢$ $\quad y = 15¢$ (Divide both sides by 6.)

The cost decreases as the number of oranges purchased decreases.

D. **Inverse Proportions**

In an inverse proportion, one quantity increases (↑) as the other decreases (↓), and vice versa. In other words, the direction of the changes is opposite. (As x increases, y decreases; or as x decreases, y increases.)

Example: A 5-pound bag of dog food lasts one week when the dog is given 2 servings per day. How long would this bag last if the dog were to receive 3 servings per day?

$$\frac{3}{2} = \frac{7}{y}$$

$3y = 14$

$y = 4.6$

(As the number of meals increases, the number of days the dog food lasts decreases.)

IV. ALGEBRA

Algebra involves the use of letters and symbols as well as numbers. Some of the introductory concepts of algebra are reviewed in this section.

A. Operations with signed numbers

For operations with signed numbers (+ or –):

1. **Addition**

   a) For numbers with the same sign, add and keep the same sign in the answer.

   b) For numbers with different signs, subtract and give the answer the sign of the higher number.

2. **Subtraction**

Combine the two signs of the subtrahend (taking the subtraction sign as a negative sign, [– and – = +] [– and + = –]. Then use the rules for addition.

Examples: $-4 - (-2) = -4 + 2 = -2$
$-4 - (+2) = -4 - 2 = -6$

3. **Multiplication**

   a) The product of an odd number of negative numbers is negative.

   b) The product of an even number of negative numbers is positive.

Example: $(-3)(-2)(-5) = -30$

$(-4)(-2)(-3)(-5) = 90$

4. **Division**

   If the two numbers have the same sign, the quotient is positive; if otherwise, the quotient is negative.

B. Algebraic Expressions

Algebraic expressions consist of a combination of variables and numbers connected by addition and subtraction signs. The parts of algebraic expressions connected by plus and minus signs are called **terms.**

1. **Combining like terms**

   Like terms are terms that contain the same variables. These variables have the same exponents.

   $2xy^2$ and $5xy^2$ are like terms.

   $3xy$ and $4x^2y$ are not like terms. The variable x in the two terms has different exponents.

   Only like terms in an algebraic expression can be combined. To combine like terms, add their numerical coefficients.

Examples: a) $7x + 2 - 4x + 3 = 3x + 5$

b) $2xy + 7x^2y - 4xy + 6y = 7x^2y - 2xy + 6y$

C. Order of Operations

When simplifying an algebraic expression:

1. First remove grouping symbols (parentheses, brackets), starting with the innermost grouping symbols. (To remove grouping symbols, perform operations inside of symbols.)

2. Perform the operations of multiplication and division, moving from left to right.

3. Perform the operations of addition and subtraction, moving from left to right.

Example: $5x - 2\,[(3x - 1) + (4 - 2x)]$

$= 5x - 2[x + 3]$

$= 5x - 2x - 6$

$= 3x - 6$

D. Evaluating Algebraic Expressions

Find the value of an algebraic expression for given values of the variable by substituting the value of the variables in the expression.

Evaluate the expression $2x^2y + 3xy$ when $x = 2$ and $y = 3$.

Example: $2x^2y + 3xy = 2(2)^2(3) + 3(2)(3)$

$= 2(4)(3) + 3(2)(3)$

$= 2 \times 4 \times 3 + 3 \times 2 \times 3$

$= 24 + 18 = 42$

E. Solving Equations with One Variable

An equation is a statement that two quantities are equal. An equation has one unknown if it has only one variable. Equations with one variable can be solved using inverse operations. One or more of the basic operations of addition, subtraction, multiplication, and division are used to solve equations.

Consider the equation, $x - 7 = 3$.

7 has been subtracted from the variable; the inverse operation for subtraction is addition. To solve the equation, add 7 to both sides of the equation.

Equivalent equations can be obtained by adding or subtracting the same number to both sides of the equation or by multiplying or dividing both sides of the equation by the same number (Do not divide by zero).

Example: 1. $3x + 5 = 17$

$3x + 5 - 5 = 17 - 5$

$3x = 12$

$\frac{3x}{3} = \frac{12}{3}$

$x = 4$

Note that to solve an equation, it is necessary to get the variable on one side of the equation and the constant on the other side.

Example: 2. $5x + 2 = x - 10$

$5x + 2 - 2 = x - 10 - 2$

$5x = x - 12$

$5x - x = x - 12 - x$

$4x = -12$

$\frac{4x}{4} = \frac{12}{4}$

$x = -3$

F. Solving Verbal (Word) Problems

The above described methods can be used to solve verbal problems once they are translated into equations. The first step in translating a verbal problem into an equation is to represent the unknown quantity by a variable. Two equivalent algebraic expressions involving the variable are then written to represent information given in the problem. The two equivalent expressions form the equation.

Examples: 1. When 3 times a number is increased by 4, the result is 19.

Let N represent the unknown number

$3N$ represents 3 times the number

$3N + 4$ represents 3 times the number increased by 4

(To increase a number means to add to it.)

Since the result is 19, the desired equation is

$3N + 4 = 19$

$3N = 15$ (4 was subtracted from both.)

$N = 5$ (Both sides were divided by 3.)

The solution to the problem is 5.

2. A number decreased by $\frac{1}{2}$ of itself equals $\frac{3}{4}$. What decimal is equivalent to the resulting fraction?

Let Y represent the unknown number.

$Y - \frac{1}{2}Y$ represents Y decreased by $\frac{1}{2}$ of itself

The desired equation is

$Y - \frac{1}{2}Y = \frac{3}{4}$

$\frac{1}{2}Y = \frac{3}{4}$

$2Y = 3$

$Y = \frac{3}{2} = 1.5$

The solution is 1.5.

G. Formulas

An equation in which a variable is expressed in terms of another variable is called a formula.

$I = PRT$ is a formula for finding interest.

P represents the principal

R represents the rate

T represents the time

$D = RT$ is the formula for finding distance.

R is the rate or speed

T is the time

$F = \frac{9}{5}C + 32$ is the formula for changing a temperature from Celsius to Fahrenheit.

C = Celsius

F = Fahrenheit

Example: How long will it take to drive a distance of 330 miles traveling at a rate of 60 mph?

Substitute in the formula

$D = R \times T$

$330 = 60 \times T$

$\frac{330}{60} = T$

$5\frac{1}{2} = T$

It will take $5\frac{1}{2}$ hours to drive the 330 miles at a rate of 60 mph.

Example: If a temperature reading on the Celsius scale is 40 degrees, we substitute 40 for C in the temperature conversion formula to get

$\text{F} = \frac{9}{5} \times 40 + 32$

$\text{F} = \frac{360}{5} + 32 = 72 + 32 = 104$ degrees Fahrenheit

H. Inequalities

The symbols "<" and ">" are used to represent the inequalities "less than" and "greater than." Various statements of inequality are expressed by the following:

Example:

1. $a < b$ means	a is less than b.
$7 < 12$	7 is less than 12.
2. $a \quad b$ means	a is either less than or equal to b.
$5 \quad 9$	5 is less than or equal to 9.
3. $a > b$ means	a is greater than b.
$18 > 14$	18 is greater than 14.
4. $a \quad b$ means	a is either greater than or equal to b.
$3 \quad 3$	3 is greater than or equal to 3.
5. $a < b \quad c$ means	a is less than b and b is less than or equal to c.
$-1 < 3 \quad 5$	−1 is less than 3 and 3 is less than or equal to 5.
$2 \quad x < 5$	x is a number that is greater than or equal to 2 and is less than 5.

I. Defined Functions

Certain questions may include a special sign such as "*" or "#" that is defined for you. The sign tells you to perform a specific function or operation. This kind of problem tests your ability to learn and apply a new concept.

Example: For all numbers, $a * b = \frac{a}{b} + 2$. What is $6 * 3$?

$6 * 3 = \frac{6}{3} + 2$

$= 2 + 2$

$= 4$

V. GEOMETRY

A. **Standard Measurements**

The following are some standard units of measurement.

Linear:
inches
feet (1 ft. = 12 in.)
yard (1 yd. = 3 ft.)
gallon (1 gal. = 4 qts.)

Capacity:
ounces
pints (16 oz. = pt.)
quart (1 qt. = 2 pts.)

Weight:
ounces
pounds (1 lb. = 16 oz.)

Area is expressed in square units and volume is expressed in cubic units (square feet, cubic inches, etc.).

1. For **literal expressions** (problems with letters instead of numbers), use the same processes as you would for numbers.

Example: How many inches are in *y* yards and *x* feet?

$y \text{ yd.} \times \frac{36 \text{ in.}}{\text{yd.}} = 36y \text{ in.}$ $x \text{ ft.} \times \frac{12 \text{ in.}}{\text{ft.}} = 12x \text{ in.}$

B. **Metric Measurements**

Metric measurements are based on powers of 10.

Problems involving metric measurements (other than conversions within the metric system) are solved using the same techniques as problems with English measurement units.

The basic metric units of measure are:

Length—Meter

Volume—Liter

Weight—Gram

Temperature—Celsius

Computations in the metric system involve multiplication and division by powers of 10. The chart below illustrates the relationship between metric units.

MILLI	CENTI	DECI	UNIT	DEKA	HECTO	KILO
.001	.01	.1	1	10	100	1000

Example: 1 gram = 1000 milligrams

2 liters = 2000 meters

1 hectometer = 100 meters

C. **Parallel and Perpendicular Lines**

1. Parallel lines are two lines that do not intersect (have no points in common). The slopes of two parallel lines are equal.
2. Perpendicular lines are two lines that intersect at right angles. The slopes of two perpendicular lines have a product of -1.

D. **Polygons**

A polygon is a simple closed plane figure made up of line segments.

1. Polygons with three sides are called **triangles.**
   a) If the lengths of two sides of a triangle are equal, the triangle is called an **isosceles** triangle.
   b) When all three sides of a triangle have the same length, the triangle is called an **equilateral** triangle.
2. Polygons with four sides are called quadrilaterals.
   a) A **square** is a quadrilateral with all four sides equal.
   b) A **rectangle** is a quadrilateral with opposite sides equal and parallel.

E. **Perimeter**

To find the **perimeter (P)** of a figure, add the lengths of all its sides.

Triangle $P =$ sum of the three sides $P = a + b + c$

Rectangle $P = 2 \times$ Length $+ 2 \times$ Width $P = 2L + 2W$

Square $P = 4 \times S$, where S = length of each side.

Circle The circumference *(C)* is the distance around a circle.

The circumference of a circle is equal to × the diameter: $C = \;\times d$.

Point O is the center of the given circle. Points P, R, and S are points on the circle.

A **chord** of a circle is any segment with its two end points on the circle. $\overline{MN}$ is a chord of the given circle.

A **radius** of a circle is a segment from the center of the circle to any point on the circle. $\overline{OP}$ is a radius of the circle.

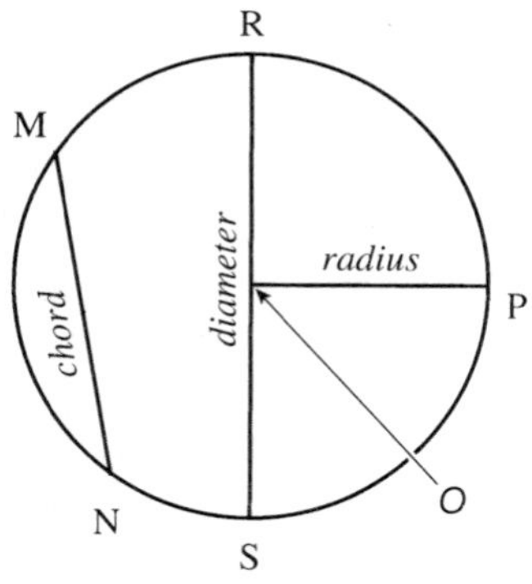

A **diameter** of a circle is a chord that passes through the center of a circle. $\overline{RS}$ is a diameter of the given circle.

All radii of a circle have the same length. A diameter of a given circle is always twice the radius of the circle.

Example: If the length of radius $\overline{OP}$ = 7 cm, the diameter $\overline{RS}$ = 14 cm.

F. **Area**

1. To find the **area (A) of plane figures:**

   Square $A = (\text{side})^2$ $A = S^2$

   Rectangle $A = \text{Base} \times \text{Height}$, or $A = L \times W$

   Triangle $A = \frac{1}{2}\text{Base} \times \text{Height}$, or $A = \frac{1}{2}bh$

   Circle $A = \ \times (\text{radius})^2$, or $A = \ r^2$

2. The **areas of other polygons** may be found by dividing the polygon into nonoverlapping triangles and/or quadrilaterals (squares, rectangles) and then adding the areas of the triangles and quadrilaterals.

Nonoverlapping triangles and quadrilaterals may be obtained by drawing diagonals of the polygon. A **diagonal** of a polygon is a line segment joining two nonconsecutive vertices of a polygon. $\overline{BE}$ is a diagonal of polygon ABCDE.

Example: Given polygon ABCDE with the measurements indicated, draw diagonal $\overline{BE}$ to divide the polygon into a triangle, ΔBAE, and a rectangle, ▭BEDC.

Area of ΔBAE = $\frac{1}{2} \times 10 \times 4 = 20$ sq. in.

Area of ▭BEDC = $2 \times 10 = 20$ sq. in.

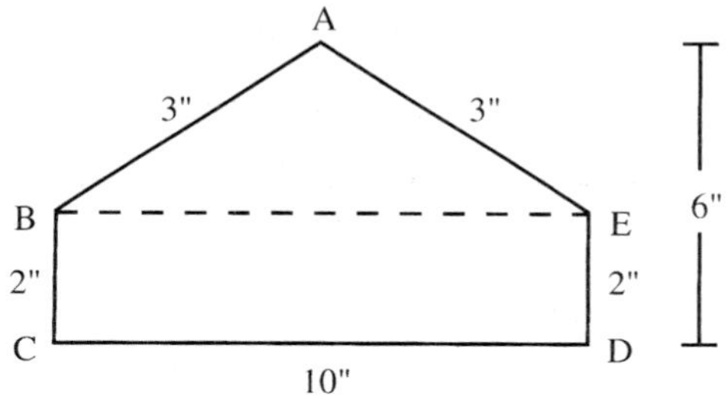

Since 20 + 20 = 40, the area of polygon ABCDE = 40 sq. in.

G. **Similar triangles** have the same shape. The angles of one similar triangle are equal to the angles of the other. The ratios of corresponding sides of similar triangles are equal.

Example: The two given triangles are similar (measures of corresponding angles are equal).

Therefore $\frac{8}{x} = \frac{y}{5}$

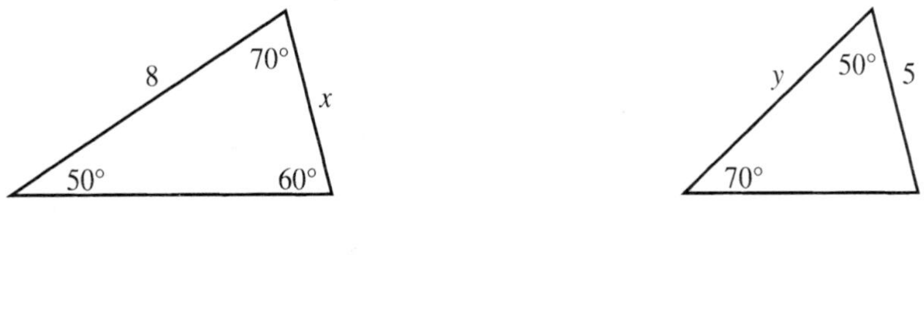

H. A **right triangle** is a triangle with a right angle. The side of the triangle that is opposite the right angle is called the **hypotenuse.**

1. **Pythagorean theorem:** The square of the hypotenuse of a triangle is equal to the sum of the squares of the other two sides.

   $c^2 = a^2 + b^2$

Example: Find the hypotenuse of the right triangle given below:

The two sides of the triangle are 5 and 12. The hypotenuse (c) can be found with the use of the Pythagorean theorem.

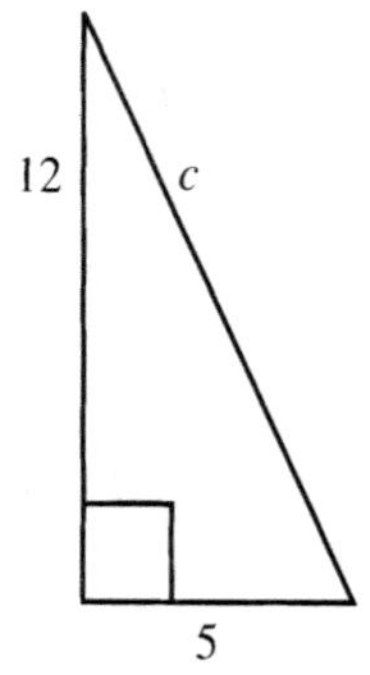

$c^2 = 5^2 + 12^2 = 25 + 144 = 169$

$c^2 = 169$ (To find c, take the square root of 169.)

$c = 13$

I. Units of measurement for angles are called **degrees.** An **acute angle** has a measure that is less than 90°.

A **right angle** has a measure of exactly 90°. (Perpendicular lines form right angles.)

An **obtuse angle** has a measure that is greater than 90°.

Two angles are **complementary** if the sum of their measures is 90°.

Two angles are **supplementary** if the sum of their measure is 180°.

If the exterior sides of a pair of adjacent angles form a straight line, the two adjacent angles are supplementary.

Example: If AB ⊥ DC (AB is perpendicular to DC), then

∠ABF and ∠FBC are complementary angles.

(The sum of the measures of ∠ABF and ∠FBC = 90°)

∠EBD and ∠EBC are supplementary angles.

(The sum of ∠EBD and ∠EBC = 180°)

∠FBC is an acute angle. ∠ABC is a right angle.

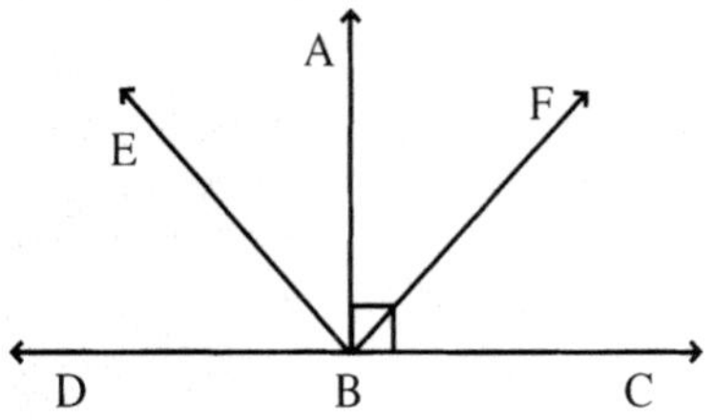

J. The sum of the measures of the three angles of a triangle is 180°. If the measures of two angles of a triangle are given, the measure of the third angle can be found by subtracting the sum of the measures of the two known angles from 180°.

Example: If $\angle A = 40°$ and $\angle B = 60°$, then $\angle C$

$= 180° - (\angle A + \angle B)$

$= 180° - (40° + 60°)$

$= 180° - 100°$

$= 80°$

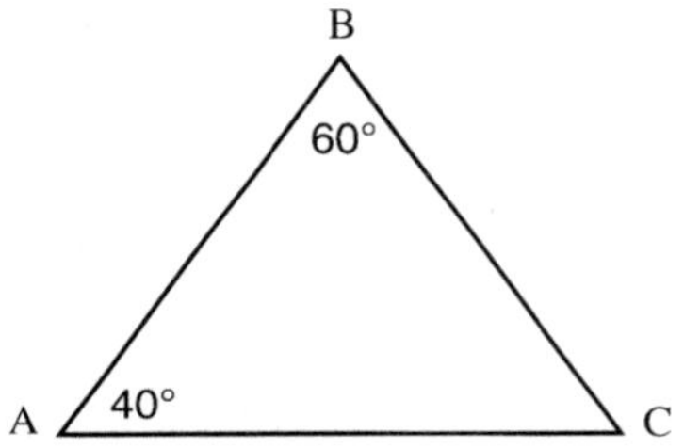

K. The total degree measure of a circle is 360°.

1. A **central angle** of a circle is an angle whose vertex is the center of the circle. If a central angle represents $\frac{1}{n}$ of a circle, the measure of the central angle is $\frac{1}{n} \times 360°$.

Angle $\angle AOB$ is a central angle in the circle below.

2. A **minor arc** of a circle consists of two points A and B where the sides of a central angle intersect the circle plus all points of the circle that lie in the interior of the central angle.

The minor arc $\overset{\frown}{AB}$ is indicated in the given circle.

3. A **major arc** of a circle consists of points A and B and all points on the circle that lie in the exterior of the central angle.

The major arc $\overset{\frown}{AB}$ is indicated in the circle below.

4. An **inscribed angle** of a circle is an angle whose vertex is on the circle and whose rays intersect the circle in two points different from the vertex. The measure of an inscribed angle equals one-half the measure of its intercepted arc.

∠ACB is an inscribed angle of the given circle. The measure of ∠ACB is one-half the measure of the central angle, ∠AOB.

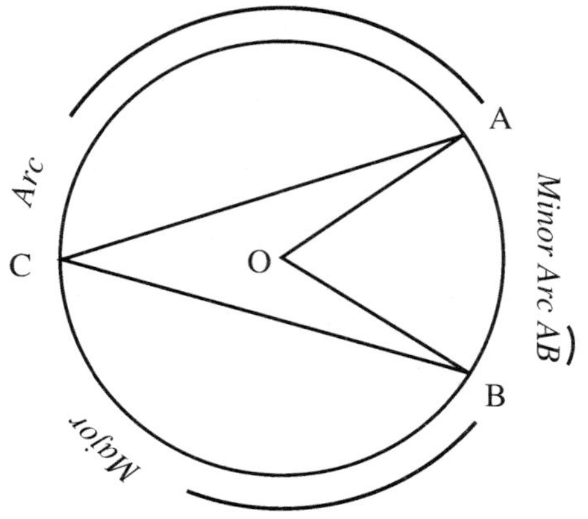

MATHEMATICS TESTS ANSWER SHEET

TEST 1: MATHEMATICS

1. Ⓐ Ⓑ Ⓒ Ⓓ	6. Ⓐ Ⓑ Ⓒ Ⓓ	11. Ⓐ Ⓑ Ⓒ Ⓓ	16. Ⓐ Ⓑ Ⓒ Ⓓ
2. Ⓐ Ⓑ Ⓒ Ⓓ	7. Ⓐ Ⓑ Ⓒ Ⓓ	12. Ⓐ Ⓑ Ⓒ Ⓓ	17. Ⓐ Ⓑ Ⓒ Ⓓ
3. Ⓐ Ⓑ Ⓒ Ⓓ	8. Ⓐ Ⓑ Ⓒ Ⓓ	13. Ⓐ Ⓑ Ⓒ Ⓓ	18. Ⓐ Ⓑ Ⓒ Ⓓ
4. Ⓐ Ⓑ Ⓒ Ⓓ	9. Ⓐ Ⓑ Ⓒ Ⓓ	14. Ⓐ Ⓑ Ⓒ Ⓓ	19. Ⓐ Ⓑ Ⓒ Ⓓ
5. Ⓐ Ⓑ Ⓒ Ⓓ	10. Ⓐ Ⓑ Ⓒ Ⓓ	15. Ⓐ Ⓑ Ⓒ Ⓓ	20. Ⓐ Ⓑ Ⓒ Ⓓ

TEST 2: MATHEMATICS

1. Ⓐ Ⓑ Ⓒ Ⓓ	6. Ⓐ Ⓑ Ⓒ Ⓓ	11. Ⓐ Ⓑ Ⓒ Ⓓ	16. Ⓐ Ⓑ Ⓒ Ⓓ
2. Ⓐ Ⓑ Ⓒ Ⓓ	7. Ⓐ Ⓑ Ⓒ Ⓓ	12. Ⓐ Ⓑ Ⓒ Ⓓ	17. Ⓐ Ⓑ Ⓒ Ⓓ
3. Ⓐ Ⓑ Ⓒ Ⓓ	8. Ⓐ Ⓑ Ⓒ Ⓓ	13. Ⓐ Ⓑ Ⓒ Ⓓ	18. Ⓐ Ⓑ Ⓒ Ⓓ
4. Ⓐ Ⓑ Ⓒ Ⓓ	9. Ⓐ Ⓑ Ⓒ Ⓓ	14. Ⓐ Ⓑ Ⓒ Ⓓ	19. Ⓐ Ⓑ Ⓒ Ⓓ
5. Ⓐ Ⓑ Ⓒ Ⓓ	10. Ⓐ Ⓑ Ⓒ Ⓓ	15. Ⓐ Ⓑ Ⓒ Ⓓ	20. Ⓐ Ⓑ Ⓒ Ⓓ

TEST 3: MATHEMATICS

1. Ⓐ Ⓑ Ⓒ Ⓓ	6. Ⓐ Ⓑ Ⓒ Ⓓ	11. Ⓐ Ⓑ Ⓒ Ⓓ	16. Ⓐ Ⓑ Ⓒ Ⓓ
2. Ⓐ Ⓑ Ⓒ Ⓓ	7. Ⓐ Ⓑ Ⓒ Ⓓ	12. Ⓐ Ⓑ Ⓒ Ⓓ	17. Ⓐ Ⓑ Ⓒ Ⓓ
3. Ⓐ Ⓑ Ⓒ Ⓓ	8. Ⓐ Ⓑ Ⓒ Ⓓ	13. Ⓐ Ⓑ Ⓒ Ⓓ	18. Ⓐ Ⓑ Ⓒ Ⓓ
4. Ⓐ Ⓑ Ⓒ Ⓓ	9. Ⓐ Ⓑ Ⓒ Ⓓ	14. Ⓐ Ⓑ Ⓒ Ⓓ	19. Ⓐ Ⓑ Ⓒ Ⓓ
5. Ⓐ Ⓑ Ⓒ Ⓓ	10. Ⓐ Ⓑ Ⓒ Ⓓ	15. Ⓐ Ⓑ Ⓒ Ⓓ	20. Ⓐ Ⓑ Ⓒ Ⓓ

TEST 4: MATHEMATICS

1. Ⓐ Ⓑ Ⓒ Ⓓ	9. Ⓐ Ⓑ Ⓒ Ⓓ	17. Ⓐ Ⓑ Ⓒ Ⓓ	25. Ⓐ Ⓑ Ⓒ Ⓓ
2. Ⓐ Ⓑ Ⓒ Ⓓ	10. Ⓐ Ⓑ Ⓒ Ⓓ	18. Ⓐ Ⓑ Ⓒ Ⓓ	26. Ⓐ Ⓑ Ⓒ Ⓓ
3. Ⓐ Ⓑ Ⓒ Ⓓ	11. Ⓐ Ⓑ Ⓒ Ⓓ	19. Ⓐ Ⓑ Ⓒ Ⓓ	27. Ⓐ Ⓑ Ⓒ Ⓓ
4. Ⓐ Ⓑ Ⓒ Ⓓ	12. Ⓐ Ⓑ Ⓒ Ⓓ	20. Ⓐ Ⓑ Ⓒ Ⓓ	28. Ⓐ Ⓑ Ⓒ Ⓓ
5. Ⓐ Ⓑ Ⓒ Ⓓ	13. Ⓐ Ⓑ Ⓒ Ⓓ	21. Ⓐ Ⓑ Ⓒ Ⓓ	29. Ⓐ Ⓑ Ⓒ Ⓓ
6. Ⓐ Ⓑ Ⓒ Ⓓ	14. Ⓐ Ⓑ Ⓒ Ⓓ	22. Ⓐ Ⓑ Ⓒ Ⓓ	30. Ⓐ Ⓑ Ⓒ Ⓓ
7. Ⓐ Ⓑ Ⓒ Ⓓ	15. Ⓐ Ⓑ Ⓒ Ⓓ	23. Ⓐ Ⓑ Ⓒ Ⓓ	31. Ⓐ Ⓑ Ⓒ Ⓓ
8. Ⓐ Ⓑ Ⓒ Ⓓ	16. Ⓐ Ⓑ Ⓒ Ⓓ	24. Ⓐ Ⓑ Ⓒ Ⓓ	

MATHEMATICS TESTS

TEST 1: MATHEMATICS

20 QUESTIONS • TIME—15 MINUTES

Directions: Each problem in this test involves a certain amount of logical reasoning and thinking on your part, besides simple computations, to help you find the solution. Read each problem carefully and choose the correct answer from the four choices that follow. Blacken the corresponding space on your answer sheet.

1. Find the interest on $25,800 for 144 days at six percent per annum. Base your calculations on a 360-day year.

   (A) $619.20
   (B) $619.02
   (C) $691.02
   (D) $691.20

2. Arthur can shovel snow from a sidewalk in 60 minutes and Jack can do it in 30 minutes. How many minutes will it take them to do the job together?

   (A) 90
   (B) 15
   (C) 30
   (D) 20

3. The visitors' section of a courtroom seats 105 people. The court is in session six hours per day. On one particular day, 485 people visited the court and were given seats. What is the average length of time spent by each visitor in the court? Assume that as soon as a person leaves his seat it is immediately filled and that at no time during the day is one of the 105 seats vacant. Express your answer in hours and minutes.

   (A) 1 hour 20 minutes
   (B) 1 hour 18 minutes
   (C) 1 hour 30 minutes
   (D) 2 hours

4. If copy paper costs $14.50 per ream and a five percent discount is allowed for cash, how many reams can be purchased for $690 cash? Do not round off cents in your calculations.

   (A) 49 reams
   (B) 60 reams
   (C) 50 reams
   (D) 53 reams

5. How many hours are there between 8:30 A.M. today and 3:15 A.M. tomorrow?

   (A) $17\frac{3}{4}$ hours
   (B) $18\frac{3}{4}$ hours
   (C) $18\frac{2}{3}$ hours
   (D) $18\frac{1}{2}$ hours

6. How many days are there from September 19 to December 25 (*inclusive*)?

   (A) 98 days
   (B) 96 days
   (C) 89 days
   (D) 90 days

7. A clerk is requested to file 800 cards. If he can file cards at the rate of 80 cards an hour, the number of cards remaining to be filed after seven hours of work is

   (A) 40
   (B) 240
   (C) 140
   (D) 260

8. If your monthly electricity bill increases from $80 to $90, the percentage of increase is, most nearly,

   (A) 10 percent
   (B) $11\frac{1}{9}$ percent
   (C) $12\frac{1}{2}$ percent
   (D) $14\frac{1}{7}$ percent

9. Fifteen nurses who work the morning shift of Get Well Hospital are responsible for 135 patients. The average number of patients served by each nurse is

(A) 120
(B) 10
(C) 9
(D) 140

10. If a nursing test contained 80 questions and you answered 72 of them correctly, what percent of the questions did you answer correctly?

(A) 90%
(B) 72%
(C) 8%
(D) 28%

11. If a patient is required to get 45 minutes of exercise each day, how many hours of exercise does he get in a week?

(A) 315 hours
(B) 5.25 hours
(C) 52 hours
(D) 6.4 hours

12. If a hospital has 120 nurses on duty during the afternoon shift and one half as many on duty for the night shift, what is the total number of nurses on duty for the two shifts?

(A) 60
(B) 180
(C) 90
(D) 120.5

13. If an inspector issued 182 summonses in the course of seven hours, his hourly average of summonses issued was

(A) 23 summonses
(B) 26 summonses
(C) 25 summonses
(D) 28 summonses

14. Last week 23 of the 76 patients admitted to Emergency Hospital had been in accidents. How many of the admitted patients had not been in accidents?

(A) 23
(B) 99
(C) 53
(D) 76

15. A truck going at a rate of 40 miles an hour will reach a town 80 miles away in how many hours?

(A) 1 hour
(B) 3 hours
(C) 2 hours
(D) 4 hours

16. If a barrel has a capacity of 100 gallons, how many gallons will it contain when it is two-fifths full?

(A) 20 gallons
(B) 60 gallons
(C) 40 gallons
(D) 80 gallons

17. If a monthly salary of $3000 is subject to a 20 percent tax, the net salary is

(A) $2000
(B) $2400
(C) $2500
(D) $2600

18. If $1000 is the cost of repairing 100 square yards of pavement, the cost of repairing one square yard is

(A) $10
(B) $150
(C) $100
(D) $300

19. If a woman's base pay is $3000 per month, and it is increased by a monthly bonus of $350 and a seniority increment of $250 this month, her total salary for the month is

(A) $3600
(B) $3500
(C) $3000
(D) $3700

20. If an annual salary of $21,600 is increased by a bonus of $7200 and by a service increment of $1200, the total pay rate is

(A) $29,600
(B) $39,600
(C) $26,900
(D) $30,000

TEST 1: MATHEMATICS ANSWER KEY

1. **A**
2. **D**
3. **B**
4. **C**
5. **B**
6. **A**
7. **B**
8. **C**
9. **C**
10. **A**
11. **B**
12. **B**
13. **B**
14. **C**
15. **C**
16. **C**
17. **B**
18. **A**
19. **A**
20. **D**

TEST 1: MATHEMATICS EXPLANATORY ANSWERS

1. **(A)** *Interest = Principal × Rate × Time*

   Note: 6% = 0.06

   144 days = $\frac{144}{360}$ year

   $I = P \times R \times T$

   $= \$25{,}800 \times 0.06 \times \frac{144}{360}$

   $= \frac{\$222{,}912}{360}$

   = \$619.20

2. **(D)** Let n = number of minutes in which they can do the job together. Arthur can do $\frac{1}{60}$ of the job in one minute, so in n minutes he can do $\frac{n}{60}$ of the job. Jack can do $\frac{1}{30}$ of the job in one minute and $\frac{n}{30}$ of the job in n minutes. Together, in n minutes they can do the complete job.

   $\frac{n}{60} + \frac{n}{30} = 1$

   $n + 2n = 60$ multiplying both sides by 60 (the lowest common denominator)

   $3n = 60$ combine like terms

   $n = 20$ divide by 3

   They can do the job together in 20 minutes.

3. **(B)** Total seats = 105

   Total time = 6 hours

   Total people involved = 486

   105 seats × 6 hours = 630 seating hours

   To find the average seating time, divide

   630 ÷ 485 = 1.3 hours

   Now change the 0.3 hours to minutes

   (1 hour = 60 minutes).

   .03 ~~hour~~ × $\frac{60 \text{ minutes}}{1 \text{ ~~hour~~}}$ = 18 minutes

   The amount is 1 hour 18 minutes.

4. **(C)** Paper per ream = \$14.50

   Discount = 5% or 0.05

   Total cash = \$690.00

   First, find the discount on the paper per ream when paying cash.

   \$14.50 × 0.05 = 0.725 cents

   Our price per ream is \$14.50 – 0.725 = \$13.775. Given \$690 to spend, divide to find how much paper can be purchased.

   \$690.00 ÷ \$13.775/ream = 50

   50 reams for \$688.75

5. **(B)** Use simple logic on this problem.

From	*To*
8:30 A.M.→	8:30 P.M. = 12 hours
8:30 P.M.→	3:30 A.M. = 7 hours

   Total = 19 hours

   But this is 15 minutes too much.

   Note: Change one of the hours to minutes (1 hour = 60 minutes.)

   45 minutes = $\frac{45}{60}$ hours or $\frac{3}{4}$ hours.

   18 hours 60 minutes
   – 15 minutes
   18 hours 45 minutes

   $18\frac{3}{4}$ is the total number of hours.

6. **(A)** Again, use logic.

Month	*Number of days/month*	
September	from 19 to 30	12 days
October	31 days	31 days
November	30 days	30 days
December	from 1 to 25	25 days
		98 days

   Note: Remember that 19 September and 25 December are included.

   Total = 98 days inclusive

7. **(B)** Total to be filed = 800 cards

   Rate cards can be filed = 80 cards per hour

   How many cards were filed in the first seven hours?

   $7 \times 80 = 560$ cards were filed

   Subtract to find the remaining cards to be filed.

   $800 - 560 = 240$

   240 cards remain unfiled

8. **(C)** From \$80 to \$90 there is a \$10 increase; the percentage of increase is found by dividing the amount of increase by the original amount:

   $10 \div 80 = 0.125$ or $12\frac{1}{2}\%$

   Note: $0.125 = 12.5\%$ or $12\frac{1}{2}\%$

   Percentage of increase $= 12\frac{1}{2}\%$

9. **(C)** To find the *average* number of patients served by each nurse, divide 135 patients by 15 nurses to get 9 patients per nurse.

10. **(A)** To find the percent of correct answers on the test, divide the number of correct answers by the total number of items on the test

    $\frac{72}{80} = .90$

    Change .90 to a percent $.90 = 90\%$

    90% of the test items were correct

11. **(B)** To find the number of hours of exercise the patient gets in a week, multiply

    45 min $\times$ 7 days = 315 minutes

    Convert the minutes to hours by dividing by 60 since there are 60 minutes in an hour.

    $\frac{315}{60} = 5.25$ hours per week

12. **(B)** To find the number of nurses on duty for the two shifts, determine the total number of nurses who worked on the night shift by finding one-half of the number who worked the afternoon shift $120 \times \frac{1}{2} = 60$

    Add the number who worked the afternoon shift to the number who worked the night shift. $120 + 60 = 180$

    180 nurses worked on the two shifts

13. **(B)** Total summonses in seven hours = 182

    To find the *average* number of summonses per hour, divide:

    182 summonses $\div$ 7 hours = 26

    Average = 26 summonses/hour

14. **(C)** To find the number of admitted patients who hadn't been in accidents, subtract the number of patients who were in accidents from the total number of patients.

    $76 - 23 = 53$

    53 of the admitted patients had not been in accidents.

15. **(C)** If it takes one truck one hour to go 40 miles, it will take two hours to go 80 miles.

    $2 \text{ hours} \times 40 \frac{\text{miles}}{\text{hour}} = 80 \text{ miles}$

16. **(C)** If the total capacity is 100 gallons, then

    $\frac{2}{5}$ of $100 = \frac{2}{5} \times 100$

    $= \frac{200}{5}$

    = 40 gallons

17. **(B)** Total salary = \$3000

    Tax= 20% or .20

    Find the amount of 20% tax by multiplying: $\$3000 \times .20 = \$600$

    Subtract the tax from the salary to find the net:

    $\$3000 - \$600 = \$2400$

    \$2400 = net pay

18. **(A)** Total cost = $1000

Total square yards = 100

Find the cost per square yard by dividing:
$1000 ÷ 100 square yards = $10

$ 10/square yard

19. **(A)**

Base pay	= $3000
Bonus	= + 350
Sr. Increment	+ 250
Total pay	= $3600

20. **(D)**

Annual salary	= $21,600
Bonus	= +7200
Increment	= +1200
Total pay	= $30,000

TEST 2: MATHEMATICS

20 QUESTIONS • TIME—15 MINUTES

Directions: Each problem in this test involves a certain amount of logical reasoning and thinking on your part, besides simple computations, to help you find the solution. Read each problem carefully and choose the correct answer from the four choices that follow. Blacken the corresponding space on your answer sheet.

1. An emergency medical technician was standing 40 feet behind his vehicle when a second emergency medical vehicle arrived and parked 90 feet from the first vehicle. If the emergency medical technician is standing between the two vehicles, how much closer is he to the first vehicle than the second?

   (A) 30 feet
   (B) 50 feet
   (C) 10 feet
   (D) 70 feet

2. If an IV bag has a capacity of 1,260 milliliters, how many milliliters does it contain when it's two-thirds full?

   (A) 809 ml
   (B) 750 ml
   (C) 630 ml
   (D) 840 ml

3. If a man's salary is $2,500 a month and there are 23 working days in the month, he earns approximately how much for each day he works that month?

   (A) $108.70
   (B) $150.00
   (C) $112.50
   (D) $186.70

4. A nursing home assistant earns $360.00 a week and has deductions of $18.00 for her retirement fund, $15.00 for medical insurance, $21.00 for social security and $72.00 for withholding taxes. How much is her take home pay?

   (A) $488.00
   (B) $296.00
   (C) $234.00
   (D) $288.00

5. A company uses 40 thirty-three-cent stamps, 25 twenty-cent stamps, and 320 sixty-cent stamps each day. The total cost of stamps used by the company in a five-day period is

   (A) $1,051.00
   (B) $210.20
   (C) $21,000.00
   (D) $105,100.00

6. A city department issued 12,000 applications in 1979. The number of applications that the department issued in 1977 was 25 percent greater than the number it issued in 1979. If the department issued 10 percent fewer applications in 1975 than it did in 1977, the number it issued in 1975 was

   (A) 16,500
   (B) 13,500
   (C) 9900
   (D) 8100

7. A secretary can add 40 columns of figures in an hour by using a calculator and 20 columns of figures an hour without using a calculator. The total number of hours it would take him to add 200 columns if he does three-fifths of the work by machine and the rest without the machine is

   (A) 6
   (B) 7
   (C) 8
   (D) 9

8. In 1995, a medical office bought 500 dozen rubber gloves at a price of $2.60 per dozen. In 1998, 25% less gloves were bought than in 1995 but the price per dozen was 20% higher than the price in 1995. The total cost of the gloves bought in 1998 was

   (A) $1,560.00
   (B) $1,170.00
   (C) $975.00
   (D) $1,040.00

9. A nurse is assigned to check the accuracy of the entries on 490 forms. He checks 40 forms an hour. After working one hour on this task, he is joined by another nurse, who checks these forms at the rate of 35 an hour. The total number of hours required to do the entire assignment is

(A) 5
(B) 6
(C) 7
(D) 8

10. Assume that there are a total of 420 employees in a medical care building. 30 percent of the employees are doctors and one-seventh are nurses. The difference between the number of nurses and the doctors is

(A) 60
(B) 66
(C) 186
(D) 360

11. Assume that a duplicating machine produces copies of a bulletin at a cost of 12 cents per copy. The machine produces 120 copies of the bulletin per minute. If the cost of producing a certain number of copies was $36, how many minutes did it take the machine to produce this number of copies?

(A) 10 minutes
(B) 6 minutes
(C) 2.5 minutes
(D) 1.2 minutes

12. The average number of medical records filed per day by a filing clerk during a five-day week was 720. She filed 610 records the first day, 720 records the second day, 740 records the third day, and 755 records the fourth day. The number of records she filed the fifth day was

(A) 748
(B) 165
(C) 775
(D) 565

13. A city department employs 1400 people, of whom 35 percent are clerks and one-eighth are stenographers. The number of employees in the department who are neither clerks nor stenographers is

(A) 640
(B) 665
(C) 735
(D) 750

14. Two nurses were assigned to take blood pressures at a health fair. They took the blood pressure of 190 people. If Nurse A took 40 more blood pressures than Nurse B, then the number of blood pressures taken by Nurse A was

(A) 75
(B) 110
(C) 115
(D) 150

15. A stock clerk had on hand the following items:

500 pads, worth $0.04 each

130 pencils, worth $0.03 each

50 dozen rubber bands, worth $0.02 a dozen

If, from this stock, he issued 125 pads, 45 pencils, and 48 rubber bands, the value of the remaining stock would be

(A) $6.43
(B) $8.95
(C) $17.63
(D) $18.47

16. Joe can paint a fence in three hours and his friend can paint the fence in four hours. How long will it take them to do the job if they work together?

(A) 7 hours
(B) $\frac{15}{7}$ hours
(C) $1\frac{5}{7}$ hours
(D) 2 hours

17. A department head hired a total of 60 temporary employees to handle a seasonal increase in the department's workload.

The following lists the number of temporary employees hired, their rates of pay, and the duration of their employment:

—One-third of the total were hired as clerks, each at the rate of $9,750 a year, for two months.

—30 percent of the total were hired as office-machine operators, each at the rate of $11,500 a year, for four months.

—22 stenographers were hired, each at the rate of $10,200 a year, for three months.

The total amount paid to these temporary employees was approximately

(A) $178,000
(B) $157,600
(C) $52,200
(D) $48,500

18. Assume that there are 2,300 employees in a city agency. Also assume that five percent of these employees are accountants; that 80 percent of the accountants have college degrees; and that one-half of the accountants who have college degrees have five years of experience. Then the number of employees in the agency who are accountants with college degrees and five years of experience is

(A) 46
(B) 51
(C) 460
(D) 920

19. If a monthly salary of $3,000 is subject to a $425 tax deduction, the net salary is

(A) $2,557.00
(B) $2,755.00
(C) $2,575.00
(D) $2,555.00

20. A sanitation worker who reports 45 minutes early for 8:00 A.M. duty will report at

(A) 7:00 A.M.
(B) 7:30 A.M.
(C) 6:15 A.M.
(D) 7:15 A.M.

TEST 2: MATHEMATICS ANSWER KEY

1. **C**
2. **D**
3. **A**
4. **C**
5. **A**
6. **B**
7. **B**
8. **B**
9. **C**
10. **B**
11. **C**
12. **C**
13. **C**
14. **C**
15. **D**
16. **C**
17. **B**
18. **A**
19. **C**
20. **D**

TEST 2: MATHEMATICS EXPLANATORY ANSWERS

1. **(C)**

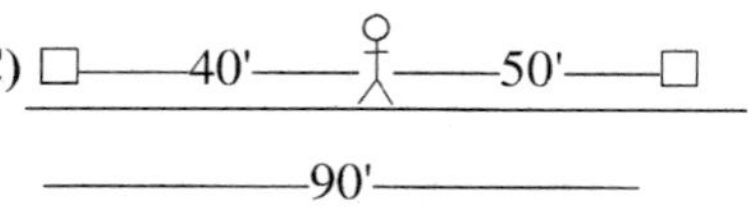

The second vehicle is 90 feet – 40 feet = 50 feet from the emergency medical technician (EMT). The first vehicle is 40 feet from the EMT. The first vehicle is 50 feet – 40 feet = 10 feet closer than the second vehicle.

2. **(D)** To find the number of milliliters the IV bag has when it's two-thirds full, multiply

$1260 \text{ milliliters} \times \frac{2}{3} = 840 \text{ milliliters}$

There are 840 milliliters in the IV bag when it's two-thirds full.

3. **(A)** Salary per month = \$2500

Days worked = 23

To find the earnings per day, divide:

$$\frac{\$2500}{\text{month}} \div \frac{23 \text{ days}}{\text{month}} = \frac{\$108.70}{\text{day}}$$

or

$$\frac{\$2500}{\text{month}} \div \frac{23 \text{ days}}{\text{month}} =$$

$$\frac{\$2500}{\text{month}} \times \frac{\text{month}}{23 \text{ days}} =$$

$$\frac{\$2500}{23 \text{ days}} = \frac{\$108.70}{\text{day}}$$

4. **(C)** To find the take home pay of the nursing home assistant, subtract the total amount of her deductions from her weekly salary.

Total deductions = \$18.00 + \$15.00 + \$21.00 + \$72.00 = \$126.00

Weekly salary = \$360.00

Salary – deductions = \$360.00 – \$126.00 = \$234.00

Take-home pay = \$234.00

5. **(A)**

Stamps per day	*Cost per day*
40/day × \$0.33	= 13.20
25/day × \$0.20	= 5.00
320/day × \$0.60	= <u>192.00</u>
Total cost/day	\$210.20

For five days, 5 × \$210.20 = \$1,051.00

Total cost = \$1,051.00

6. **(B)** Number of applications issued in 1979 = 12,000
In 1977, 25 percent more were issued, or:
0.25 × 12,000 = 3000 more in 1977

So there were 3000 + 12,000 = 15,000 issued in 1977.

In 1975, ten percent fewer were issued than in 1977, or:

0.10 × 15,000 = 1500 fewer were issued in 1975.

The number issued in 1975 is

15,000 – 1500 = 13,500

13,500 issued

7. **(B)** If three-fifths of the 200 are done by calculator, then:

$$\frac{3}{5} \times 200 = \frac{600}{5} = 120$$

columns will be done by the machine. To find the number done by hand, subtract:

200 – 120 = 80 will be done by hand.

To find the time it takes to do the 120 columns by machine and the 80 columns by hand, divide:

120 columns ÷ 40 columns per hour = 3 hours

80 columns ÷ 20 columns per hour = 4 hours

Total time = 7 hours

8. **(B)** To find the total cost of the rubber gloves bought in 1998, first determine the amount of the 20% increase for a dozen gloves in 1998.

.20 × \$2.60 = 0.52

Add the cost in 1995 to the amount of the increase to get the cost of the gloves in 1998.

\$2.60 + 0.52 = \$3.12

In 1998 a dozen gloves cost \$3.12

The number of gloves purchased in 1998 was 25% less than the number purchased in 1995.

To find how many dozens of gloves were purchased in 1999, find 25% of 500 dozen and subtract the result from 500 dozen.

500 dozen – .25 × 500 dozen = 500 dozen – 125 dozen = 375 dozen

375 dozen gloves were purchases in 1998.

Multiply the price per dozen $3.12 × 375 dozen = $1,170.00

The total cost of the gloves bought in 1998 was $1,170.00

9. **(C)** During the first hour, 40 forms were checked, leaving 450 to be checked:

   490 – 40 = 450

   The two nurses working together can check 75 forms.

   Now find the time it takes to do the 450 forms. Do this by dividing:

   450 forms ÷ 75 forms/hour = 6 hours

   It takes six hours to do the 450 and one hour for the first 40 forms:

   6 hours + 1 hour = 7 hours to do the job.

   A total of 7 hours is needed

10. **(B)** Total employed = 420

    If 30 percent are nurses,

    420 × 0.30 = 126 nurses

    $\frac{1}{7}$ are doctors:

    $420 \times \frac{1}{7} = 60$ doctors

    The difference is 126 – 60 = 66

11. **(C)** Cost = 12¢ per copy

    Time = 120 copies per minute

    To find the number of copies produced, divide:

    36 ÷ 0.12 = 300 copies

    To find the number of minutes, divide:

    300 copies ÷ 120 copies/minute = 2.5 minutes

12. **(C)** If the average number of medical records filed for five days was 720 then

    5 days × 720 records/day = 3600 records for the five-day period

    For four days:

    610 + 720 + 740 + 755 = 2825 medical records were filed

    Subtract:

    3600 – 2825 = 775 need to be filed the fifth day to get an average of 720 for the five-day period

13. **(C)** Total employees = 1400

    35% clerks = 1400 × .35 = 490 clerks

    $\frac{1}{8}$ stenos = $1400 \times \frac{1}{8}$ = 175 stenos

    Together (490 + 175 = 665), there are 665 clerks and stenographers. To find how many employees are neither, subtract:

    1400 – 665 = 735

    Answer = 735 other employees

14. **(C)** If Nurse A takes 40 more blood pressures than Nurse B, let x represent the number of blood pressures taken by Nurse B. Then $x + 40$ = the number of blood pressures taken by Nurse A. Add the number of blood pressures taken by Nurse A to the number taken by Nurse B to get the total number of blood pressures taken.

    $x + x + 40 = 190$

    $2x + 40 = 190$

    $2x = 150$

    $x = 75$ the number of blood pressures taken by Nurse B

    $x + 40 = 75 + 40 = 115$ the number of blood pressures taken by Nurse A

15. **(D)** Stock on hand and cost per item:

	cost
500 pads × 0.04/pad	= $20.00
130 pencils × 0.03/pencil	= $3.90
50 dozen rubber bands × 0.02/dozen	= $1.00
value of stock on hand =	$24.90

    If we issue the items below,

125 pads × $0.04	= 5.00
45 pencils × .03	= 1.35
48 rubber bands or 4 dozen × .02	= .08
	$6.43

    To find the value of the remaining stock, subtract:

    $24.90 – $6.43 = $18.47

    Value = $18.47

16. **(C)** Let t be the amount of time for both to do the job. If Joe does $\frac{t}{3}$ part of the job, and his friend does $\frac{t}{4}$ part of the job, then

$\frac{t}{3} + \frac{t}{4} = 1$ (the whole job)

$4t + 3t = 12$ multiply lowest common denominator by 12

$7t = 12$ combine like terms

$t = \frac{12}{7}$ divide by 7

$t = 1\frac{5}{7}$ hours

17. **(B)** Total employees = 60

$\frac{1}{3} \times = 20$ clerks

$30\% \times 60$,

or $0.30 \times 60 = \frac{18}{38}$ office machine operators

$60 - 38 = 22$ stenos

To find their *rate per month*, divide their monthly salaries by 12, because there are 12 months in a year:

clerks $\frac{\$9750}{12} = \$812.50$

OMOs $\frac{\$11,500}{12} = \$958.33$

stenos $\frac{\$10,200}{12} = \$850.00$

Now find the salary for all employees for the time they worked:

If 20 clerks worked two months, total pay equals:

$20 \times 2 \times \$812.50 = \$32,500.00$

If 18 OMOs worked four months, total pay equals:

$18 \times 4 \times \$958.33 = \$68,999.76$

If 22 stenos worked three months, total pay equals:

$22 \times 3 \times \$850.00 = \$56,100.00$

Total salaries = \$157,599.76. This amount can be rounded off to \$157,600.00.

18. **(A)** 5 percent of 2300 are accountants:

$0.05 \times 2300 = 115$

80 percent of the 115 accountants have college degrees:

$0.80 \times 115 = 92$

One-half of the 92 have five years' experience:

$\frac{1}{2} \times 92 = 46$

46 employees have all three qualifications

19. **(C)** \$3000 is subject to \$425 tax. The net can be found by subtracting:

$\$3000 - \$425 = \$2575$

20. **(D)** A sanitation worker who reports 45 minutes early for 8:00 A.M. duty reports

7 hours 60 minutes
– 45 minutes
7 hours 15 minutes

Note: 1 hour = 60 minutes

8 hours = 7 hours 60 minutes

This worker reports at 7:15 A.M.

TEST 3: MATHEMATICS

20 QUESTIONS • TIME—15 MINUTES

Directions: Each problem in this test involves a certain amount of logical reasoning and thinking on your part, besides simple computations, to help you find the solution. Read each problem carefully and choose the correct answer from the four choices that follow. Blacken the corresponding space on your answer sheet.

1. If the average cost of sweeping a square foot of a small town's street is $0.75, the cost of sweeping 100 square feet is

   (A) $7.50
   (B) $750
   (C) $75
   (D) $70

2. After his car broke down while he was on his way to a conference, a nurse had the car towed to his home 90 miles away. If the car was towed at a rate of 36 miles per hour, how many hours did it take to tow the car to his home?

   (A) .4 hours
   (B) 54 hours
   (C) 2.5 hours
   (D) 25 hours

3. A man is standing between a bank and a drug store. He is 60 feet away from the bank and the drug store is 100 feet away from the bank. How many feet nearer is the man to the bank than the drug store is to the bank?

   (A) 60 feet
   (B) 40 feet
   (C) 50 feet
   (D) 20 feet

4. A clerk divided his 35-hour work week as follows:

   One-fifth of his time in sorting mail; one-half of his time in filing letters; and one-seventh of his time in reception work.

   The rest of his time was devoted to messenger work. The percentage of time spent on messenger work by the clerk during the week was most nearly

   (A) 6 percent
   (B) 10 percent
   (C) 14 percent
   (D) 16 percent

5. A city department has set up a computing unit and has rented five computing machines at a yearly rental of $1400 per machine. In addition, the cost to the department for the maintenance and repair of each of these machines is $100 per year. Five computing machine operators, each receiving an annual salary of $30,000 and a supervisor, who receives $38,000 a year, have been assigned to the unit. This unit will perform the work previously performed by ten employees whose combined salary was $324,000 a year. On the basis of these facts, the savings that will result from the operation of this computing unit for five years will be most nearly

   (A) $500,000
   (B) $947,500
   (C) $640,000
   (D) $950,000

6. Joe can do a certain job in eight days. After working alone for four days, he is joined by Mary, and together they finish the work in two more days. How long would it take Mary alone?

   (A) 5 days
   (B) 6 days
   (C) 7 days
   (D) 8 days

7. Eighty dozen pairs of rubber gloves were purchased for a medical facility. If the gloves are used at a rate of 32 pairs a day, what is the maximum number of days the gloves will last?

   (A) 2.5 days
   (B) 48 days
   (C) 30 days
   (D) 360 days

8. At a certain health care facility, the average cost of providing care for 3 patients for 5 days is $7,200.00. What is the average cost of providing care for 24 patients for 5 days?

   (A) $43,200.00
   (B) $36,000.00
   (C) $34,560.00
   (D) $57,600.00

9. Typist A can do a job in three hours. Typist B can do the same job in five hours. How long would it take both, working together, to do the job?

   (A) 5 hours
   (B) $3\frac{1}{2}$ hours
   (C) $1\frac{7}{8}$ hours
   (D) $1\frac{5}{8}$ hours

10. After gaining 50 percent of his original capital, a man had capital of $18,000. Find the original capital.

    (A) $12,200.00
    (B) $13,100.00
    (C) $12,000.00
    (D) $12,025.00

11. To work off 60 calories, Brenda needs to walk the treadmill for 15 minutes. How long will it take her to work off 100 calories?

    (A) 25 minutes
    (B) 55 minutes
    (C) 40 minutes
    (D) 45 minutes

12. A student worked 30 days at a part-time job. He paid two-fifths of his earnings for room and board and had $81 left. What was his daily wage?

    (A) $4.50
    (B) $5.00
    (C) $5.50
    (D) $6.25

13. A dealer bought motorcycles for $4,000. He sold them for $6,200, making $50 on each motorcycle. How many motorcycles were there?

    (A) 40
    (B) 38
    (C) 43
    (D) 44

14. An organization had one-fourth of its capital invested in goods, two-thirds of the remainder in land, and the remainder, $1,224, in cash. What was the capital of the firm?

    (A) $4,986.00
    (B) $4,698.00
    (C) $4,896.00
    (D) $4,869.00

15. A and B together earn $2,100. If B is paid one-fourth more than A, how many dollars should B receive?

    (A) $1,166.66
    (B) $1,162.66
    (C) $1,617.66
    (D) $1,167.66

16. If a boat is bought for $21,500 and sold again for $23,650, what is the percentage of gain?

    (A) 8 percent
    (B) 15 percent
    (C) 20 percent
    (D) 10 percent

17. A person owned five-sixths of a piece of property and sold three-fourths of her share for $1,800. What was the value of the property?

    (A) $2,808.00
    (B) $2,880.00
    (C) $2,088.00
    (D) $2880.80

18. A lot costing $21,250 leases for $1,900 a year. The taxes and other expenses are $300 per year. Find the percentage of net income on the investment.

    (A) $7\frac{1}{2}$ percent
    (B) 6 percent
    (C) 4 percent
    (D) 10 percent

19. B owned 75 shares of stock in a building association worth $50 each. The association declared a dividend of eight percent, payable in stock. How many shares did he then own?

    (A) 81 shares
    (B) 80 shares
    (C) 90 shares
    (D) 85 shares

20. It requires four men three days to take an inventory; the weekly salary of each is as follows:

    A—$250, B—$130, C—$120, D—$90.

    Calculate the cost of taking the inventory, assuming that there are five full working days in a week.

    (A) $119.00
    (B) $196.00
    (C) $354.00
    (D) $588.00

TEST 3: MATHEMATICS ANSWER KEY

1. **C**
2. **C**
3. **B**
4. **D**
5. **C**
6. **D**
7. **C**
8. **D**
9. **C**
10. **C**
11. **A**
12. **A**
13. **D**
14. **C**
15. **A**
16. **D**
17. **B**
18. **A**
19. **A**
20. **C**

TEST 3: MATHEMATICS EXPLANATORY ANSWERS

1. **(C)** If it cost \$0.75 to sweep one square foot, to find the cost for 100 square feet, multiply:

   100 square feet × 0.75 square foot = \$75

   Total cost = \$75

2. **(C)** To determine how many hours it will take to tow the car 90 miles at a rate of 36 mph, divide

   $90 \div 32 = 2.5$

   It will take 2.5 hours = $2\frac{1}{2}$ hours to tow the car 90 miles.

3. **(B)** To determine how many feet nearer the man is to the bank than the drug store is to bank, use a diagram

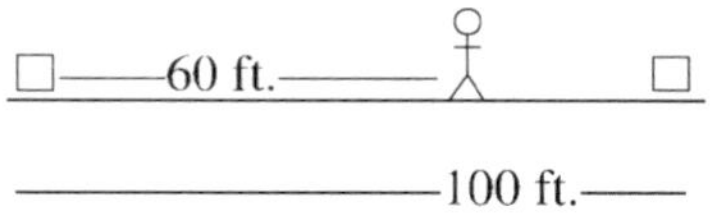

   The total distance from the bank to the drug store is 100 feet. Subtract to find the distance from the man to the drug store.

   100 feet – 60 feet = 40 feet

   The man is 40 feet nearer to the bank than the drug store is to the bank.

4. **(D)** A clerk works 35 hours per week. $\frac{1}{5}$ of his time is used to sort mail:

   $\frac{1}{5} \times 35 = 7$ hours

   $\frac{1}{2}$ of his time is used to file letters:

   $\frac{1}{2} \times 35 = 17\frac{1}{2}$ hours

   $\frac{1}{7}$ of his time is used for reception work.

   $\frac{1}{7} \times 35 = 5$ hours

   Total = $29\frac{1}{2}$ hours

   $29\frac{1}{2}$ hours were used for the above. To find the time left for messenger work, subtract $35 - 29\frac{1}{2} = 5\frac{1}{2}$ hours.

   Now to find what percentage of 35 is $5\frac{1}{2}$, divide:

   $5.5 \div 35 = 0.16$ or 16%

   Note: $5\frac{1}{2} = 5.5$

   16% remains for messenger work.

5. **(C)** *Item*

5 machines—		
\$1400/year	5 × 1400	\$7000
Maintenance, repairs—		
\$100/machine	5 × 100	\$500
5 operators' annual salary—		
\$30,000	5 × \$30,000	\$150,000
Supervisor's annual salary—		
\$38,000	1 × \$38,000	\$38,000
total cost		\$195,500

   If ten employees were paid a total of \$324,000, find the savings by subtracting:

   \$324,000 – \$195,500 = \$128,500 one year's savings

   To find the savings for five years, multiply:

   \$128,500 × 5 = \$642,500

   This amount *rounds off* to (is nearest) \$640,000

6. **(D)** If Joe can do the job alone in eight days, then he can do $\frac{1}{8}$ in one day and $\frac{6}{8}$ or $\frac{3}{4}$ in six days.

   Let n be the number of days it would take Mary to do the job alone. Then:

   $\frac{1}{n}$ is the part of the job she can do in one day and $\frac{2}{n}$ is the part of the job she can do in the two days she works with Joe.

   Now, the sum of parts done by Joe and Mary equals one whole job:

   $\frac{3}{4} + \frac{2}{n} = 1$

   $3n + 8 = 4n$ multiply by the lowest common denominator (LCD), $4n$

   $8 = 4n - 3n$ subtract $3n$ from both sides of the equation

$8 = n$ subtract like term

$n = 8$

Mary alone could do the job in 8 days.

7. **(C)** Eighty dozen = $80 \times 12 = 960$

   960 pairs of gloves were purchased.

   To find the maximum number of days the gloves will last,

   Divide $960 \div 32 = 30$

   If the gloves are being used at a rate of 32 pairs a day, they will last 30 days.

8. **(D)** To determine the cost of caring for 24 patients for 5 days, find the cost of caring for one patient by dividing.

   $7,200.00 ÷ 3 = $ 2,400.00

   To get the cost for caring for 24 patients, multiply

   24 × $2,400.00 = $57,600.00

   The cost for caring for 24 patients is $57,600.00.

9. **(C)** A can do one-third of the job in one hour. B can do one-fifth of the job in one hour.

   Together they can do $\frac{1}{3} + \frac{1}{5}$ of the job in one hour. Let t be the time it takes for both to do the job. Together, they can do $\frac{1}{t}$ of the job in one hour. Thus:

   $\frac{1}{3} + \frac{1}{5} = \frac{1}{t}$

   $5t + 3t = 15$ multiply lowest common denominator by the $15t$ or $3 \times 5 \times t$

   $8t = 15$ add like terms

   $t = \frac{15}{8}$ divide both sides by 8 hour

   $t = 1\frac{7}{8}$

10. **(C)** Let x be the unknown original capital and $0.50x$ be 50 percent of the unknown capital.

    Therefore: sides by 1.50

    $x + .50x = \$18,000$

    $1.50x = \$18,000$ add like terms

    $\frac{150\ x}{1.50} = \frac{\$18,000}{1.50}$ divide both

    $x = \$12,000$

    $12,000 is the original amount of the capital

11. **(A)** Let x represent the amount of time it takes to walk off 100 calories.

    The ratio of the amount of time it takes to work off 60 calories equal the ratio of the amount of time it takes to work off 100 calories.

    15 minutes/60 calories = x minutes/100 calories

    $60x = 15 \times 100$

    $60x = 1500$

    $x = 25$ minutes

    It will take 25 minutes on the treadmill to work off 100 calories.

12. **(A)** If two-fifths of his salary was used, then three-fifths was left; three-fifths of his salary is $81. Now, since his salary is unknown, let x represent it:

    $\frac{3}{5} \times x = \$81$

    $x = \$81 \div \frac{3}{5}$ divide both sides by $\frac{3}{5}$

    $x = \$81 \times \frac{5}{3}$ invert and multiply

    $x = \$135$

    His salary is $135 for 30 days of work. To find the *daily wage*, divide the salary by 30:

    $135 ÷ 30 days = $4.50/day

    Daily wage = $4.50

13. **(D)** To find the number of motorcycles purchased, first subtract his original purchase price from the selling price:

    $6200 – $4000 = $2200 profit

    Since the profit was $2200, and the profit on each motorcycle was $50, the number of motorcycles sold is:

    $2200 profit ÷ 50 profit/motorcycle = 44 motorcycles sold

14. **(C)** $\frac{1}{4}$ in *goods* (given)

    $\frac{2}{3} \times \frac{3}{4} = \frac{1}{2}$ in *land* (because $\frac{3}{4}$ is the remainder after the goods are invested)

    $\frac{1}{4}$ is left in *cash*, because if, $\frac{1}{4}$ is in goods + $\frac{1}{2}$ is in land, $\frac{3}{4}$ is invested, leaving $\frac{1}{4}$ for cash

If $\frac{1}{4}$, which is the cash, is valued at \$1,224,

$\frac{1}{4}$ in goods = \$1,224

$\frac{1}{2}$ is twice as much as $\frac{1}{4}$

$\frac{1}{2}$ in land = \$2,448

$\frac{1}{4}$ in cash = $\frac{\$1,224}{\$4,896}$

Total capital = \$4,896

15. **(A)** Let A equal the amount A earned, and B equal the amount B earned.

Together, they earned $A + B = \$2,100$.

If B is paid $\frac{1}{4}$ more than A, then A's salary plus $\frac{1}{4}$ of A's salary is equal to B's salary. Express this as follows:

$B = A + \frac{1}{4}A$

$4B = 4A + A$ multiply by 4

$-5A + 4B = 0$ transpose the A terms

Now you have two equations with two unknowns. Use the elimination method to find B's salary:

$A + B = \$2,100$	multiply
$-5A + 4B = 0$	the first
$5A + 5B = \$10,500$	equation
$-5A + 4B = 0$	by 5
$9B = \$10,500$	add the two equations
$B = \$1,166.67$	now divide
or \$1,166 $\frac{2}{3}$	by 9

Note: $0.67 = \frac{2}{3}$

16. **(D)** The boat costs \$21,500 and was sold for \$23,650. Subtract:

\$23,650 – \$21,500 = \$2,150

\$2,150 was gained. To find the percentage gained, divide the amount gained by the original amount:

\$2150 ÷ \$21,500 = 0.10 or 10%

Percentage gained = 10%

17. **(B)** $\frac{5}{6} \times \frac{3}{4} = \frac{5}{8}$ of the property costs \$1,800

Then, letting y represent the value of the property,

$\frac{5}{8} \times y = \$1800$

$y = \$1,800 \div \frac{5}{8}$ divide both sides by $\frac{5}{8}$

$y = \$1,800 \times \frac{8}{5}$ invert and multiply

Therefore, \$2,880 is the price of the property.

18. **(A)** A lot costs \$21,250.

\$1,900	is received for lease
– 300	is deducted for expenses
\$1,600	is net income

To find what percentage \$1,600 is of the cost of the lot, divide:

$1600 \div 21,250 = 0.075$ or $7\frac{1}{2}\%$

$7\frac{1}{2}\%$ = percentage of cost

19. **(A)** Total shares currently owned = 75

Values per share = \$50

To find the value of the stock, multiply 75 × \$50 = \$3,750

To find 8%, multiply the stock value by 0.08

\$3,750 × 0.08 = \$300 (dividend)

Given \$300, divide by \$50 to see how many additional shares of stock can be purchased:

\$300 ÷ 50 = 6 shares

Therefore, he now owns 75 + 6 = 81 shares.

20. **(C)** First, find the salary each man is paid for one day. To do so, divide their salaries by 5 days:

			salary/ day	salary/ 3 days
A	$\frac{\$250}{5}$	=	\$50.00 × 3 =	\$150
B	$\frac{\$130}{5}$	=	\$26.00 × 3 =	\$78
C	$\frac{\$120}{5}$	=	\$24.00 × 3 =	\$72
D	$\frac{\$90}{5}$	=	\$18.00 × 3 =	$\frac{\$54}{354}$

Total salaries for 3 days = \$354

TEST 4: MATHEMATICS

31 QUESTIONS • TIME—22 MINUTES

Directions: Each problem in this test involves a certain amount of logical reasoning and thinking on your part, besides simple computations, to help you find the solution. Read each problem carefully and choose the correct answer from the choices that follow. Blacken the corresponding space on your answer sheet.

1. In simplest form, –11 – (–2) is

(A) 7
(B) 9
(C) –11
(D) –9

2. Find the average of 6.47, 5.89, 3.42, 0.65, and 7.09.

(A) 5.812
(B) 4.704
(C) 3.920
(D) 4.705

3. $\frac{456.3}{0.89}$ equals

(A) $513\frac{13}{89}$
(B) 512.70
(C) 513.89
(D) $512\frac{59}{89}$

4. Add 5 hours 13 minutes; 3 hours 49 minutes; and 24 minutes. The sum is

(A) 9 hours 26 minutes
(B) 8 hours 16 minutes
(C) 9 hours 76 minutes
(D) 8 hours 6 minutes

5. Two numbers are in the ratio of 18:47. If the smaller number is 126, the larger number is

(A) 376
(B) 144
(C) 235
(D) 329

6. Change 0.3125 to a fraction.

(A) $\frac{3}{64}$
(B) $\frac{1}{16}$
(C) $\frac{1}{64}$
(D) $\frac{49}{64}$

7. Divide $\frac{7}{8}$ by $\frac{7}{8}$.

(A) 1
(B) 0
(C) $\frac{7}{8}$
(D) $\frac{49}{64}$

8. In the series 5, 8, 13, 20, the next number should be

(A) 23
(B) 26
(C) 29
(D) 32

9. What is the interest on $300 at 6 percent for ten days? (Assume year = 360 days)

(A) $0.50
(B) $1.50
(C) $2.50
(D) $5.50

10. If the scale on a map indicates that one and one-half inches equals 500 miles, then five inches on the map will represent approximately

    (A) 1800 miles
    (B) 1700 miles
    (C) 1300 miles
    (D) 700 miles

11. $\frac{1}{2}$ percent equals

    (A) 0.002
    (B) 0.020
    (C) 0.005
    (D) 0.050

12. If 20% of an employee's bonus was $260.00, what was her entire bonus?

    (A) $2,300
    (B) $2,600
    (C) $1,600
    (D) $1,300

13. If a kilogram equals about 35 ounces, the number of grams in one ounce is approximately

    (A) 29
    (B) 30
    (C) 31
    (D) 32

14. An IV pump delivers medication at a constant rate of 24 milligrams per hour. How long does it take to deliver 90 milligrams?

    (A) 3 hours 15 minutes
    (B) 3 hours 45 minutes
    (C) 3 hours 75 minutes
    (D) 4 hours 15 minutes

15. If sound travels at the rate of 1100 feet per second, in one-half minute it will travel about

    (A) 6 miles
    (B) 8 miles
    (C) 10 miles
    (D) 3 miles

16. If a kilometer is about five-eighths of a mile, two miles are about

    (A) 1.6 kilometers
    (B) 3.2 kilometers
    (C) 2.4 kilometers
    (D) 3.75 kilometers

17. A lecture hall which is 25 feet wide and 75 feet long has a perimeter equal to

    (A) 1750 feet
    (B) 200 yards
    (C) $66\frac{2}{3}$ yards
    (D) 1875 feet

18. After deducting a discount of $16\frac{2}{3}$ percent, the price of a blouse was $35. The list price was

    (A) $37.50
    (B) $38
    (C) $41.75
    (D) $42

19. The number of decimal places in the product of 0.4266 and 0.3333 is

    (A) 8
    (B) 4
    (C) 14
    (D) none of these

20. What is the cost of 5,500 bandages at $50 per thousand?

    (A) $385
    (B) $550
    (C) $275
    (D) $285

21. 572 divided by 0.52 is

    (A) 1100
    (B) 110
    (C) 11.10
    (D) 11,000

22. 200 percent of 800 equals

    (A) 2500
    (B) 16
    (C) 1,600
    (D) 4

23. The average of a seventh-grade baseball team that won ten games and lost five games is

 (A) 0.667
 (B) 0.500
 (C) 0.333
 (D) 0.200

24. The number of cubic feet of soil needed for a flower box three feet long, eight inches wide, and one foot deep is

 (A) 24
 (B) 12
 (C) $4\frac{2}{3}$
 (D) 2

25. At $1,250 per hundred, 228 watches will cost

 (A) $2,850
 (B) $36,000
 (C) $2,880
 (D) $360

26. The area of the shaded portion of the rectangle below is

 (A) 54 square inches
 (B) 90 square inches
 (C) 45 square inches
 (D) 36 square inches

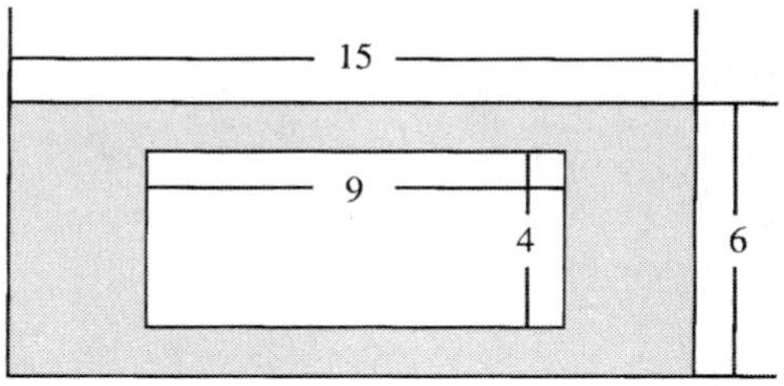

27. On February 12, 1989, the age of a boy who was born on March 15, 1979, will be

 (A) 10 years 10 months 3 days
 (B) 9 years 9 months 27 days
 (C) 10 years 1 month 3 days
 (D) 9 years 10 months 27 days

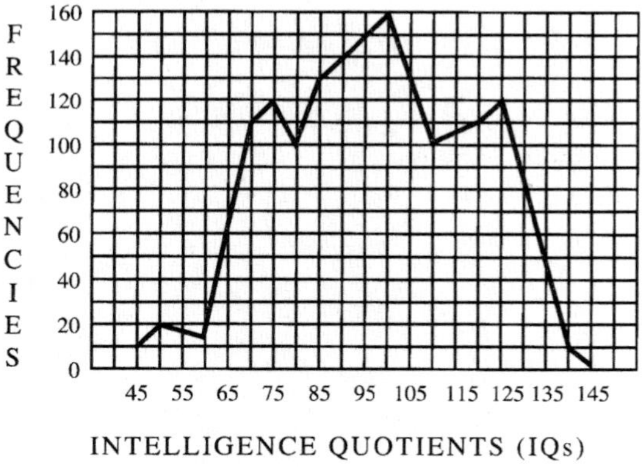

Questions 28 to 31 are based on the above graph.

28. The number of pupils having the highest IQ is about

 (A) 5
 (B) 160
 (C) 145
 (D) 20

29. The number of pupils having an IQ of 75 is about

 (A) 130
 (B) 100
 (C) 120
 (D) 110

30. The number of pupils having an IQ of 80 is identical with the number of pupils having an IQ of

 (A) 100
 (B) 68
 (C) 110
 (D) 128

31. The IQ that has the greatest frequency is

 (A) 100
 (B) 95
 (C) 105
 (D) 160

TEST 4: MATHEMATICS ANSWER KEY

1. **D**
2. **B**
3. **B**
4. **A**
5. **D**
6. **D**
7. **A**
8. **C**
9. **A**
10. **B**
11. **C**
12. **D**
13. **A**
14. **B**
15. **A**
16. **B**
17. **C**
18. **D**
19. **A**
20. **C**
21. **A**
22. **C**
23. **A**
24. **D**
25. **A**
26. **A**
27. **D**
28. **A**
29. **C**
30. **C**
31. **A**

TEST 4: MATHEMATICS EXPLANATORY ANSWERS

1. **(D)** – 11 – (–2)

   = –11 + 2

   = –9

2. **(B)** 6.47 + 5.89 + 3.42 + .65 + 7.09 = 23.52

   To find the average, divide the sum by five (the number of terms involved).

   23.52 ÷ 5 = 4.704

   Average = 4.704

3. **(B)**

$$\begin{array}{r} 512.69\frac{59}{89} \\ .89\overline{)456.30.00} \\ \underline{445} \\ 113 \\ \underline{89} \\ 240 \\ \underline{178} \\ 620 \\ \underline{534} \\ 860 \\ \underline{801} \\ 59 \text{ remainder} \end{array}$$

$512.69\frac{59}{89}$ rounds off to 512.70.

4. **(A)**

	5 hours 13 minutes
	3 hours 49 minutes
+	24 minutes
	8 hours 86 minutes

   Since there are 60 minutes in one hour, then 86 minutes = 60 minutes + 26 minutes or 1 hour and 26 minutes.

   So, 8 hours and 86 minutes = 9 hours and 26 minutes.

5. **(D)** $\frac{18}{47} \times \frac{126}{x}$

   $18x = 47(126)$ cross-multiply

   $18x = 5922$

   $x = 329$ divide by 18

6. **(D)** $0.3125 = \frac{3125}{1,000} = \frac{5}{16}$

7. **(A)** $\frac{7}{8} \div \frac{7}{8}$

   $= \frac{7}{8} \times \frac{8}{7}$ invert the second term and multiply

   = 1

8. **(C)** 5, 8, 13, 20. To each number, add the next odd number to determine the next number in the series.

Series		*Odd Number*	
5	+	3	= 8
8	+	5	= 13
13	+	7	= 20
20	+	9	= 29

   29 will be the next number.

9. **(A)** *Interest = Principal × Rate × Time*

   $= \$300 \times 0.06 \times \frac{10}{360}$

   $= \frac{\$180}{360} = \frac{\$1}{2}$

   = $.50

10. **(B)** First, find the number of $1\frac{1}{2}$ inch units there are in five inches. Do this by dividing:

   $5 \div 1\frac{1}{2}$

   $= 5 \div \frac{3}{2}$ (change $1\frac{1}{2}$ to $\frac{3}{2}$)

   $= 5 \times \frac{2}{3}$ (invert and multiply)

   $= \frac{10}{3}$

   Now find the total miles by multiplying:

   $500 \times \frac{10}{3} = 1666.67$

   Five inches represents approximately 1700 miles.

11. **(C)** $\frac{1}{2}\% = 0.5\%$ or $\frac{0.5}{100} = 0.005$

12. **(D)** \$260 is 20% of the bonus. Write this in equation form. Let the bonus be x.

$\$260 = .20x$

$\frac{260}{.20} = \frac{.20\,x}{.20}$ divided by 0.20

$\$1{,}300 = x$

Her entire bonus was \$1,300.

13. **(A)** 1 kilogram = 35 ounces

Find how many grams there are in 1 ounce.

Note: 1 kilogram = 1000 grams

1000 grams = 35 ounces

$1 \text{ ounce} \times \frac{1000 \text{ grams}}{35 \text{ ounces}}$

$= \frac{1000 \text{ grams}}{35}$

= 28.6 or 29 grams in one ounce

14. **(B)** To find the amount of time it takes to deliver the 90 milligrams at a rate of 24 milligrams per hour, divide

Amount of Time = 90 milligrams ÷ 24 milligrams per hour = 3.75 hours

3.75 hours = $3\frac{3}{4}$ hours = 3 hours and 45 minutes

15. **(A)** First, find the number of seconds there are in one-half minute:

$\frac{1}{2} \times 60$ sec/min = 30 seconds

Since sound travels 1,100 feet per second, it will travel:

30 sec. × 1,100 ft. = 33,000 ft.

Change the 33,000 feet to miles (1 mile = 5,280 feet).

$33{,}000 \text{ feet} \times \frac{1 \text{ mile}}{5280 \text{ feet}}$

= 6.25

Round off: 6.25 miles = about 6 miles

16. **(B)** 1 kilometer = $\frac{5}{8}$ mile

x kilometers = 2 miles

$\frac{1 \text{ kilometer}}{\frac{5}{8} \text{ mile}} = \frac{x}{2}$

$\frac{5}{8}x = 2$

$5x = 16$

$x = 3.2$

Two miles = about 3.2 kilometers

17. **(C)** Perimeter of a rectangle (the hall is shaped like a rectangle) is:

Perimeter = 2 *length* + 2 *width*

= 2(75) + 2(25)

= 150 + 50

= 200 feet

The perimeter is 200 feet.

Now change 200 feet to yards (3 feet = 1 yard).

$200 \text{ feet} \times \frac{1 \text{ yard}}{3 \text{ feet}} = 66\frac{2}{3}$ yards

18. **(D)** Let the price of a blouse be x. Then:

$x - 16\frac{2}{3}\%x = 35$

$\frac{2}{3} = 0.67$, so 16.6770% = 0.1667

$x - 0.1667x = \$35$ change the percent to a decimal

$0.8333x = \$35$ combine like terms

$x = \$42$ divide by 0.8333

List price was \$42.

19. **(A)** To find the number of decimal places in the product of two numbers, find the sum of the number of digits to the right of the decimal of each number.

0.4266 has 4 digits to the right.

0.3333 has 4 digits to the right.

There should be 8 digits in the product.

20. **(C)** 5.5 thousand × \$50 thousand = \$275

21. **(A)**

$$
\begin{array}{r}
1100. \\
.52.\overline{)572.00.} \\
\underline{52} \\
52 \\
\underline{52} \\
00 \\
\underline{00}
\end{array}
$$

Answer: 1100

22. **(C)** 200 percent of 800

   $2.00 \times 800 = 1600$

23. **(A)** The total games played was 15. To find their average, divide games won by total played:

   $10 \div 15 = 0.667$

   Their average is 0.667.

24. **(D)** To find the soil needed, first change the 8 inches to feet, so all units will be the same.

   $8 \text{ inches} \times \frac{1 \text{ foot}}{12 \text{ inches}} = 0.67 \text{ feet}$

   Now multiply all units.

   $3 \text{ feet} \times 0.67 \text{ feet} \times 1 \text{ foot} = 2 \text{ cubic feet}$

   2 cubic feet of soil will be needed to fill the box.

25. **(A)** Find the price for one watch by dividing:

   $1,250 (per hundred) ÷ 100 = $12.50 (price of one watch)

   To find the cost of 228, multiply the number of watches by the price per watch.

   228 watches × $12.50 per watch = $2,850

   The cost of the watches will be $2,850.

26. **(A)** Find the area of the small rectangle and subtract its area from the large rectangle to determine the shaded area.

   Large rectangle

   A = *length* × *width*

   = 6 × 15

   = 90 square inches

   Small rectangle

   A = length × width

   = 4 × 9

   = 36 square inches

   90 – 36 = 54 square inches

   The area of the shaded area is 54 square inches.

27. **(D)**

From	*To*
March 15, 1979	March 15, 1988
March 15, 1988	Jan. 15, 1989
Jan. 15, 1989	Feb. 12, 1989

Time

9 years

10 months

27 days

His age will be 9 years, 10 months, 27 days.

28. **(A)** On the chart, each line represents ten units. The highest IQ is about halfway on the first line, which is half of ten.

   So the answer is five.

29. **(C)** Locate IQ on base and trace to horizontal intersection.

30. **(C)** There are 100 students with an IQ of 80. Looking across the chart we see that there are also 100 students with an IQ of 110.

31. **(A)** Highest point on the graph, an IQ of 100.

MATHEMATICS—QUANTITATIVE COMPARISONS ANSWER SHEET

TEST 5: QUANTITATIVE COMPARISONS

1. Ⓐ Ⓑ Ⓒ Ⓓ	8. Ⓐ Ⓑ Ⓒ Ⓓ	15. Ⓐ Ⓑ Ⓒ Ⓓ	22. Ⓐ Ⓑ Ⓒ Ⓓ
2. Ⓐ Ⓑ Ⓒ Ⓓ	9. Ⓐ Ⓑ Ⓒ Ⓓ	16. Ⓐ Ⓑ Ⓒ Ⓓ	23. Ⓐ Ⓑ Ⓒ Ⓓ
3. Ⓐ Ⓑ Ⓒ Ⓓ	10. Ⓐ Ⓑ Ⓒ Ⓓ	17. Ⓐ Ⓑ Ⓒ Ⓓ	24. Ⓐ Ⓑ Ⓒ Ⓓ
4. Ⓐ Ⓑ Ⓒ Ⓓ	11. Ⓐ Ⓑ Ⓒ Ⓓ	18. Ⓐ Ⓑ Ⓒ Ⓓ	25. Ⓐ Ⓑ Ⓒ Ⓓ
5. Ⓐ Ⓑ Ⓒ Ⓓ	12. Ⓐ Ⓑ Ⓒ Ⓓ	19. Ⓐ Ⓑ Ⓒ Ⓓ	26. Ⓐ Ⓑ Ⓒ Ⓓ
6. Ⓐ Ⓑ Ⓒ Ⓓ	13. Ⓐ Ⓑ Ⓒ Ⓓ	20. Ⓐ Ⓑ Ⓒ Ⓓ	27. Ⓐ Ⓑ Ⓒ Ⓓ
7. Ⓐ Ⓑ Ⓒ Ⓓ	14. Ⓐ Ⓑ Ⓒ Ⓓ	21. Ⓐ Ⓑ Ⓒ Ⓓ	28. Ⓐ Ⓑ Ⓒ Ⓓ

TEST 6: MATHEMATICS

1. Ⓐ Ⓑ Ⓒ Ⓓ	7. Ⓐ Ⓑ Ⓒ Ⓓ
2. Ⓐ Ⓑ Ⓒ Ⓓ	8. Ⓐ Ⓑ Ⓒ Ⓓ
3. Ⓐ Ⓑ Ⓒ Ⓓ	9. Ⓐ Ⓑ Ⓒ Ⓓ
4. Ⓐ Ⓑ Ⓒ Ⓓ	10. Ⓐ Ⓑ Ⓒ Ⓓ
5. Ⓐ Ⓑ Ⓒ Ⓓ	11. Ⓐ Ⓑ Ⓒ Ⓓ
6. Ⓐ Ⓑ Ⓒ Ⓓ	12. Ⓐ Ⓑ Ⓒ Ⓓ

TEST 5: QUANTITATIVE COMPARISONS

28 QUESTIONS • TIME—35 MINUTES

Common Information: In each question, information concerning one or both of the quantities to be compared is given in the ITEM column. A symbol that appears in any column represents the same thing in Column A as it does in Column B.

Figures: Assume that the position of points, angles, regions, and so forth, are in the order shown; that the lines shown as straight are indeed straight; that figures lie in a plane unless otherwise indicated. Figures accompanying questions are intended to provide information you can use in answering the questions. However, unless a note states that a figure is drawn to scale, you should solve the problems by using your knowledge of mathematics, NOT by estimating sizes by sight or by measurement.

Directions: For each of the following questions, two quantities are given: one in Column A and one in Column B. Compare the two quantities and mark your answer sheet with the correct, lettered conclusion. These are your options:

A: the quantity in Column A is the greater;

B: the quantity in Column B is the greater;

C: the two quantities are equal;

D: the relationship cannot be determined from the information given.

	Item	Column A	Column B
1.	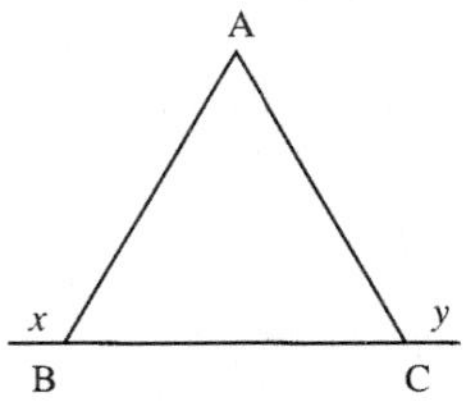 Isosceles ΔABC ∠CAB = ∠ACB	∠x	∠y
2.	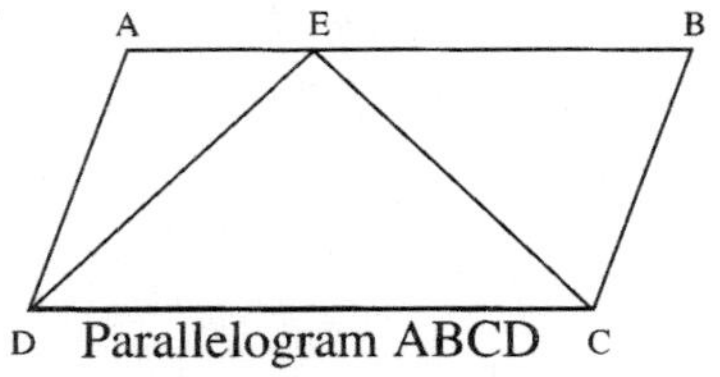 Parallelogram ABCD E is a point on AB	Area of ΔDEC	Area of ΔAED + Area of ΔEBC

Item	Column A	Column B
3. $x = -1$	$x^3 + x^2 - x + 1$	$x^3 - x^2 + x - 1$
4.	The edge of a cube whose volume is 27.	The edge of a cube whose total surface area is 54.
5.	$\frac{\frac{1}{2} + \frac{1}{3}}{\frac{2}{3}}$	$\frac{\frac{2}{3}}{\frac{1}{2} + \frac{1}{3}}$
6. x is a given number.	Area of a circle radius $= x^3$	Area of a circle radius $= 3x$
7.	$\frac{1}{4} - 2$	4^2
8.	0.02	$\sqrt{0.02}$
9. 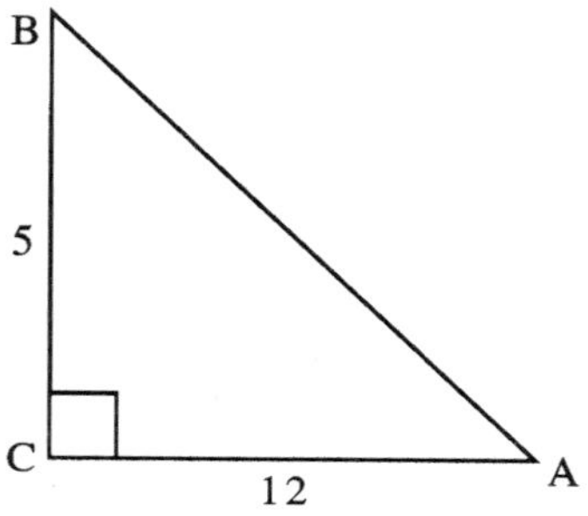 Right ΔABC	$(AB)^2$	$(AC)^2 + 5(CB)$
10.	Area of circle with radius 7.	Area of equilateral triangle with side 14.
11. 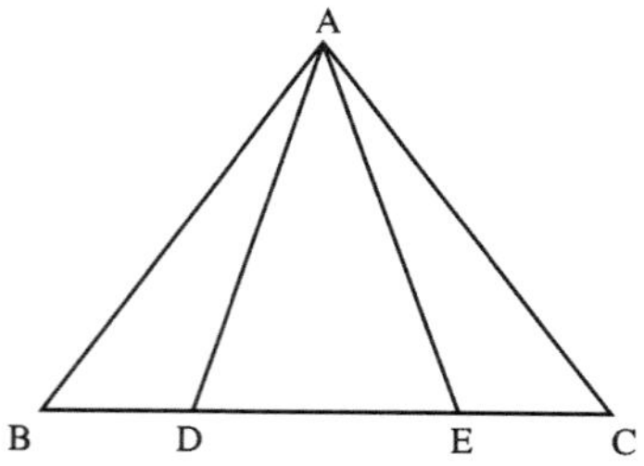 $\angle ADE > \angle AED$	$\angle B$	$\angle C$

Item	Column A	Column B

12.

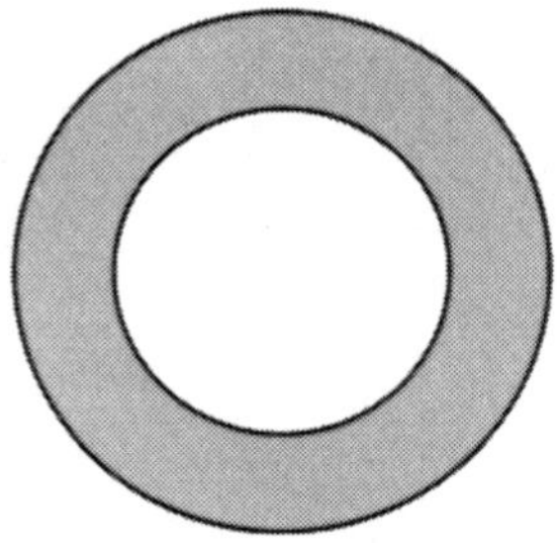

Radius of large circle = 10
Radius of small circle = 7

Area of shaded portion. · Area of small circle.

13.m ‖ n ‖ o ‖ p and q ‖ r

$\angle x$ · $\angle y$

14. $a < 0 < b$ · a^2 · $\frac{b}{2}$

15. $t < 0 < r$ · t^2 · r

Diagram for problems 16–20

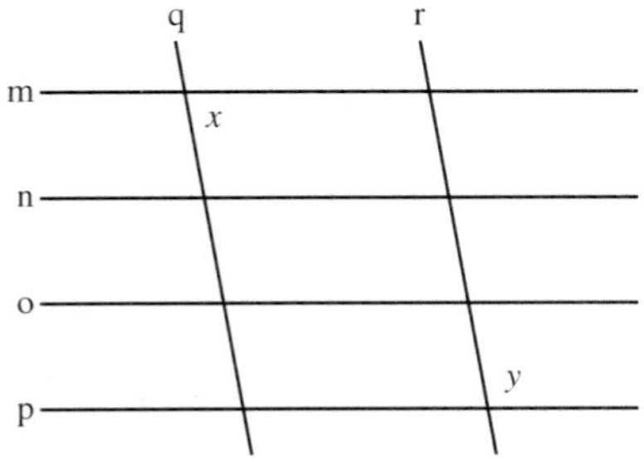

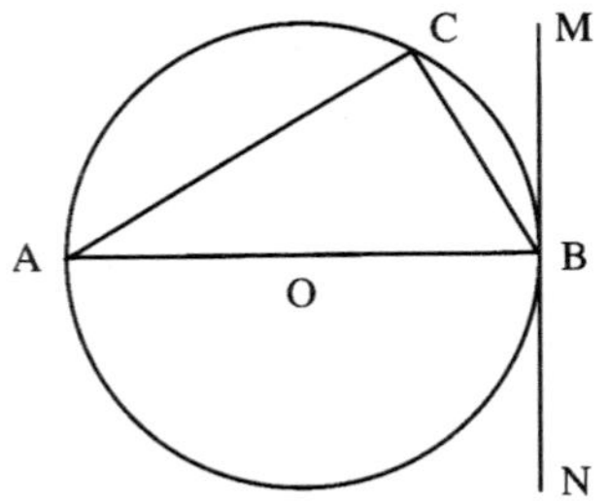

MN tangent to circle O at point B and $\angle A = 30°$

16. · m $\angle ACB$ · m $\angle NBO$

17. · $\overset{\frown}{CB}$ · $\overset{\frown}{AC}$

18. · m $\angle CBM$ · m $\angle CAB$

19. · m $\angle CBA$ · m $\angle CBM$

20. · $\overline{AO} + \overline{AC}$ · $\overline{BO} + \overline{BC}$

Item	Column A	Column B

Diagram for problems 21–25

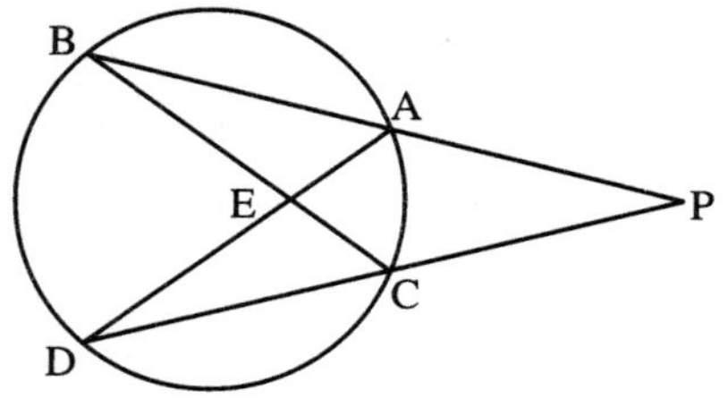

$\overline{AB}$ + $\overline{CD}$

$\widehat{BD} = 160°$

$\widehat{AC} = 40°$

Item	Column A	Column B
21.	m ∠APC	m ∠ABC
22.	m ∠BED	m ∠BEA
23.	m ∠BAD	m ∠DCB
24.	m ∠BCP	m ∠AEC + m ∠ADC
25.	$\widehat{DC}$ + $\widehat{AC}$	$\widehat{BD}$
26.	75% of $\frac{3}{4}$	0.09 × 6
27.	4% of 0.003	3% of 0.004
28.	∠BCA	∠FEG

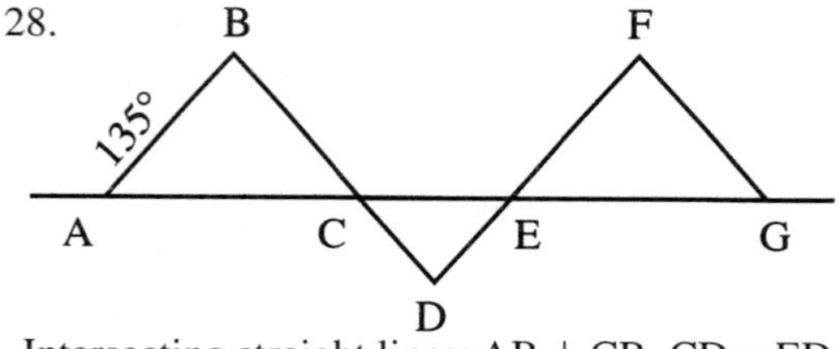

Intersecting straight lines; AB ⊥ CB, CD = ED

TEST 5: QUANTITATIVE COMPARISONS ANSWER KEY

1. **D**
2. **C**
3. **A**
4. **C**
5. **A**
6. **D**
7. **C**
8. **C**
9. **C**
10. **A**
11. **D**
12. **A**
13. **D**
14. **D**
15. **D**
16. **C**
17. **B**
18. **C**
19. **A**
20. **A**
21. **A**
22. **A**
23. **C**
24. **B**
25. **B**
26. **A**
27. **C**
28. **C**

TEST 5: QUANTITATIVE COMPARISONS EXPLANATORY ANSWERS

1. **(D)** The value of $\angle x$ or $\angle y$ cannot be determined unless the measure of at least one angle is known.

2. **(C)** Area of Δ DEC = $\frac{1}{2}$ *base* × *height*

   Area of parallelogram = *base* × *height*

   Area of Δ ADE + Δ EBC = area of the whole parallelogram − Δ DEC = *base* × *height* − $\frac{1}{2}$ *base* × *height* = $\frac{1}{2}$ *base* × *height*

3. **(A)** $x^3 + x^2 - x + 1 = (-1)^3 + (-1)^2 - (-1) + 1$

   $= -1 + 1 + 1 + 1$

   $= 2$

   $x^3 - x^2 + x - 1 = (-1)^3 - (-1)^2 + (-1) - 1$

   $= -1 - 1 - 1 - 1$

   $= -4$

4. **(C)** A cube has six surfaces, each one's area e^2

   $e^3 = 27$

   $e = 3$

   $6e^2 = 54$

   $e^2 = 9$

   $e = 3$

5. **(A)** $\dfrac{\frac{1}{2} + \frac{1}{3}}{\frac{2}{3}} = \dfrac{3 + \frac{2}{6}}{\frac{2}{3}}$

   $= \dfrac{\frac{5}{6}}{\frac{2}{3}}$

   $= \dfrac{\frac{15}{12}}{1}$

   $= \dfrac{15}{12}$

   $\dfrac{\frac{2}{3}}{\frac{1}{2} + \frac{1}{3}} = \dfrac{\frac{2}{3}}{3 + \frac{2}{6}}$

   $= \dfrac{\frac{2}{3}}{\frac{5}{6}}$

   $= \dfrac{\frac{12}{15}}{1}$

   multiply numerator and denominator by $\frac{6}{5}$

   $= \dfrac{12}{15}$

   $\dfrac{15}{12} > \dfrac{12}{15}$

6. **(D)** Area of circle $x^3 = (x^3)^2$

   $= x^6$

   Area of circle radius $3x = (3x)^2$

   $= 9x^2$

   We cannot know whether x^6 or $9x^2$ is larger unless we know the value of x.

7. **(C)** $(\frac{1}{4})^{-2} = \dfrac{1}{(\frac{1}{4})^2}$ $4^2 = 16$

   $= \dfrac{1}{\frac{1}{16}}$

   $= 16$

8. **(B)** $0.02 = \sqrt{0.0004}$

   $\sqrt{0.02} > \sqrt{0.0004}$

9. **(C)** By the Pythagorean theorem, $(AB)^2 = (AC)^2 + (BC)^2$

   However, $(BC)^2 = 5^2 = 25$ and $5CB = 5 \bullet 5 = 25$

   Therefore, $(BC)^2 = 5CB$

   $(AB)^2 = (AC)^2 + 5CB$ (Substituting 5CB for $(BC)^2$ in the Pythagorean theorem)

10. **(A)** Area of circle radius 7 = $r^2 = (7)^2 = 49$

    Area of equilateral Δ with side of 14:

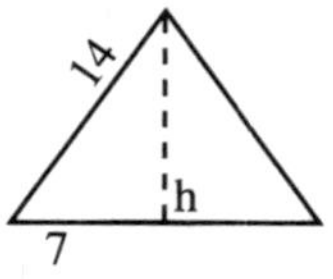

A line from one vertex to the mid-point of the opposite side is perpendicular to the opposite side. It is, therefore, the height of the triangle.

Let the length of this line be h. Then, by the Pythagorean theorem, $7^2 + h^2 = 14^2$.

$h^2 = 14^2 - 7^2 = 14$

$h^2 = 3 \times 7 \times 7$

$h = 7\sqrt{3}$

Area of $\Delta = \frac{1}{2}\, base \times height$

$= \frac{1}{2}(14)\,(7\sqrt{3})$

Area of $\Delta = (7)7\sqrt{3}$

$= 49\sqrt{3}$

Is 49 bigger than 49 $\sqrt{3}$?

= 3.14

Therefore, $> \sqrt{3}$

Therefore, 49 $> 49\sqrt{3}$ and A > B

11. **(D)** Not enough information is given to determine the values of the angles.

12. **(A)** (Area of shaded portion) = (Area of larger circle) – (Area of smaller circle)

$= (10^2) - (7^2)$

$= 100 - 49$

$= 51$

(Area of smaller circle) = r^2

$= (7^2)$

$= 49$

$51 > 49$

13. **(D)**

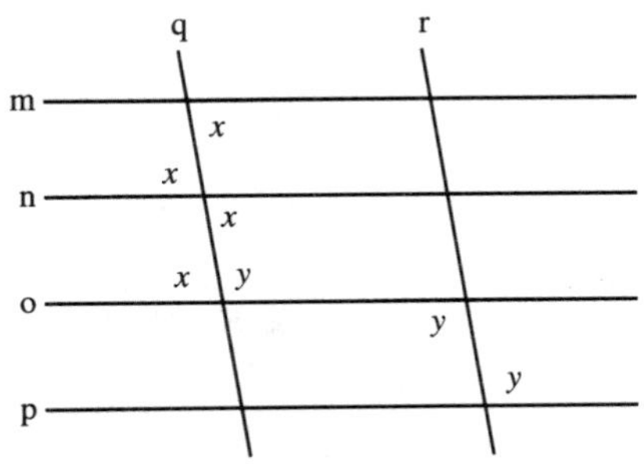

All that can be determined is that x and y are supplementary.

14. **(D)** There is insufficient information to determine an answer.

15. **(D)** There is insufficient information to determine an answer.

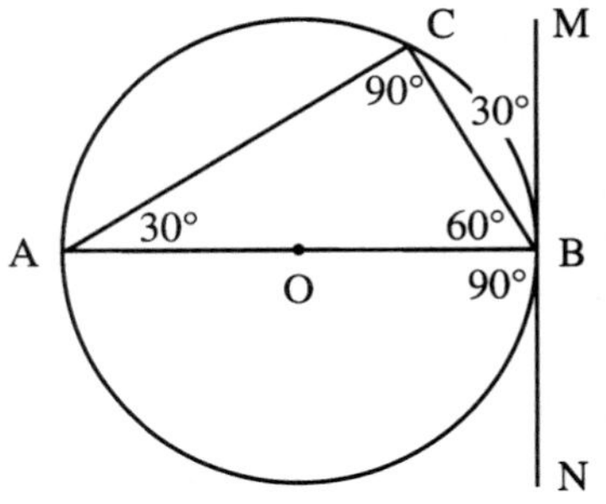

16. **(C)** m $\angle$ACB = 90° m $\angle$NBO = 90°

A tangent to a circle is perpendicular to the radius of the circle at their point of contact. An inscribed angle is equal to one-half its intercepted arc. Therefore m $\angle$ACB = 90°.

17. **(B)** $\overset{\frown}{AC}$ = 120° $\overset{\frown}{CB}$ = 60°

An inscribed angle is equal to one-half its intercepted arc.

18. **(C)** m $\angle$CBM = 30° m $\angle$CAB = 30°

19. **(A)** m $\angle$CBA = 60° m $\angle$CBM = 30°

20. **(A)** $\overline{AO}$ = $\overline{BO}$ all radii in the same circle are equal.

$\overline{AC} > \overline{BC}$ in a triangle the greater side lies opposite the greater angle

$\overline{AO} + \overline{AC} > \overline{BO} + \overline{BC}$

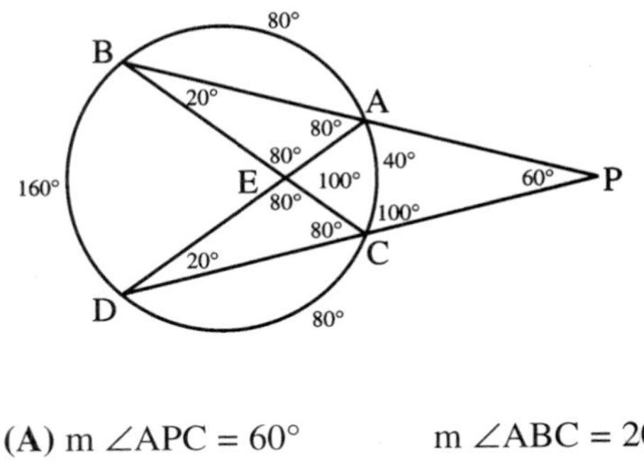

21. **(A)** m $\angle$APC = 60° m $\angle$ABC = 20°

22. **(A)** m $\angle$BED = 100° m $\angle$BEA = 80°

23. **(C)** m $\angle$BAD = 80° m $\angle$DCB = 80°

24. **(B)** m $\angle BCP = 100°$

m $\angle AEC$ + m $\angle ADC = 100° + 20°$

$= 120°$

25. **(B)** $\overset{\frown}{DC} + \overset{\frown}{AC} = 80° + 40° = 120°$

$\overset{\frown}{BD} = 160°$

26. **(A)** 75% of $\frac{3}{4} = .75 \times .75$ $\quad .09 \times 6 = .54$

$= .5625$

27. **(C)** 4% of $0.003 = 0.04 \times .003$

$= 0.00012$

3% of $0.004 = 0.03 \times 0.004$

$= 0.00012$

28. **(C)**

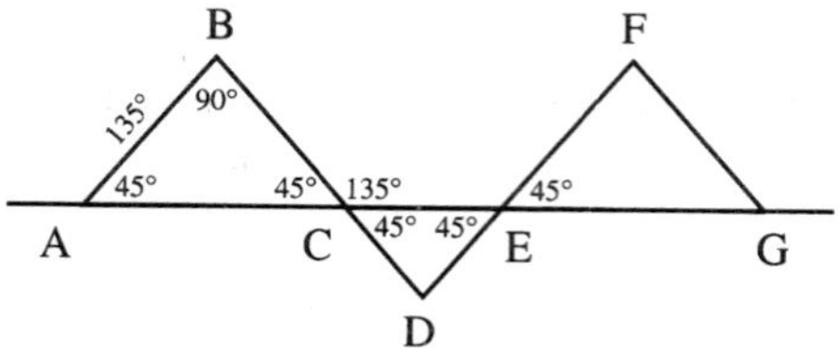

$\angle BCA = 45°$ $\qquad \angle FEG = 45°$

TEST 6: QUANTITATIVE COMPARISONS

12 QUESTIONS • TIME—15 MINUTES

Common Information: In each question, information concerning one or both of the quantities to be compared is given in the ITEM column. A symbol that appears in any column represents the same thing in Column A as it does in Column B.

Figures: Assume that the position of points, angles, regions, and so forth, are in the order shown; that the lines shown as straight are indeed straight; that figures lie in a plane unless otherwise indicated. Figures accompanying questions are intended to provide information you can use in answering the questions. However, unless a note states that a figure is drawn to scale, you should solve the problems by using your knowledge of mathematics, and NOT by estimating sizes by sight or by measurement.

Directions: For each of the following questions, two quantities are given: one in Column A and one in Column B. Compare the two quantities and mark your answer sheet with the correct lettered conclusion. These are your options:

A: the quantity in Column A is the greater;

B: the quantity in Column B is the greater;

C: the two quantities are equal;

D: the relationship cannot be determined from the information given.

	Item	Column A	Column B
1.	$a > 0; x > 0$	$a + x$	$a - x$
2.		The average of: 17, 19, 21, 23, 25	The average of: 16, 18, 20, 22, 24
3.	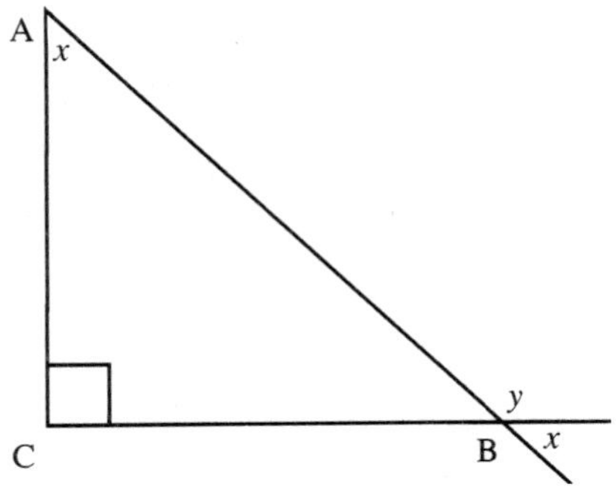	$2x$	y
4.	$0 < a < 12; 0 < b < 12$	a	b
5.	$4a - 4b = 20$	a	b

Item	Column A	Column B
6.	angle A	angle B

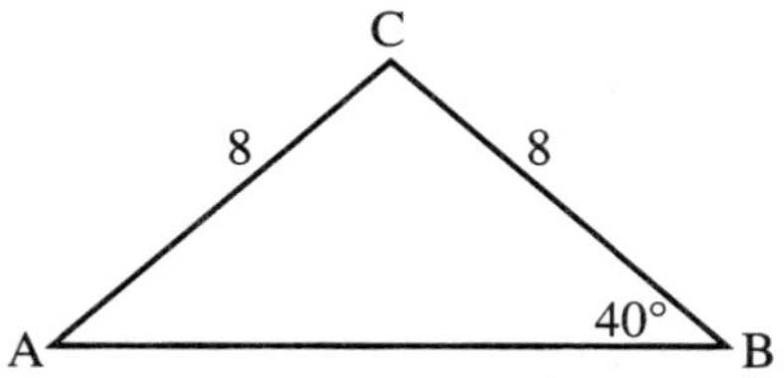

Item	Column A	Column B
7. $\frac{a}{9} = b^2$	a	b
8.	a	b

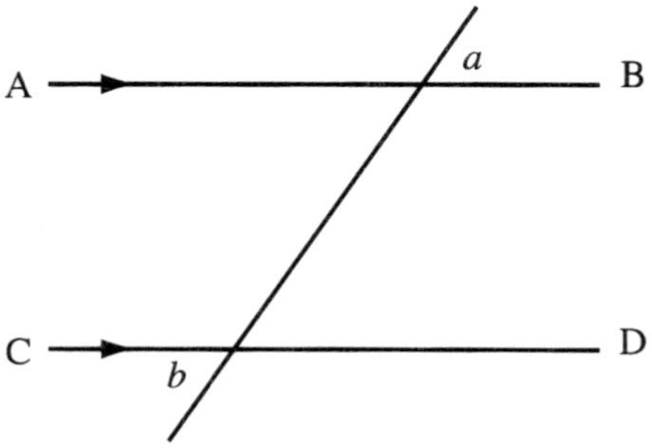

AB || CD

Item	Column A	Column B
9.	$3 + 24(3 - 2)$	$27 + 5(0)(5)$
10.	AM	BM

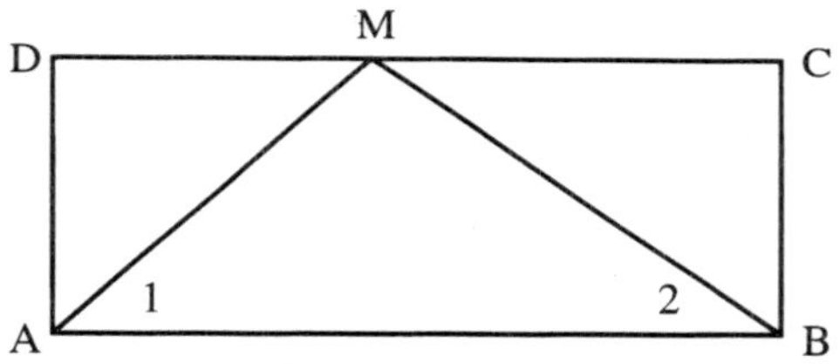

$\angle 1 > \angle 2$

Item	Column A	Column B
11.	angle A + angle B	angle ACD

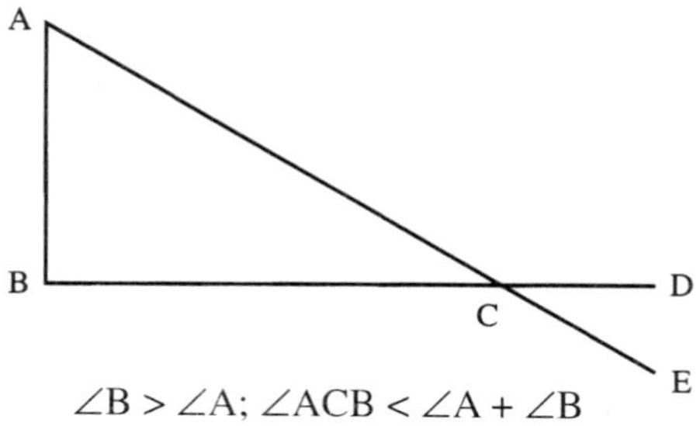

$\angle B > \angle A$; $\angle ACB < \angle A + \angle B$

Item	Column A	Column B
12.	$(\frac{2}{3})^2(3)^3$	$(3)^2(\frac{2}{3})^3$

TEST 6: QUANTITATIVE COMPARISONS ANSWER KEY

1. **A**	7. **D**
2. **A**	8. **C**
3. **B**	9. **C**
4. **D**	10. **B**
5. **A**	11. **C**
6. **C**	12. **A**

TEST 6: QUANTITATIVE COMPARISONS EXPLANATORY ANSWERS

1. **(A)** The statement $a > 0$ and $x > 0$ implies both a and x are positive. The sum of two positive numbers is always greater than their difference.
2. **(A)** The averages of Column A and Column B are 21 and 20 respectively.
3. **(B)** Angle ABC = x (vertical angles are equal). Since $\angle C = 90°$, $\angle A + \angle ABC = 90°$ (180° in a triangle). Therefore, $2x = 90°$, and $x = 45°$. Angle ABC and $\angle y$ are supplementary; hence $y = 135°$. Therefore, $y > 2x$.
4. **(D)** Impossible to determine because a could be any number between 0 and 12 and b any number between 0 and 10.
5. **(A)** $4a - 4b = 20$

   $a - b = 5$

   $a - 5 = b$

   For all values of a and b, $a > b$.
6. **(C)** Angles opposite equal sides of a triangle are equal.
7. **(D)** Impossible to determine because b could be positive or negative.
8. **(C)** If two parallel lines are cut by a transversal, the alternate exterior angles are equal.
9. **(C)** Column A and Column B both equal 27.
10. **(B)** The greater side lies opposite the greater angle.
11. **(C)** The exterior angle of a triangle is equal to the two interior nonadjacent angles.
12. **(A)** The value of Column A is 12 and the value of Column B is $2\frac{2}{3}$. Therefore, A > B.

FINAL MATHEMATICS EXAMINATION ANSWER SHEET

Part 1: General Mathematics

1. Ⓐ Ⓑ Ⓒ Ⓓ	12. Ⓐ Ⓑ Ⓒ Ⓓ	23. Ⓐ Ⓑ Ⓒ Ⓓ	34. Ⓐ Ⓑ Ⓒ Ⓓ
2. Ⓐ Ⓑ Ⓒ Ⓓ	13. Ⓐ Ⓑ Ⓒ Ⓓ	24. Ⓐ Ⓑ Ⓒ Ⓓ	35. Ⓐ Ⓑ Ⓒ Ⓓ
3. Ⓐ Ⓑ Ⓒ Ⓓ	14. Ⓐ Ⓑ Ⓒ Ⓓ	25. Ⓐ Ⓑ Ⓒ Ⓓ	36. Ⓐ Ⓑ Ⓒ Ⓓ
4. Ⓐ Ⓑ Ⓒ Ⓓ	15. Ⓐ Ⓑ Ⓒ Ⓓ	26. Ⓐ Ⓑ Ⓒ Ⓓ	37. Ⓐ Ⓑ Ⓒ Ⓓ
5. Ⓐ Ⓑ Ⓒ Ⓓ	16. Ⓐ Ⓑ Ⓒ Ⓓ	27. Ⓐ Ⓑ Ⓒ Ⓓ	38. Ⓐ Ⓑ Ⓒ Ⓓ
6. Ⓐ Ⓑ Ⓒ Ⓓ	17. Ⓐ Ⓑ Ⓒ Ⓓ	28. Ⓐ Ⓑ Ⓒ Ⓓ	39. Ⓐ Ⓑ Ⓒ Ⓓ
7. Ⓐ Ⓑ Ⓒ Ⓓ	18. Ⓐ Ⓑ Ⓒ Ⓓ	29. Ⓐ Ⓑ Ⓒ Ⓓ	40. Ⓐ Ⓑ Ⓒ Ⓓ
8. Ⓐ Ⓑ Ⓒ Ⓓ	19. Ⓐ Ⓑ Ⓒ Ⓓ	30. Ⓐ Ⓑ Ⓒ Ⓓ	41. Ⓐ Ⓑ Ⓒ Ⓓ
9. Ⓐ Ⓑ Ⓒ Ⓓ	20. Ⓐ Ⓑ Ⓒ Ⓓ	31. Ⓐ Ⓑ Ⓒ Ⓓ	42. Ⓐ Ⓑ Ⓒ Ⓓ
10. Ⓐ Ⓑ Ⓒ Ⓓ	21. Ⓐ Ⓑ Ⓒ Ⓓ	32. Ⓐ Ⓑ Ⓒ Ⓓ	
11. Ⓐ Ⓑ Ⓒ Ⓓ	22. Ⓐ Ⓑ Ⓒ Ⓓ	33. Ⓐ Ⓑ Ⓒ Ⓓ	

Part 2: Quantitative Comparisons

1. Ⓐ Ⓑ Ⓒ Ⓓ	7. Ⓐ Ⓑ Ⓒ Ⓓ
2. Ⓐ Ⓑ Ⓒ Ⓓ	8. Ⓐ Ⓑ Ⓒ Ⓓ
3. Ⓐ Ⓑ Ⓒ Ⓓ	9. Ⓐ Ⓑ Ⓒ Ⓓ
4. Ⓐ Ⓑ Ⓒ Ⓓ	10. Ⓐ Ⓑ Ⓒ Ⓓ
5. Ⓐ Ⓑ Ⓒ Ⓓ	11. Ⓐ Ⓑ Ⓒ Ⓓ
6. Ⓐ Ⓑ Ⓒ Ⓓ	12. Ⓐ Ⓑ Ⓒ Ⓓ

FINAL MATHEMATICS EXAMINATION

54 QUESTIONS • TIME—60 MINUTES

PART 1: GENERAL MATHEMATICS

42 QUESTIONS • TIME—40 MINUTES

1. Jane Doe borrowed $225,000 for five years at $13\frac{1}{2}$ percent. The annual interest charge was

   (A) $1,667
   (B) $6,000
   (C) $30,375
   (D) $39,375

2. A junior salesman gets a commission of 14 percent on his sales. If he wants his commission to amount to $140, he will have to sell merchandise totaling

   (A) $1,960
   (B) $10
   (C) $1,000
   (D) $100

3. On a list price of $200, the difference between a single discount of 25 percent and successive discounts of 20 percent and 5 percent is

   (A) $0
   (B) $48
   (C) $8
   (D) $2

4. A worked five days on overhauling an old car. B worked four days more to finish the job. After the sale of the car, the net profit was $243. They wanted to divide the profit on the basis of the time spent by each. A's share of the profit was

   (A) $108
   (B) $135
   (C) $127
   (D) $143

5. If cloth costs $42\frac{1}{2}$ cents per yard, how many yards can be purchased for $76.50?

   (A) 220
   (B) 180
   (C) 190
   (D) 230

6. A fashionable dress shop offers a 20 percent discount on selected items. For a dress marked at $280, what is the discount price?

   (A) $224.00
   (B) $232.00
   (C) $248.00
   (D) $261.00

7. If A takes six days to do a task and B takes three days to do the same task, working together they should do the same task in

   (A) $2\frac{2}{3}$ days
   (B) 2 days
   (C) $2\frac{1}{3}$ days
   (D) $2\frac{1}{2}$ days

8. The area of a mirror 40 inches long and 20 inches wide is approximately

   (A) 8.5 square feet
   (B) 5.5 square feet
   (C) 8.0 square feet
   (D) 2.5 square feet

9. $\frac{2}{3}$ plus $\frac{1}{8}$ equals

   (A) $\frac{37}{72}$
   (B) $\frac{82}{72}$
   (C) $\frac{3}{11}$
   (D) $\frac{19}{24}$

10. A student has received two grades of 90 and two grades of 80 in an English course. Assuming the grades are weighed equally, what is the student's average for the course?

    (A) 90
    (B) 87
    (C) 85
    (D) 84

11. If a man has only quarters and dimes totaling \$2.00, the number of quarters *cannot* be

(A) 2
(B) 4
(C) 6
(D) 3

12. The number that increased by one-sixth of itself yields 182 is

(A) 156
(B) 176
(C) 148
(D) 160

13. $0.16\frac{3}{4}$ written as a percent is

(A) $16\frac{3}{4}$ percent
(B) $16.\frac{3}{4}$ percent
(C) $0.016\frac{3}{4}$ percent
(D) $0.0016\frac{3}{4}$ percent

14. If 4 ounces of protein provide 448 calories, how much protein is needed to provide 392 calories?

(A) 2.8 ounces
(B) 3.5 ounces
(C) 4.57 ounces
(D) 56 ounces

15. \$1,296.53 minus \$264.87 is

(A) \$1,232.76
(B) \$1,032.76
(C) \$1,031.66
(D) \$1,132.53

16. $12\frac{1}{2}$ minus $6\frac{1}{4}$ is

(A) $5\frac{3}{4}$
(B) $6\frac{1}{4}$
(C) $6\frac{1}{2}$
(D) $5\frac{1}{2}$

17. Men's handkerchiefs cost \$1.29 for three. The cost per dozen handkerchiefs is

(A) \$7.74
(B) \$3.87
(C) \$14.48
(D) \$5.16

18. Add: $\frac{1}{4}, \frac{7}{12}, \frac{3}{8}, \frac{1}{2}, \frac{5}{6}$

(A) $2\frac{1}{2}$
(B) $2\frac{13}{24}$
(C) $2\frac{3}{4}$
(D) $2\frac{15}{24}$

19. A floor is 25 feet wide by 36 feet long. To cover this floor with carpet will require

(A) 100 square yards
(B) 300 square yards
(C) 900 square yards
(D) 25 square yards

20. 72 divided by 0.0009 is

(A) 0.125
(B) 800
(C) 80,000
(D) 80

21. 345 safety pins at \$4.15 per hundred will cost

(A) \$0.1432
(B) \$1.4320
(C) \$14.32
(D) \$143.20

22. The number that decreased by one-fifth of itself yields 132 is

(A) 165
(B) 198
(C) 98
(D) 88

23. 285 is 5 percent of

(A) 1,700
(B) 7,350
(C) 1,750
(D) 5,700

24. A store sold jackets for \$65 each. The jackets cost the store \$50 each. The percentage of increase of selling price over cost is

(A) 40 percent
(B) $33\frac{1}{2}$ percent
(C) $33\frac{1}{3}$ percent
(D) 30 percent

25. The denominator of a fraction is 20 more than the numerator. What is the numerator if the fraction is equivalent to $\frac{3}{5}$.

    (A) 12
    (B) 30
    (C) –50
    (D) 10

26. Which statement below is true about the inequality of $2 < x \quad 7$

    (A) $x < 2$
    (B) $x = 2$
    (C) x is greater than 7
    (D) $x > 2$

27. $\frac{x}{5} - 4 = 11$. Find the value of x.

    (A) 75
    (B) 3
    (C) 35
    (D) 59

28. A punch recipe for a half gallon (64 ounces) of punch requires one pint (16 ounces) of grape juice. How many quarts (1 quart = 32 ounces) of grape juice are required for $2\frac{1}{2}$ gallons of the punch.

    (A) 5 quarts
    (B) 10 quarts
    (C) $1\frac{1}{4}$ quarts
    (D) $2\frac{1}{2}$ quarts

29. Mrs. Bowler got up at 7:00 A.M. last Wednesday morning and went to bed at 11:00 P.M. Wednesday night. During the time that she was up, she spent $\frac{1}{2}$ her time at work, $\frac{1}{8}$ her time bowling with friends, and $\frac{1}{4}$ her time with her family. How much time did she have left for other activities?

    (A) 2 hours
    (B) 4 hours
    (C) 1 hour
    (D) 8 hours

30. If 24 percent of the students who enrolled in an algebra class of 50 students dropped the course before the semester ended, how many students remained in the class?

    (A) 27
    (B) 76
    (C) 12
    (D) 38

31. How many $\frac{3}{4}$ gram tablets are needed for a dosage of $4\frac{1}{2}$ grams?

    (A) 3.75
    (B) 1.5
    (C) 6
    (D) 3

32. $3.6 - 1.2(.8 - .3) + 8 \div .4 =$

    (A) 23
    (B) 20.5
    (C) 50
    (D) 3.2

33. Find .2 percent of 400.

    (A) 80
    (B) 800
    (C) .8
    (D) 2000

34. An eight-ounce bottle of fruit juice provides 200 calories. What percent of the 200 calories is provided by three ounces of the fruit juice?

    (A) 12.5%
    (B) 22.5%
    (C) 37.5%
    (D) 75%

35. Find the length of the hypotenuse in the triangle below.

    (A) 7
    (B) 5
    (C) 25
    (D) 6

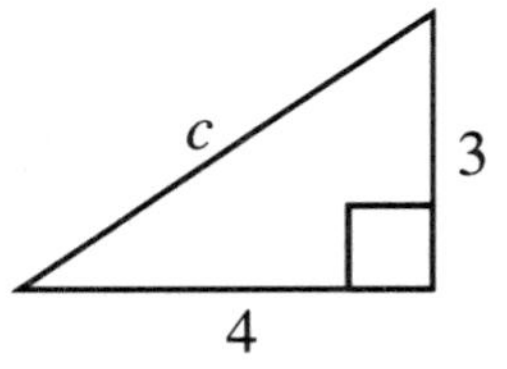

36. What is the width of a rectangle with an area of 63 square feet and a length of 9 feet?

    (A) 22.5 feet
    (B) 7 feet
    (C) 567 feet
    (D) 144 feet

37. If the triangles below are similar, find the length of side x.

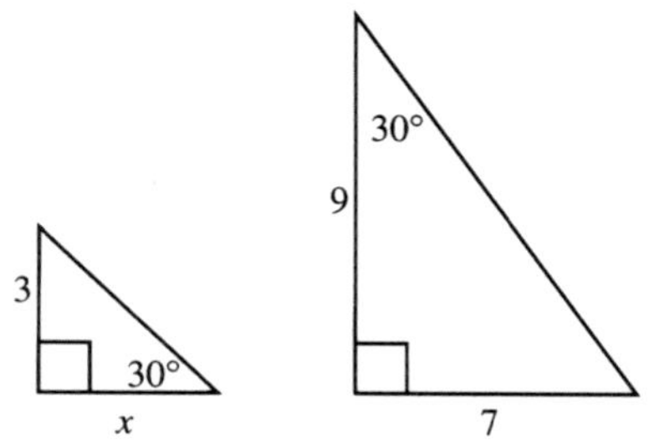

(A) 21 inches
(B) 11 inches
(C) 13 inches
(D) $3\frac{6}{7}$ inches

38. If two lines are parallel, the following statements are true:

(A) The two lines have equal slopes.
(B) The two lines have one point in common.
(C) The product of the slopes of the lines is −1.
(D) The two lines form right angles.

39. If the area of a square is 144 m^2, what is the length of a side of the square?

(A) 12m
(B) $12m^2$
(C) 72m
(D) $72m^2$

40. Find the area of the figure below.

(A) 40m
(B) 46m
(C) $80m^2$
(D) $96m^2$

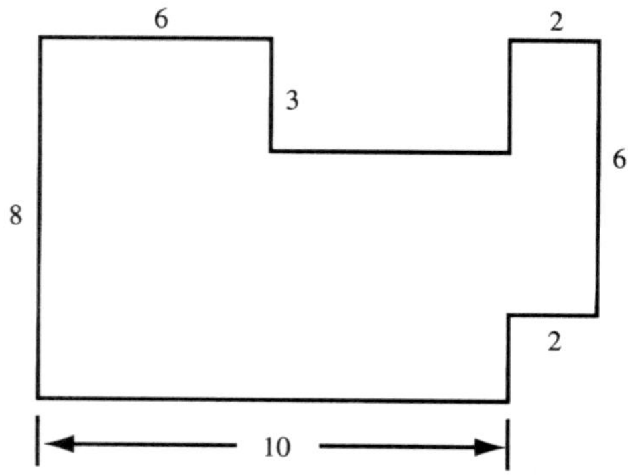

41. Consider the circle with central angles shown below:

What percent of the circle does the central angle of 60° represent? (give answer to the nearest degree.)

(A) 6%
(B) 60%
(C) 17%
(D) 25%

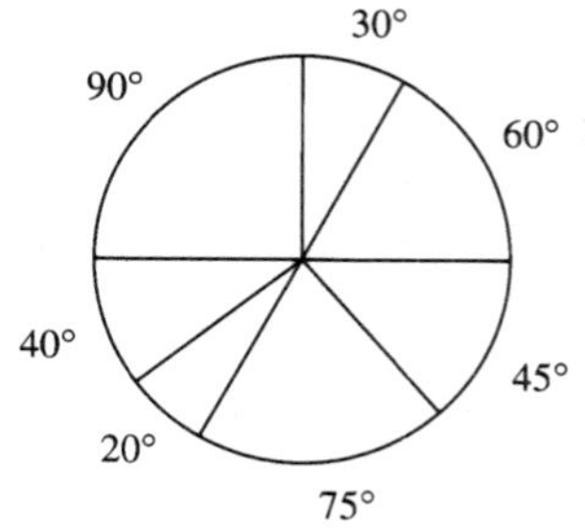

42. If $\frac{1}{12}$ of a family's weekly budget is spent on entertainment and $\frac{1}{8}$ of the budget is spent on gasoline, which central angle represents the total spent on entertainment and gasoline?

(A) 20
(B) 45
(C) 90
(D) 75

PART 2: QUANTITATIVE COMPARISONS

12 QUESTIONS • TIME—15 MINUTES

Common Information: In each question, information concerning one or both of the quantities to be compared is given in the ITEM column. A symbol that appears in any column represents the same thing in column A as it does in column B.

Figures: Assume that the position of points, angles, regions, and so forth, are in the order shown; that the lines shown as straight are indeed straight; that figures lie in a plane unless otherwise indicated. Figures accompanying questions are intended to provide information you can use in answering the questions. However, unless a note states that a figure is drawn to scale, you should solve the problems by using your knowledge of mathematics, and NOT by estimating sizes by sight or by measurement.

Directions: For each of the following questions two quantities are given: one in Column A and one in Column B. Compare the two quantities and mark your answer sheet with the correct, lettered conclusion. These are your options:

A: the quantity in Column A is the greater;

B: the quantity in Column B is the greater;

C: the two quantities are equal;

D: the relationship cannot be determined from the information given.

	Item	Column A	Column B
1.	$n < 0; a < 0$	$n + a$	$n - a$
2.		The average of: 22, 24, 26, 28, 30	The average of: 17, 19, 21, 23, 25, 27, 29, 31, 33
3.	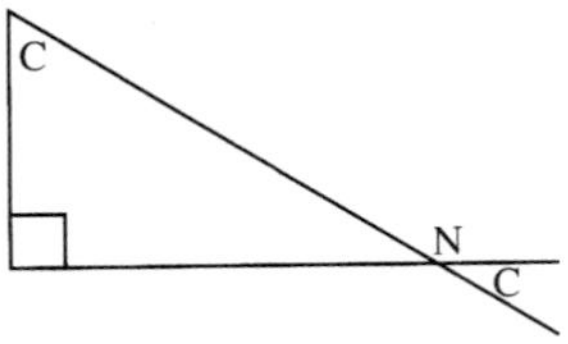	∠N – ∠C	90°
4.	$0 < y < 5; 0 < n < 7$	y	n
5.	$5n - 5a = 25$	n	a
6.	In isosceles ΔNCY: 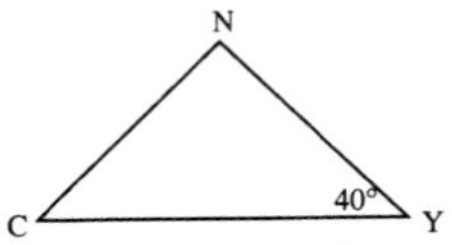	∠C	∠Y

Item		Column A	Column B
7.	$\frac{m}{2} = c^2$	m	c
8.	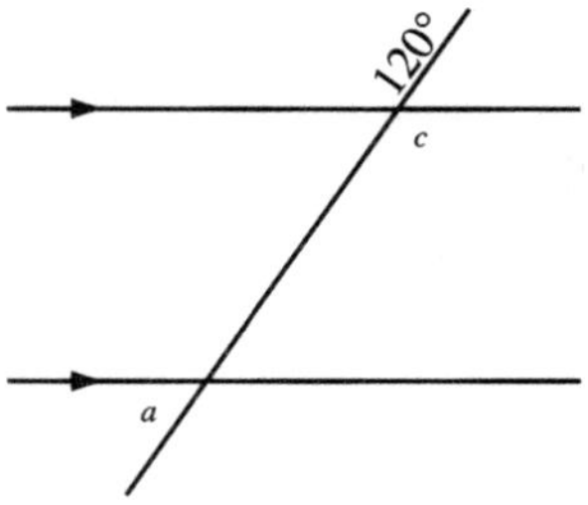	c	a
9.	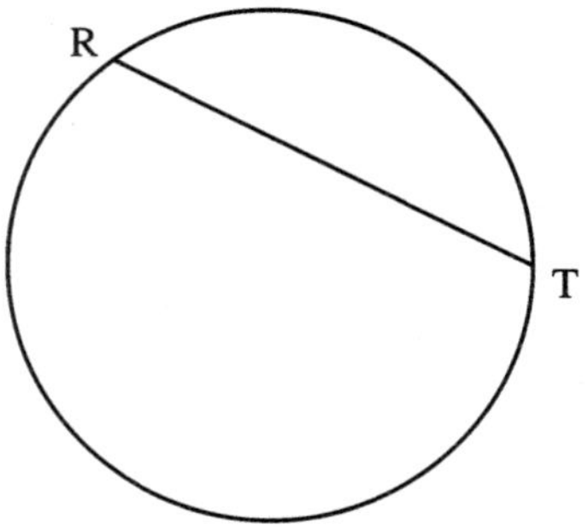	arc $\overset{\frown}{RT}$	chord $\overline{RT}$
10.		$5 + 16(3 - 2)$	$21 + 5 - 3(4 - 3)(0)$
11.		$8[2x - 3(4x - 6) - 9]$	$6[3x - 2(6x - 3) + 2]$
12.	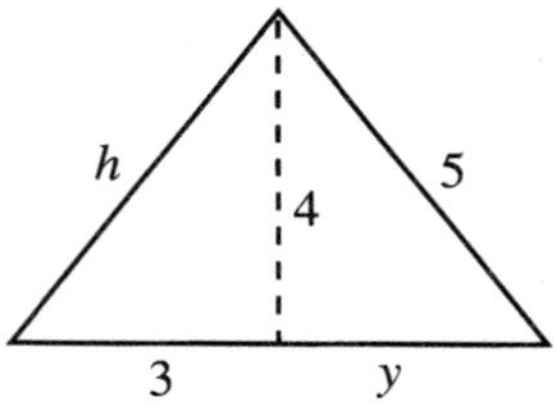	h	y

FINAL MATHEMATICS EXAMINATION ANSWER KEY

PART 1: GENERAL MATHEMATICS

1. **C**	10. **C**	19. **A**	27. **A**	35. **B**
2. **C**	11. **D**	20. **C**	28. **D**	36. **B**
3. **D**	12. **A**	21. **C**	29. **A**	37. **D**
4. **B**	13. **A**	22. **A**	30. **D**	38. **A**
5. **B**	14. **B**	23. **D**	31. **C**	39. **A**
6. **A**	15. **C**	24. **D**	32. **A**	40. **C**
7. **B**	16. **B**	25. **B**	33. **C**	41. **C**
8. **B**	17. **D**	26. **D**	34. **C**	42. **D**
9. **D**	18. **B**			

PART 2: QUANTITATIVE COMPARISONS

1. **B**	5. **A**	9. **A**
2. **A**	6. **D**	10. **B**
3. **C**	7. **D**	11. **D**
4. **D**	8. **A**	12. **A**

FINAL MATHEMATICS EXAMINATION EXPLANATORY ANSWERS

PART 1: GENERAL MATHEMATICS

1. **(C)** $I = P \times R \times T$

   $= \$225{,}000 \times 0.135 \times 1$ (year)

   $= \$30{,}375$

2. **(C)** 14% of x = \$140 (Let x be the total sales)

   $0.04 \times x = \$140$

   $x = 1000$ (divide by 0.04)

3. **(D)** 25% of \$200 = .25 × \$200 = \$50

   Next, find the 20% discount on \$200:

   $0.20 \times \$200 = \$40$

   The list price is \$200 – \$40 = \$160

   Now take 5% of \$160:

   $0.05 \times \$160 = \$8$

   The discount is \$48 when taken at 20% and 5% successively.

   $\$50 - \$48 = \$2$

4. **(B)** The job took 9 days to complete.

   A worked 5 days: he completed $\frac{5}{9}$ of the work.

   B worked 4 days: he completed $\frac{4}{9}$ of the work.

   If the net profit was \$243, then A received $\frac{5}{9} \times \$243 = \$135$

5. **(B)** \$76.50 ÷ $42\frac{1}{2}$¢/yard

   ($42\frac{1}{2}$¢ = \$0.425)

   = \$76.50 ÷ \$0.425/yard

   = 180 yards

6. **(A)** Discount = 20%

   Sale price = 80%

   $0.80 \times \$280.00 = \$224.00$

7. **(B)** $\frac{n}{6} + \frac{n}{3} = 1$

   $n + 2n = 6$ multiply by 6

   $3n = 6$ combine like terms

   $n = 2$ divide by 3

8. **(B)** Area of a rectangle is

   $A = length \times width$

   = 40 inches × 20 inches

   = 800 square inches

   Note: 1 square foot = 144 square inches

   $\frac{800 \text{ square inches}}{144 \text{ square inches}} = 5.5$ square feet

9. **(D)** $\frac{2}{3} \times \frac{8}{8} = \frac{16}{24}$ (lowest common

   $+\ \frac{1}{8} \times \frac{3}{3} = \frac{3}{24}$ denominator is 24)

   $= \frac{19}{24}$

10. **(C)** To arrive at the average, add all numbers and divide by total number of grades.

    80
    80
    90
    +90
    $340 \div 4 = 85$

11. **(D)** The number of quarters must be even; otherwise, adding dimes will not give \$2.00 *exactly*. So the answer cannot be 3, choice (D)

    3 × 25¢ = 75¢ or 0.75

    \$2.00 – 0.75 = \$1.25

    \$1.25 cannot be changed to all dimes.

12. **(A)** Let the *number* be x. A *number* increased by $\frac{1}{6}$ of itself is 182. To put this in equation form:

$x + \frac{1}{6}x = 182$

$6x + x = 1092$ multiply each term by 6

$7x = 1092$ combine like terms

$x = 156$ divide by 7

13. **(A)** $.16\frac{3}{4} = 16\frac{3}{4}\%$

When changing decimals to percents, move the decimal to the right two places.

14. **(A)** Let p represent the amount of protein needed for 392 calories. Use a proportion

4 ounces/448 calories = p ounces/392 calories

$448p = 4 \times 392$

$448p = 1568$

$p = 3.5$ ounces of protein

3.5 ounces of protein are needed for 392 calories

15. **(C)**

$$\begin{array}{r} \$1296.53 \\ -\ 264.87 \\ \hline \$1031.66 \end{array}$$

16. **(B)**

$$\begin{array}{rr} 12\frac{1}{2} = & 12\frac{2}{4} \\ -6\frac{1}{4} = & -6\frac{1}{4} \\ \hline & 6\frac{1}{4} \end{array}$$

Note: $\frac{1}{2} \times \frac{2}{2} = \frac{2}{4}$

17. **(D)** Price per dozen can be found by multiplying the $1.29 by 4. (There are 4 groups of 3 in a dozen.)

$\$1.25 \times 4 = \$5.16$

18. **(B)** $\frac{1}{4} + \frac{7}{12} + \frac{3}{8} + \frac{1}{2} + \frac{5}{6}$

Note: The lowest common denominator is 24. Each fraction needs to be rewritten to an equivalent fraction, so the denominator will be 24.

$= \frac{6 + 14 + 9 + 12 + 20}{24} = \frac{61}{24}$

Divide:

$$= 24\overline{)61} \quad 2 \text{ or } 2\tfrac{13}{24}$$

$$\begin{array}{r} 48 \\ \hline 13 \end{array}$$

19. **(A)** 25 feet × 36 feet = 900 square feet

Now change 900 square feet to square yards.

Note: 9 square feet = 1 square yard

$900 \text{ square feet} \times \frac{1 \text{ square yard}}{9 \text{ square feet}}$

= 100 square yards

20. **(C)**

$$.0009\overline{)72.000} \quad 80000. \text{ or } 80{,}000$$

21. **(C)** One safety pin costs:

$\$4.15 \div 100 = \$.0415$

So 345 cost:

$345 \times 0.0415 = \$14.32$

22. **(A)** A number, x, that decreased by $\frac{1}{5}$ of itself equals 132, can be expressed as:

$x - \frac{1x}{5} = 132$

$5x - x = 660$ multiply each term by 5

$4x = 660$ combine like terms

$x = 165$ divide by 4

23. **(D)** $285 = 0.05y$ y is the unknown value

$5700 = y$ divide by 0.05

24. **(D)** $65 – $50 = $15 is the increase, but to find the percentage of increase, we divide the increase by the original amount:

$\$15 \div \$50 = 0.30$ or 30%

25. **(B)** Let x represent the numerator of the fraction, then the denominator will be $x + 20$.

Since the fraction is equivalent to $\frac{3}{5}$, we get

$$\frac{x}{x+20} = \frac{3}{5}$$

$$5x = 3(x + 20)$$

$$5x = 3x + 60$$

$$2x = 60$$

$$x = 30$$

26. **(D)** $2 < x$ 7 means that x is greater than 2 and it is less than or equal to 7.

27. **(A)** $\frac{x}{5} - 4 = 11$

$$\frac{x}{5} - 4 + 4 = 11 + 4$$

$$\frac{x}{5} = 15$$

$$5 \bullet \frac{x}{5} = 5 \bullet 15$$

$$x = 75$$

28. **(D)** Note that one gallon of punch contains 128 ounces (one-half gallon contains 64 ounces). Hence $2\frac{1}{2}$ gallons equals 320 ounces. A direct proportion can be used to solve the problem.

Let x = the number of ounces of grape juice needed.

$$\frac{16 \text{ ounces grape}}{64 \text{ ounces punch}} = \frac{x}{320 \text{ ounces punch}}$$

$$\frac{1}{4} = \frac{x}{320}$$

$$4x = 320$$

$$x = 80 \text{ ounces grape juice}$$

Since the answer is to be given in quarts, change 80 ounces to quarts by dividing 80 by 32. (There are 32 ounces in a quart.)

$80 \div 32 = 2.5$, thus 2.5 quarts of grape juice are needed to make $2\frac{1}{2}$ gallons of punch.

29. **(A)** There are 16 hours from 7:00 A.M. until 11:00 P.M. Hence Mrs. Bowler was up 16 hours.

Let x = the time Mrs. Bowler had left for other activities, then

$$\frac{1}{2}(16) + \frac{1}{8}(16) + \frac{1}{4}(16) + x = 16$$

$$8 + 2 + 4 + x = 16$$

$$14 + x = 16$$

$$x = 2$$

30. **(D)** 24 percent of the 50 students dropped the class.

24 percent of 50 = $.24 \times 50 = 12$

Since 12 students dropped, 50 – 12 or 38 students remained in the class.

31. **(C)** Divide $4\frac{1}{2}$ by $\frac{3}{4}$. (First change $4\frac{1}{2}$ to $\frac{9}{2}$)

$$4\frac{1}{2} \div \frac{3}{4} = \frac{9}{2} \times \frac{4}{3} = \frac{36}{6} = 6$$

32. **(A)** $3.6 - 1.2(.8 - .3) + 8 \div .4$

$$= 3.6 - 1.2(.5) + 8 \div .4$$

$$= 3.6 - .6 + 8 \div .4$$

$$= 3.6 - .6 + 20$$

$$= 3 + 20$$

$$= 23$$

Note: Operations must be performed in the correct order. (Parentheses first, then multiplication and division before addition and subtraction.)

33. **(C)** Change .2 percent to a decimal and multiply .2 percent by 400.

$.002 \times 400 = .800$ or $.8$

34. **(C)** Find the number of calories provided by 3 ounces of fruit juice.

$$\frac{8}{200} = \frac{3}{c}$$

$$8c = 600$$

$$c = 75$$

75 calories are provided by 3 ounces of fruit juice.

Now determine what percent 75 is of 200.

$$n\% \text{ of } 200 = 75$$

$$200n = 75$$

$$n = .375 = 37.5\%$$

Three ounces of the fruit juice provides 37.5% of the calories in the eight ounces.

35. **(B)** Use the Pythagorean theorem

$c^2 = a^2 + b^2$

$c^2 = 3^2 + 4^2$

$c^2 = 9 + 16$

$c^2 = 25$

$c = \sqrt{25}$

$c = 5$

36. **(B)** The formula for the area of a rectangle is $A = LW$. We know the area of the rectangle is 63 and the length is 9 feet. Thus,

63 square feet = $9W$ feet

$$\frac{63 \text{ square feet}}{9 \text{ feet}} = \frac{9 \text{ W feet}}{9 \text{ feet}}$$

7 ft. = W

37. **(D)** The corresponding sides of similar triangles are proportional. Therefore,

$\frac{3}{7} = \frac{x}{9}$

$7x = 27$

$x = 3\frac{6}{7}$

38. **(A)** Parallel lines have equal slopes, they do not intersect.

39. **(A)** The area of a square is found by squaring a side of the square.

If $A = 144\ m^2$

$144\ m^2 = s^2$ where s is a side of the square

$\sqrt{144\ m^2} = s$

$12\ m = s$

40. **(C)** Divide the figure into nonoverlapping rectangles. Find the area of each rectangle. Add the areas of the rectangles to get the total area of the figure.

$A = 48m^2 + 20m^2 + 12m^2 = 80m^2$

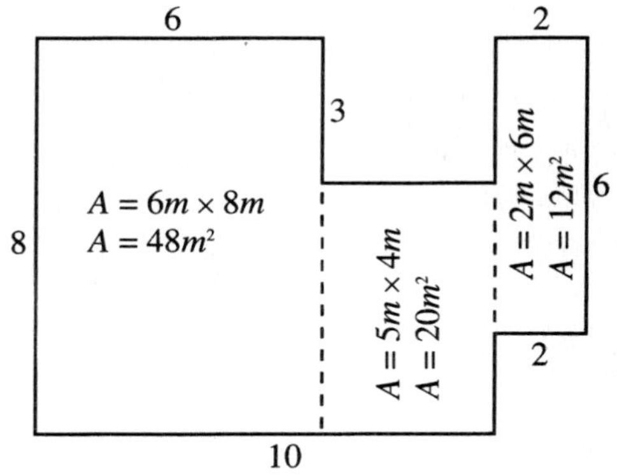

41. **(C)** The entire circle contains 360°. The central angle of 60° represents $\frac{60}{360} = \frac{1}{6}$. Change $\frac{1}{6}$ to a percent by dividing the denominator into the numerator. Thus $\frac{1}{6} = 16\frac{2}{3}\%$. We get 17 when we express $16\frac{2}{3}$ to the nearest whole percent.

42. **(D)** The weekly budget is represented by the entire circle, $\frac{1}{12}$ of the circle represents $\frac{1}{12} \times 360 = 30°$, which is the measure of the central angle for the amount spent on entertainment. $\frac{1}{8}$ of the circle represents $\frac{1}{8} \times 360 = 45°$, which is the measure of the central angle for the amount spent on gasoline. A central angle which represents the total spent on entertainment and gasoline is $30° + 45° = 75°$. (Alternatively, $\frac{1}{8} + \frac{1}{12} = \frac{5}{24}$ and $\frac{5}{24} \times 360° = 75°$.)

PART 2: QUANTITATIVE COMPARISONS

1. **(B)** Both n and a are negative because they are both less than 0. Hence $(n - a)$ must be greater than $(n + a)$ because a negative minus a negative is greater than a negative plus a negative.

   $-a > +a$ ($-a$ = positive, $+a$ = negative)

   $n - a > n + a$ (adding n to both sides)

2. **(A)** The average of Column A is 26, while the average of Column B is 25.

3. **(C)**

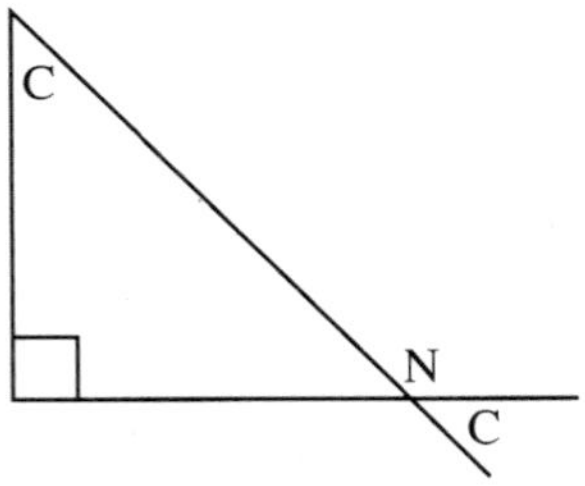

   $\angle N = \angle C + 90°$ An exterior angle is equal to the sum of the interior remote angles.

   $\angle N - \angle C = 90°$ When equals are subtracted from equals, the differences are equal.

4. **(D)** It is impossible to determine because y could be any number from 0 to 5 and n any number from 0 to 7.

5. **(A)** $5n - 5a = 25$

   $n - a = 5$ equals divided by equals are equals

   $n = a + 5$ equals plus equals are equal

   n is five greater than a.

6. **(D)** An isosceles triangle has two equal angles, but from the information given it is impossible to determine which two angles are actually equal.

7. **(D)** There is insufficient information to determine whether m or c is the greater. By substituting numbers for m and c, we see that either quantity could be greater—for example (1) $m = 2$, $c = 1$; (2) $m = \frac{1}{8}$, $c = \frac{1}{4}$.

8. **(A)**

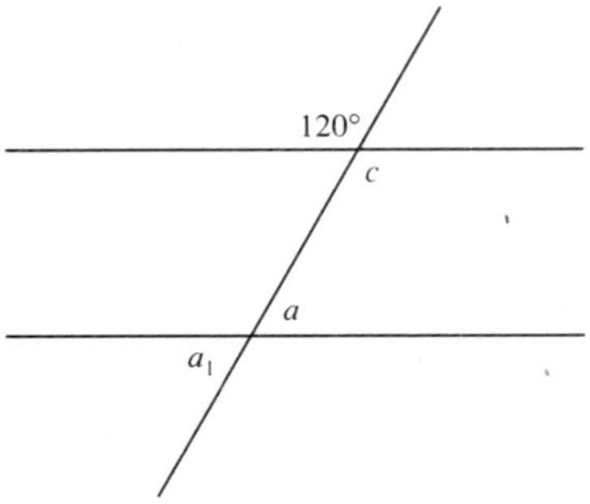

   $\angle c = 120°$ and $\angle a = \angle a_1$ since all vertical angles are equal.

   $\angle c + \angle a_1 = 180°$ since the two interior angles on the same side of a transversal are supplementary.

   $\angle a_1 = 60°$

   $\angle a = 60° < \angle c = 120°$

9. **(A)** The shortest distance between two points is a straight line. Therefore the chord, a straight line, must be shorter than the arc.

10. **(B)** $5 + 16(3 - 2) = 5 + 16(1)$

    $= 5 + 16$

    $= 21$

    $21 + 5 - 3(4 - 3)(0) = 21 + 5 - 0$

    $= 26$

11. **(D)** Since the value of x cannot be determined, the value of Columns A and B remain unknown.

12. **(A)** It can be readily seen that the figure consists of two 3, 4, 5 right triangles. Therefore, $h = 5$ and $y = 3$.

UNIT III: SCIENCE

INTRODUCTION

Living organisms used to be placed into either a plant kingdom or animal kingdom. However, modern classification systems are more sophisticated, and more than two kingdoms are recognized in them. The most widely accepted classification system includes five kingdoms of organisms, as presented below:

MONERA

Prokaryotic (cells without a nucleus bounded by a membrane or true, membrane-bounded organelles in the cytoplasm), unicellular or colonial, autotrophic or saprotrophic.

Includes bacteria and cyanobacteria (formerly called "blue-green algae").

PROTISTA

Eukaryotic (cells with a nucleus bounded by a membrane and with membrane-bound organelles, such as mitochondria or chloroplasts, in the cytoplasm), unicellular or with a simple multicellular body lacking distinct tissues, autotrophic or saprotrophic or phagotrophic.

Includes amoebae, flagellates, ciliates, algae (except cyanobacteria), and slime molds.

FUNGI

Eukaryotic, usually with a simple multicellular body in the form of a mass of slender filaments (mycelium), sometimes unicellular (e.g., yeasts), lacking chlorophyll, saprophytic, often parasitic.

Includes mushrooms and many types of molds.

ANIMALIA

Eukaryotic, multicellular, body usually complex and with many types of true tissues, phagotrophic, sometimes parasitic, usually motile, cells lacking a cell wall.

Includes all types of animals such as sponges, worms, arthropods, and vertebrates.

PLANTAE

Eukaryotic, multicellular, body usually complex and usually with many types of true tissues, possessing chlorophyll, autotrophic, rarely parasitic, never motile, cells always surrounded by a cell wall made of cellulose.

Includes flowering plants, conifers, ferns, and mosses.

Regardless of the kingdom in which organisms are classified, all living things have certain characteristics in common. These characteristics sometimes are used to describe life: We can say that any object that exhibits all of these characteristics is alive. Organisms are always made of cells; they respond to stimuli: they reproduce; they exhibit growth and development; they obtain food and metabolize it for the generation of energy and the synthesis of materials for growth and life; they possess nucleic acid(s); and they exhibit some adaptation to environmental conditions.

Organisms are interdependent. This can be exhibited by an indirect relationship, in which two species are adapted to occupying the same habitat, or a direct relationship, such as predation or symbiosis. In addition, organisms may have an effect on the environment, and the environment, in turn, can affect the organisms and the species that are able to live within it.

Organisms are composed of matter; all matter, whether organic or inorganic, obeys certain physical and chemical laws. Thus, the life sciences and the physical sciences are interrelated. The sciences may be described as follows:

LIFE SCIENCES

The study of living things, including cellular activities; structure and function of tissues; structure and function of organs and of organ systems; and psychological behavior and factors affecting all of these, such as heredity, nutrition, and environmental interaction.

PHYSICAL SCIENCES

The study of matter and all of the interacting physical and chemical forces that affect matter, life, and the use of the earth's resources for living.

The outline below indicates some of the basic principles of the sciences with special emphasis on the descriptions of the "activities or characteristics of life" as related to humans.

I. The cell is the basic structural and functional unit of an organism.

- A. All cells have cytoplasm and a cell membrane.
    1. *Prokaryotic cells* lack a nuclear membrane surrounding the DNA.
    2. *Eukaryotic cells* possess a nuclear membrane that surrounds the DNA and separates it from the cytoplasm, creating a well-defined nucleus.
    3. Some types of eukaryotic cells, such as red blood cells of man, lack a nucleus at maturity for functional reasons, but these cells always possess a nucleus during their development.
- B. Typical plant cells lack a centriole, but have plastids and a cell wall, while typical animal cells lack a cell wall and plastids, but possess a centriole.
- C. Reproduction of cells normally involves mitosis, a nuclear process during which nuclear materials, including DNA, are distributed equally to daughter nuclei.
    1. Mitosis may occur without division of the cell, leading to a multinucleate cell.
    2. DNA replicates itself during interphase, before the nucleus enters the mitotic process.
- D. The sum total of cellular functions comprises the functions of the tissues or organ.
    1. The cellular functions are accomplished by one or more parts, or *organelles,* of the cell.
        - a) The cell membrane is differentially permeable and functions in regulating the passage of materials into and out of the cell.
            - (1) Materials may pass through the membrane by osmosis, by diffusion, by active transport, or by some other mechanism.
        - b) *Mitochondria* are cellular organelles in which food is oxidized for the release of energy.
        - c) *Plastids* (in plants) are of different types and vary in function.
            - (1) *Chloroplasts* are green plastids in which photosynthesis occurs.
            - (2) *Chromoplasts* and *leucoplasts* function in storage and other processes.

d) The *endoplasmic reticulum* is a network of branching tubules composed of membrane that functions as an intracellular transport system for many types of materials. It extends through out the cytoplasm of the cell.

e) *Ribosomes* are organelles in which protein synthesis occurs. They are typically associated with the rough endoplasmic reticulum of the cell; RNA passes over the ribosomes to "line up" the amino acids to form the protein.

f) The *Golgi apparatus* functions in collecting and preparing secretions of the cell for export outside the cell.

g) *Contractile vacuoles* are membranous sacs that maintain a proper concentration of water inside the cell by draining excess water from the cytoplasm and expelling it. They are found in many protists and some animal cells.

h) *Cilia* and *flagella* are slender projections of the cell used for movement. Flagella are longer thancilia, but both have the same internal arrangement of microtubules, the 9 + 2 pattern, and are formed by the same kind of organelle, a *kinetosome*.

i) *Centrioles* are tiny, barrel-shaped organelles similar to kinetosomes that form the *spindle apparatus* that pulls chromosomes to opposite poles of the cell during mitosis or meiosis.

j) *Phagocytic vacuoles,* also called *food vacuoles,* are membranous sacs used by some types of cells to engulf and digest food material. Cells form similar organelles called *autophagic vacuoles* to engulf, digest, and recycle worn-out cytoplasmic organelles.

k) The *nucleus* is the control center of the cell; the nuclear membrane is porous, and materials pass into and out of the nucleus through the nuclear membrane.

(1) In eukaryotes, DNA is stored in the nucleus.

(2) *Transcription,* or the biosynthesis of RNA from the DNA, occurs within the nucleus; the RNA travels to the ribosomes where *translation,* or the synthesis of a polypeptide, occurs.

(3) The *nucleolus,* located within the nucleus, is the site where RNA is manufactured.

II. Animals and plants exhibit organizational levels.

A. Unicellular organisms are composed of one cell, which accomplishes all of the functions necessary for life.

1. Unicellular organisms may be prokaryotic, as with bacteria, or eukaryotic, as with protistans.

a) The first indication of "division of labor" is seen in some colonial unicellular forms, in which specific cells are concerned with the specific functions.

B. Organisms at the tissue level of organization have well-developed tissues, some of which may be specialized for certain functions, but do not have well-developed organs.

C. The organ level of organization indicates the presence of well-developed organs.

D. Most animals, from round and segmented worms to vertebrates, are characterized by the system level of organization in which organs are arranged to accomplish a multiphase process.

III. All organisms exhibit response to stimuli.

A. Response involves reception of a stimulus, transmission of the impulse, and reaction to the stimulus.

1. In higher animals, such as humans, well-developed sense organs may be involved in the reception of stimuli; these include the skin, eye, and ear.

a) Primitive sense organs may be seen in lower animals; in some lower animals, the sense organs may be well developed.

b) Sensory organelles may be seen in some unicellular forms, such as the eyespot of *Euglena.*

2. The transmission of impulses involves nerves or nerve fibers; in humans and other animals, a nervous system is involved in the transmission of impulses.

a) Transmission of nerve impulses is electrical, and involves a difference in the concentration of certain ions, especially potassium and sodium, along the nerve fibers.

b) Nerve impulses are transmitted from one nerve fiber to another across a tiny gap, called a *synapse,* that separates the two cells. Passage of a nerve impulse along the presynaptic fiber causes it to release into the synaptic space a substance called a *neurotransmitter* that either stimulates or blocks the generation of a nerve impulse in the postsynaptic neuron. This enables synapses to function as points of control in nerve pathways.

3. Reaction to stimuli may involve a change in position, in movement, and in secretory activities. Thus, the skeletal system, muscle system, endocrine glands, and digestive glands may be involved in reactions, as exhibited by humans and other higher animals.

a) Other systems that may be indirectly involved in reactions are the circulatory system, the respiratory system, and the excretory system.

IV. All organisms exhibit reproduction; this maintains continuity of the species or population extant.

Reproduction may be sexual or asexual.

A. Asexual reproduction occurs by means of mitosis and does not involve a union of reproductive cells (gametes) or gametic nuclei.

1. The following are types of asexual reproduction:

a) *Sporulation* involves the production of asexual reproductive cells (or multicellular units) called spores; these spores develop directly into new individuals.

b) *Binary fission* involves the division of the organism (usually unicellular) into two organisms. In the case of unicellular eukaryotes, binary fission usually involves mitosis.

c) *Multiple fission,* or *fragmentation,* as seen in lower organisms such as filamentous algae, involves the breaking of the organism into smaller units, each of which can develop into a new organism.

d) *Budding* involves the production of an outgrowth or miniature organism that breaks away from the parent and develops into a new adult.

B. Sexual reproduction involves meiosis followed by fertilization, meaning the union of the nuclei of reproductive cells.

1. Several types of sexual reproduction may be described, depending on the morphology of the gametes.

a) *Isogamy* is reproduction involving fusion of morphologically identical gametes; this is more common among lower plants.

b) *Heterogamy* is sexual reproduction involving fusion of gametes that differ in size and/or structure.

(1) One type of heterogamy involves motile gametes differing only in size; this is *anisogamy.*

(2) The other type of heterogamy involves gametes differing in size and in structure: this is *oogamy.*

(a) Oogamy is exhibited by man; the gamete produced by the male is the spermatozoon; the gamete produced by the female is the ovum or egg.

(b) In animals such as man, gametes are produced in gonads: the male gonads are the testes; the female gonads are the ovaries.

i. Gonads in higher animals, such as man, also have an endocrine function, producing hormones involved with the appearance of secondary sex characteristics and with reproductive cycles.

c) *Conjugation* is sexual reproduction involving a temporary union of cells for exchange or transmission of nuclei or DNA.

2. Meiosis is involved in the production of gametes or of spores in the case of most plants.

a) Gametes are haploid, having one-half the chromosome number characteristic of the zygote of the species.

b) The diploid number is restored to the zygote (the cells resulting from gametic union, or *syngamy*) when fertilization occurs.

c) The zygote typically develops mitotically into the embryo; thus, there is no further change in chromosome number.

d) Because of meiosis and syngamy, the individual developing from the zygote receives one-half of its DNA from each parent; thus, the chromosome number for the species remains constant.

e) Sexual reproduction allows the spread of changes through a population.

V. Growth and development allow for the characteristic size range of a species to be maintained and for the differentiation of organs and tissues to be accomplished.

A. In multicellular organisms, growth may involve an increase in the number of cells, an increase in the size of cells, or both.

B. The zygote develops mitotically into a multicellular organism. In man and other multicellular organisms, development, or differentiation, accompanies growth.

C. In higher animals, such as man, the basic development patterns are similar.

1. The zygote undergoes cleavage to produce a cluster of cells known as a *morula.*

2. The morula develops into a *blastula* or *blastocyst;* this is a hollow ball of cells with a cavity known as a *blastocoel.*

3. The blastula develops into a two-layered *gastrula* with a cavity known as a *gastrocoel* or *archenteron.*

a) The outer germ layer of the gastrula is the *ectoderm.*

b) The inner germ layer of the gastrula is the *endoderm.*

c) The third germ layer, *mesoderm,* develops between the ectoderm and the endoderm.

4. Each germ layer gives rise to definite body structures and tissues.

a) From the ectoderm develops the nervous system, some sense organs such as the eye, and the outer skin.

b) From the mesoderm develops the muscle system, skeletal system, muscle of the viscera, mesenteries, and circulatory system.

c) From the endoderm develops the lining of the digestive tract, the lungs, much of the liver and pancreas, the thyroid, parathyroid, and thymus glands.

VI. Nutritional processes, involving the obtaining and utilizing of food, are exhibited by all organisms.

A. Food may be defined as any substance that can be used by the organism as a source of energy and as a source of materials for growth and maintenance of the body.

1. Most food is organic; the process involving the conversion of inorganic materials into organic foods is photosynthesis.

a) This process occurs only in green plants, in the presence of the chlorophylls and in the presence of light as an energy source.

(1) The chloroplast is the cellular organelle in which photosynthesis occurs.

b) All organisms (except for a few algae and prokaryotes that may exhibit similar processes) depend directly or indirectly on photosynthesis for food.

2. Some food consists of inorganic minerals necessary for the maintenance of bodily processes. Examples of essential minerals are sodium, potassium, iron, calcium, zinc, and cobalt.

B. Organisms must obtain food in some way to live.

1. *Autotrophs,* such as green plants, manufacture food within their bodies from inorganic environmental materials.

2. *Heterotrophs* receive organic food from the environment.

a) *Saprotrophs* digest food externally and absorb the digested food into the body; most bacteria and fungi are saprotrophs.

b) *Parasites* live on and at the expense of a host.

c) *Phagotrophs,* such as man and most animals, ingest solid food into a digestive cavity of some sort.

(1) The digestive cavity of phagotrophic protozoa may be a *food vacuole;* this is characteristic of the cellular level of organization.

(2) The digestive cavity of simple animals such as coelenterates and flatworms is a *gastro vascular cavity* with a mouth as its only opening; this is characteristic of the tissue level of organization or simpler versions of the system level.

(3) The digestive cavity of humans and most other animals is a complete *digestive tract* (digestive system) with a mouth at one end and an anus at the other end; this is characteristic of the system level of organization.

C. Food that has been obtained must be digested, changed into a usable, absorbable state. This occurs in the digestive system in humans.

1. In lower animals, digestion occurs in a food vacuole (as in protozoa), a gastrovascular cavity, or a simple gut.

D. The digested food is distributed throughout the body to the cells.

1. In humans, the circulatory or vascular system distributes the food to the cells.

E. Utilization of food, or *metabolism,* occurs in the cells.

1. Oxidation of glucose within the cells (in the mitochondria) yields energy for life and for life's activities.

a) Aerobic oxidation is most common, involving the use of free, molecular oxygen. Enzymes control each step of oxidation.

(1) Oxygen is made available by means of respiratory organs, or, in the case of humans, the respiratory system.

(2) Oxygen is absorbed from air inhaled into the lungs of man and transported to the cells by means of the circulatory system.

(a) In man, oxygen is transported in combination with hemoglobin of the red blood cells.

(3) Carbon dioxide resulting from the oxidation of glucose is transported by the blood stream to the lungs for elimination through exhalation.

(4) As a result of oxidation of glucose, the energy transporting substance, adenosine triphosphate (ATP) is formed. ATP transfers energy to the areas that need it or to specialized areas and compounds for energy storage.

(5) Liquid waste from metabolism is collected, concentrated, and eliminated by the excretory system.

2. The synthesis of other compounds, proteins, and secretory products occurs in the cell.

F. Solid indigestible wastes are eliminated from the digestive system; in humans, elimination occurs through the anus.

VII. Organisms must adapt to the environment in which they live in order to survive.

A. Organisms may possess or develop certain traits that enable them to live or thrive in a specific environment.

1. Changes in populations may originate and spread throughout the population, making survival and thriving a greater possibility.

a) Changes that are conducive to survival are conserved, accumulate, and may eventually lead to a new variety or race.

B. Organisms, by their presence and exploitation of an environment, may change the environment to the extent that it becomes suitable for a different group or species. Thus, succession occurs as the environment continues to change under the influence of different species, causing other species to adapt to or invade the environment.

VIII. Two types of nucleic acids are known; all organisms possess one or both types. Most organisms possess both.

A. Deoxyribonucleic acid (DNA) functions as the genetic information of an individual. Different parts of the genetic information contained in the structure of DNA can be used for the following purposes: day to day regulation of cellular processes (metabolism), development of a new individual (heredity), or manufacture of RNA. DNA is contained within the nucleus of eukaryotic cells and is attached to the inner side of the cell membrane in prokaryotic cells.

1. DNA is a long, double-stranded, chain-like molecule that is twisted into the form of a helix (double helix). Each strand is a chain of "building units," which are smaller molecules called nucleotides.

a) A nucleotide consists of a sugar (deoxyribose), a phosphate, and a purine or pyrimidine base.

(1) The purine bases are guanine and adenine.

(2) The pyrimidine bases are cytosine and thymine.

2. DNA is the pattern or template from which complementary RNA (ribonucleic acid) is synthesized.

a) RNA is similar in structure to DNA except that it is much smaller and consists of only one strand. Like DNA, the single strand of RNA is a chain of nucleotides.

(1) The purine bases of RNA nucleotides are guanine and adenine.

(2) The pyrimidine bases of RNA nucleotides are cytosine and uracil.

b) There are three types of RNA and all of them play essential roles in protein synthesis. Together, DNA and RNA form a system for the storage and use of information needed to make the proper structure of each of the many different types of proteins used by an individual organism.

(1) Messenger RNA serves as the actual pattern or template for the sequential arrangement of amino acids into a chain to make a protein. The information in a molecule of messenger RNA is copied from part of a DNA molecule (transcription); this information is equivalent to a *gene* or a group of related genes.

(2) Transfer RNA carries amino acids to specific complementary spots on the messenger RNA template, insuring that amino acids are placed in the correct sequence for a particular protein (translation).

(3) Ribosomal RNA is the key component of ribosomes, which are the cellular sites for the synthesis of proteins.

Of major concern in the health sciences is an understanding of how humans function biologically, psychologically, and socially. Man's behavior is influenced by his environment; thus, the "laws of nature" apply to man as well as to other organisms and to the matter making up his environment. It is necessary, therefore, for a person involved in the health sciences to have knowledge of the physical sciences as well as of the life sciences.

CONCEPTS RELATED TO HEALTH SCIENCES

Concepts	**Related Topics**
I. Concepts about man	Cell structure
A. Develops from a single cell (zygote)	Similarities and differences in animal and plant cellular activities
1. Reproduction is a basic function of life.	
a) Humans reproduce by sexual reproduction (mating), the union of male and female sex cells.	Animal cell division
b) Humans transmit like characteristics to offspring.	Plant cell division
2. Heredity, the transmission of traits, can be explained in terms of	Mutations
a) Mendel's Law	Dominant and recessive genes
b) Gene theory	Hybrids
c) Blending	Punnett Square
d) Meiosis	
e) Chromosomal influence in sex determination.	Role of RNA and DNA
3. Deoxyribonucleic acid (DNA) is the only known type of self-duplicating molecule that plays a central role in heredity by ensuring the orderly development of offspring into a form similar to that of their parents.	Fetal development
4. Fertilization produces a zygote, which then begins to grow by mitosis, the first stage of life of the embryo.	
5. Mature cells group together in distinct patterns to form tissues. Tissues unite to form organs, and organs unite to form the lifesystems of the body.	
B. Life processes based on metabolism	Energy transfer mechanisms in living cells
1. All human cells must utilize oxygen through respiration, receive nutrition through digestive processes, eliminate wastes, and grow to their potential stage of maturity.	ATP cycle Aerobic and anaerobic respiration
2. These life processes involve chemical changes (called *metabolism*) that are controlled by enzymes.	Oxidation of carbohydrates Photosynthesis
3. The energy needed for life-processes in man comes from food: proteins, carbohydrates, and fats. Energy from food is used to make adenosine triphosphate (ATP), which is used as a universally available source of energy in all cells of the body.	Protein and lipid synthesis Classification systems for living organisms
4. The cell constantly interacts with its environment through the processes of osmosis and diffusion.	

Concepts	Related Topics
5. All cellular functions depend on specific types of proteins, especially enzymes. By controlling the manufacture of specific proteins, DNA (with the help of RNA) is able to control all cellular functions.	
6. The maintenance of internal balance (called *homeostasis*) is a major part of metabolism. Internal conditions such as concentrations of substances in cells or body fluids, pH, and temperature are kept within narrow ranges by constant regulation. These regulatory activities always require a major expenditure of energy by the organism. Much of homeostasis is done to satisfy the requirements of enzymes, which are always sensitive to physical conditions.	
C. Life processes conducted through bodily systems.	Gills, lungs, and tracheae
1. The function of the respiratory system is to transport oxygen to the blood and eliminate carbon dioxide from the blood.	Oxygen and carbon dioxide exchange
a) The quantity of available oxygen determines the effectiveness of respiration.	Positive and negative pressure breathing; basal metabolic rates
b) Oxygen consumption is directly proportional to the rate of bodily activity and energy use.	Energy production from metabolic processes
c) Metabolic processes of the body are directly affected by oxygen supply.	Factors affecting metabolic rate
d) Changes in oxygen consumption caused by an increase or decrease in activity temporarily affect the concentration of oxygen in the blood, which is then restored to normal by an increase or decrease in respiratory rate.	
2. The circulatory system transports all nutrients to the cells and wastes from the cells.	Rhythmic beating of heart Structure of arteries and veins
a) The force of the circulatory flow (blood pressure) is created by the pumping of the heart. This force delivers blood to the capillaries where exchange of materials between the blood and tissues takes place.	Location of major blood vessels
b) The stimulation of the heart comes from within the heart muscle, but the rate of beating is modified by chemicals (hormones) and nerve transmissions from the brain.	Capillary as medium for exchange
c) The rate of blood flow through the vessels is directly proportional to blood pressure and is partially maintained by the closed nature of the cardiovascular circuit.	Electrolytes Acids and bases
d) The volume of blood pumped through the cardiovascular circuit per unit of time is directly proportional to blood pressure.	Hyper- and hypothermia Blood typing—Rh factor

Concepts	Related Topics
e) Arteries are able to change their internal diameter by constriction or dilation; blood pressure is inversely proportional to the diameter of arteries.	Clotting mechanism
f) In capillaries, exchange of materials between the blood and tissues is accomplished by a combination of blood pressure, diffusion, and osmosis.	Body defenses in blood and lymph
g) Blood is returned to the heart through veins by the passive mechanisms of pushing from behind, squeezing of veins by skeletal muscles, and gravity.	Distribution of body fluids
3. The digestive system breaks down foods and delivers the nutrients to the circulatory system.	Solid and liquid components of blood
a) Food must be ingested into the system, mixed with digestive substances, broken down chemically (digestion), and selectively absorbed into the blood stream.	Materials required for plant growth (auxins, vitamins, etc.) Variations in digestive systems of living organisms.
b) The rate of digestion is directly related to the quantity of food. c) The lining of the alimentary tube provides mucus to lubricate the passage of food and protect the lining itself from enzymes or acid.	a. Utilization of large quantities of food. b. Utilization of fluids and soft tissues.
d) Chemical breakdown is the result of enzymes and activators. e) Nutrients are stored in the liver for reserve supply.	Chemical digestion of carbohydrates, proteins, and fats Role of vitamins and minerals Hydrolysis
f) Waste products are eliminated through the colon.	Structure formula and isomerism a. hydrocarbons b. halogen derivatives c. alcohols and phenols d. aldehydes and phenols e. amino acids f. heterocyclics g. lipids h. organometallics i. nucleic acid
4. The excretory (renal) system removes metabolic wastes and excess substances from the body.	Invertebrate mechanisms for excretion
a) The kidneys selectively absorb wastes and excess substances from the blood to form urine.	Role of nephron unit in homeostasis
b) The kidneys selectively reabsorb substances needed by the body and return them to the blood.	Filtration and dialysis
c) Selective reabsorption conserves water and electrolytes, which balances their concentrations in the blood and tissues.	Artificial kidney Excretion of wastes through skin

Concepts	Related Topics
d) The circulating volume of the blood has a direct affect on kidney activity.	
e) The ureters connect the kidneys to the bladder, a receptacle for holding urine.	
f) Micturition (urination) is a reflex action.	
5. The endocrine system regulates body activities.	Interrelationships of endocrine glands
a) Endocrine glands secrete hormones into the blood and tissues.	Function of insulin, thyroxin, parathyrin
b) Hormonal secretion is activated by chemical and neural factors.	Role of pituitary gland Sex hormones
c) Hormones regulate primary metabolic processes.	Steroids
d) Hypo- or hyperactivity of endocrine glands results in disorders.	Release of energy by adrenalin
6. The musculoskeletal system generates motion and maintains posture.	Location of bones in the skeleton and functional relationships of bones to one another Ligaments and joints
a) The bones and muscles are combined into individual lever systems to produce motion.	
b) In the human body, a lever system consists of a muscle (force), joint (fulcrum), and a bone (lever). The arrangement of a lever system permits movement with a minimal expenditure of energy.	Function of red and yellow marrow
c) Joints act as points of balance and are also sculptured to regulate the extent or direction of movement.	Smooth and striated muscles
d) Change in position is produced by a shift of weight accomplished by muscular force.	Major muscles of the body and functional relationships of muscles to bones
e) The longer the axis of the lever (bone) being moved, the greater the extent of movement.	Principles of energy and work
f) The use of muscular force consumes a large amount of energy and results in much waste heat, used to maintain body temperature, as a byproduct.	
7. The nervous system provides a means of internal bodily communication that controls and coordinates all activities in response to environmental stimuli.	Plant stimulus-response systems Responses to light, temperature, touch, and other physical conditions
a) Impulses travel along neurons (nerve cells).	Sensory and motor organs
b) Neurons are grouped together to form the central nervous system (brain and spinal cord) and nerves that connect the central nervous system to all parts of the body.	Brain centers Spinal nerves

Concepts

c) Stimuli are changes in either the external or internal environment.

d) The central nervous system receives stimuli and ensures that a proper response is given to each one.

e) Responses are initiated through the central nervous system and consist of either a muscular movement or secretion of a substance by a gland.

II. Human potential for adaptation

A. Interdependent relationships with other living forms

1. Humans, like other living things, form complex relationships with the environment.
2. The kinds and amount of life found in different environments is determined by temperature, moisture, sunlight, and soil.
3. Humans, like other animals, depend on animal and plant sources of food (food chains).
4. Only organisms with chlorophylls, such as plants, can make food.
5. Food chains exist because all living things need energy.
6. The survival of humankind (and species in general) is influenced by other species in the same environment.
7. Living organisms in the same environment form an interrelated community in which many species out of the total number live in close associations with one another (symbiosis). Most of these symbiotic associations constitute mutualism (benefit to both partners) or parasitism (benefit to one partner at the expense of the other).

B. Conservation of resources

1. Supplies of natural resources are finite.
2. Population growth reduces the amount of resource available to individual humans.
3. Supplies of natural resources can be expanded to some extent by new ways of increasing food production, development of new sources of energy, recycling of waste materials, conservation of natural habitats, and soil conservation.
4. Ultimately, population control is the only way to ensure adequate amounts of food. energy, and other resources for individual humans.

Related Topics

Cranial nerves

Autonomic nervous system

Ecological balance

Producers, consumers, decomposers

Movement of energy through ecosystems

Biomes

Climatic effects on life processes

Composition of sea water
- a. sodium chloride
- b. magnesium
- c. calcium
- d. sulfur
- e. oxygen

Classification of matter
- a. organic and inorganic
- b. elements, compounds, mixtures

Structure of matter
- a. atoms
- b. molecules

Forms of matter
- a. liquid
- b. gas
- c. solid

Changes in form
- a. physical
- b. chemical

Concepts	**Related Topics**
III. Human interaction with the environment A. Environmental regulation of life processes 1. Inorganic matter is synthesized into food for plants; plants provide food for animals. 2. The physiological phenomena (assimilation, respiration, and growth) are controlled by temperature, light, moisture, nutrient supplies, and general atmospheric conditions. B. Use and modification of the environment 1. Humans must protect themselves from biological, physical, and radiological hazards. 2. Humans must discover and develop new ways of using natural resources to minimize or reverse environmental destruction; conservation, recycling, and avoidance of "disposable" products are central elements in this strategy.	Physiology of plants Nitrogen cycle Photosynthesis Vaporization, distillation Carbon-oxygen cycle Magnetism Light, sound, electricity Pollution and pest control Gamma, Beta, Alpha rays Causative organisms of disease Koch's postulates Natural and acquired immunity Antibiotics and disinfectants Sterilization, pasteurization, refrigeration Community characteristics, principle of succession Solar energy, heat production, transfer convection Nuclear fission

SCIENCE GLOSSARY

Items in capitals have a special entry in the glossary.

A

absolute zero	The lowest temperature that a gas can attain. This is 460 degrees below zero on the FAHRENHEIT scale and 273 degrees below zero on the CELSIUS scale.
absorption	The movement of water and/or dissolved substances into a cell, tissue, or organism.
acceleration	A change in the speed of an object. If the object speeds up, this is called *positive acceleration*. If the object goes slower, it is called *negative acceleration.*
acid	A compound with a pH less than 7, which means that it releases hydrogen ions when dissolved in water. An acid changes blue litmus paper to red and tastes sour.
acquired immunity	Immunity that is not natural or congenital; obtained after birth.
active immunity	Immunity brought about by activity of certain cells of the body as a result of being exposed to an antigen.
active transport	An energy-requiring process by means of which materials are moved across a cell membrane.
adsorption	The gathering of molecules of a substance on a surface.
aerobe	Any organism living in the presence of and utilizing free, molecular oxygen (that is, oxygen not in chemical combination) in its oxidative processes.
alchemy	The science of transforming less valuable metals into gold or silver, and the philosophy behind this idea. The theories of the alchemists of the Middle Ages were false, but their experiments laid the foundation of modern chemistry.
alkali	A compound with a pH greater than 7. An alkaline substance changes red litmus paper to blue. It can combine with hydrogen. *See* BASE.
alkaline	A substance having the properties of an ALKALI.
allantois	One of four extraembryonic membranes attached to the body of the embryo or fetus of a land-dwelling vertebrate. In humans it is modified to form part of the placenta and umbilicus.
amino acid	An organic molecule containing an amino group (NH_2) and a carboxyl group (COOH) bonded to the same carbon atom; the "building blocks" of proteins.
amnion	The innermost of four extraembryonic membranes attached to the body of the embryo or fetus of a land-dwelling vertebrate. It forms a fluid-filled sac around the body that provides an aqueous environment and cushions the embryo from shocks.
ampere	A measurement of electric current, abbreviated *amp*. It was named after French scientist ANDRÉ MARIE AMPÈRE.
Ampère, André Marie	A French scientist (1775–1836) whose work and theory laid the foundation for the Andre Marie science of electrodynamics. His name lives on in the electrical measurement AMPERE.
amphipods	A crustacean group that includes sand fleas.
anaerobe	Any organism not requiring free, molecular oxygen for its cellular oxidative processes. Some anaerobes are *obligate,* and cannot survive in the presence of oxygen; others are *facultative,* and can survive with or without oxygen.
anatomy	The study of the structure of living things. Usually, "anatomy" refers to the structure of the human body.
anemone	A sea animal (a coelenterate) that resembles the flower of the same name.

antibiotic A substance derived from lower organisms that can be used to prevent growth of certain pathogens, thus combating infection.

antibody A specific type of protein molecule that is manufactured in the tissues, blood, or lymph in response to the presence of viruses or foreign cells. Each variety of antibody will attach to the surface of only one type of invader, enabling it to be recognized and marked for destruction by the immune system.

antigens Protein molecules on the surface of viruses or foreign cells that provoke the manufacture of matching antibodies, enabling invaders to be recognized as such so they can be destroyed.

apolipoprotein (apo E) a gene which codes for a protein that facilitates the transports cholesterol and influence human longevity.

ATP Adenosine triphosphate; the energy-transport compound of a cell.

atrium The anterior chamber(s) of the heart of vertebrates.

attenuated The state of being weakened, as in the case of pathogens used to induce active immunity.

auricle The projecting outer portion, or pinna, of the ear.

autotroph An organism, such as a green plant, capable of manufacturing its food from inorganic environmental materials.

B

bacteria Unicellular. microscopic, PROKARYOTIC organisms, mostly SAPROTROPHIC or PARASITIC.

base A compound with a pH greater than 7 that can react with an acid to accept a hydrogen ion and form a salt. *See* ALKALI.

biochemistry The study of the chemical makeup of organisms. This science is a branch of both chemistry and biology.

biology The study of living things, a major science.

biome A type of community recognized by certain characteristics of plants and climate, such as the plains of the Midwest.

bond The force of attraction that holds two atoms together in a molecule. There are two major types of chemical bonds, COVALENT BONDS and IONIC BONDS.

botany The study of plant life. Botany is a branch of BIOLOGY.

Brahe, Tycho A Danish astronomer (1546–1601) who made a systematic study of the movement of celestial bodies. He is often referred to only as *Tycho*.

C

carbohydrate A food substance made up of carbon, hydrogen, and oxygen.

carbon An important chemical element that forms the basic skeleton of all ORGANIC compounds. Atoms of other elements are bonded to the carbon skeleton to form the many different varieties of organic compounds.

carbon dioxide A compound made up of one atom of carbon and two atoms of oxygen. It exists in the form of a gas and is one of the principle waste byproducts resulting from CELLULAR RESPIRATION.

carcinogen A cancer causing substance that may be physical, chemical or biological.

catalyst A chemical substance that lowers the energy necessary for a chemical reaction to take place and makes the reaction proceed more rapidly. ENZYMES act as catalysts in living organisms.

celestial An adjective referring to the sky.

cell The basic structural and functional unit of organisms.

cellular respiration The oxidation of glucose into carbon dioxide and water (or into other products, in the case of anaerobic respiration), leading to the release of energy.

Celsius A system of measurement of temperature, often referred to as *centigrade.* On the Celsius scale the freezing point for water is 0 degrees and the boiling point is 100 degrees.

centriole A cellular organelle characteristic of animal cells but not plant cells that migrates to the poles during mitosis; spindle fibers and astral rays arise from it.

centromere The portion of the chromosome that holds the chromatids together and to which spindle fibers apparently attach.

chelicerae The claw-like head appendages on certain arthropods, such as spiders.

chemistry The science that studies the composition and transformation of matter; a major science.

Chlamydiae Small intracellular obligate parasites closely related to the *Rickettsiae.*

chlorophylls The green pigments of plants, produced in the presence of light and essential for photosynthesis.

chromosomes Small cellular bodies containing tightly bound and packaged DNA that are formed during MITOSIS and MEIOSIS from loosely packaged DNA (chromatin). The hereditary determinants called GENES are carded on chromosomes.

colloid A type of mixture intermediate between a SOLUTION and a SUSPENSION. It consists of liquid plus particles that are too small to settle out of the mixture and too large to dissolve. Colloids can exist in the form of a gel and pass through membranes either slowly or not at all.

commensalism A symbiotic relationship in which one member is benefited, and the other member is neither benefited nor harmed.

compound The combination of two or more elements into a single unit.

condensation The transition of water vapor to liquid water due to a lowering of temperature.

conduction The transfer of heat from one object or physical medium to another by direct contact.

conservation of energy The principle that energy changes its form but cannot be created or destroyed.

conservation of matter The principle that matter can change its form but cannot be created or destroyed.

constellation A particular grouping of stars.

copepod A small aquatic crustacean.

Copernicus, Nicholas A Polish astronomer (1473–1543) who proposed the theory that the earth moves through space. It was generally believed up to that time that the earth was the immobile center of the universe.

cosmic year The time it takes the sun to go around its galaxy.

covalent bond A type of chemical bond created by the sharing of electrons between two atoms to achieve the maximum number of electrons in the outer electron orbit of each atom. Covalent bonds are the strongest type of chemical bonds.

crop rotation An agricultural method by which crops in an area are changed each year. This helps maintain the fertility of the soil.

crustaceans A group of aquatic animals with a hard outside covering. They are often included with MOLLUSKS in the group of "shellfish."

crystal A form of solid in which the constituent atoms or molecules are arranged in a very regular, repeating pattern.

cytoplasm In a prokaryotic cell, the entire contents of the cell contained within the plasma membrane. In a eukaryotic cell, the region of the cell lying within the plasma membrane but exterior to the nucleus.

D

Dalton, John An English chemist and physicist (1766–1844) who introduced the theory that matter is made up of atoms.

Darwin, Charles An English naturalist (1809–1883) who developed a theory of EVOLUTION.

deforestation The process by which land is cleared of forests.

density Mass per unit volume, often expressed as grams per milliliter.

dictyosome The *Golgi apparatus* of a cell, which serves as a collecting and packaging center for secretions.

diffusion The spontaneous movement of dissolved molecules from an area where they are in high concentration to an area where they are in lower concentration. This process requires no energy and, in living organisms, often takes place across semi-permeable membranes.

distillation The purification of a liquid substance by heating it until it vaporizes and then cooling it to cause it to condense into liquid again.

DNA Deoxyribonucleic acid; a large, helical, double-stranded molecule in which the chromosomes code hereditary information.

dorso-ventral An adjective referring to a back-to-front plane.

Down syndrome A genetic disorder of humans caused by the presence of an extra, third, copy of chromosome 21. Individuals with Down syndrome are mentally retarded and possess characteristic physical features.

E

eclipse The obscuring of a celestial body that takes place when one celestial object moves in front of another. When the moon comes between the earth and the sun, it casts a shadow, or *umbra,* on part of the earth. Since during this time the sun cannot be seen on that part of the earth, this is known as a *solar* eclipse. When the earth comes between the sun and the moon, it casts a shadow on the moon. Since the moon cannot be seen during this time, this is called a *lunar* eclipse.

Einstein, Albert A German physicist (1879-1955) who lived the last years of his life in the United States. His theories changed the field of PHYSICS. He, more than any other scientist, was responsible for nuclear fission.

electron A negatively charged particle in the atom that moves in an orbit around the NUCLEUS of the atom.

electronics The study of the motion or movement of free electrons and ions, and the application of these phenomena to radio and television.

electrophoresis A biochemical technique used to separate organic molecules such as PROTEINS or NUCLEIC ACIDS out of a mixture. In the most commonly used version of the technique, a sample of the mixture is placed at one end of a slab-shaped gel immersed in a buffer solution. An electric current is passed through the chamber containing the gel, and molecules travel through the gel for different distances according to their size and electrical charge. Each type of molecule accumulates in its own distinct zone or band in the gel.

element One of more than 100 known basic substances. These substances and their combinations make up all matter as far as is known.

embryology The study of development of organisms from the time of conception.

energy The capacity to do work.

enthalpy The heat content of the reactants and products in a chemical reaction.

entropy The concept that closed system move to a state of maximum disorder unless energy enters from the surroundings.

enzyme An organic CATALYST; specific types of proteins produced by cells that govern or otherwise affect all biological reactions. *Exoenzymes* act outside the cells that produce them, and *endoenzymes* act within the cells that produce them. Enzymes are sensitive to the pH and temperature of their environment, and deviations from the optimal pH and temperature for an enzyme will lessen its activity. The maintenance of optimal internal environments for enzymes is a major objective of HOMEOSTASIS.

erg A unit of work or energy.

erythrocytes Red blood cells.

eugenics A science that deals with the improvement of hereditary qualities of a race or breed.

eukaryote An organism characterized by cells containing a true or visible nucleus.

evaporation The process by which liquids change to gases.

evolution, theory of Usually refers to Darwin's theory that changes occur in populations because natural selection favors the survival of those organisms best fitted for their environment.

exergonic reaction Downhilll reaction whose products have less energy than the reactant.

experiment A test to see if an idea is true or false.

F

Fahrenheit The system of measurement of temperature generally used in the United States. It was developed by Gabriel Fahrenheit (1686–1736), a German scientist. On the Fahrenheit scale, 32 degrees is the freezing point of water, 212 degrees is the boiling point of water, and 98.6 degrees is the average temperature of the human body. Another widely used temperature measurement is the CELSIUS scale.

Faraday, Michael An English physicist and chemist (1791–1867) who developed the first dynamo and discovered that a magnet could induce an electric current in a conductor such as metal.

fertility The ability to reproduce. *See* REPRODUCTION.

force That which stops or creates motion, or changes the velocity of motion.

friction The resistance created to the movement of an object when it rubs or collides with other objects.

fungi A group of organisms, typically SAPROTROPHIC (or *parasitic*), many of which have a MYCELIUM. A few fungi, such as yeasts, do not have a mycelial body. *See* SAPROTROPH.

G

galaxy A grouping of stars. Our sun is a star in the galaxy called the *Milky Way.*

Galileo An Italian astronomer and physicist (1564–1642) who made many contributions to science. He discovered that objects of different weights and shapes fall to the ground at the same rate of speed, attracted by GRAVITY. He was a strong believer in COPERNICUS' theory that the earth moved in space and was persecuted for this belief.

gene A hereditary determinant consisting of a segment of a DNA molecule that contains the coded information necessary for assembling a specific type of protein molecule. Each gene occupies a fixed locus on a specific CHROMOSOME, enabling the transmission of hereditary determinants from one generation to the next.

genetic code The sequence of NUCLEOTIDE bases in a molecule of DNA or RNA that, when translated by a RIBOSOME, specifies the sequence of AMINO ACIDS in a PROTEIN molecule.

genetic disorder A metabolic disorder caused by inheritance of a damaged gene, a damaged chromosome, or an incorrect number of chromosomes. *See* DOWN SYNDROME, HEMOPHILIA, PHENYLKETONURIA, and SICKLE CELL ANEMIA.

genetics The study of HEREDITY, or the manner in which hereditary traits are passed on from one generation to the next.

genome The genetic makeup of an individual; the genotype.

geology The study of the formation, structure, and history of the earth.

geriatrics The science of the diseases of aged persons.

glycolysis The anaerobic decomposition of a glucose into two molecules of pyruric acid, with the production of two net molecules of ATP.

golgi Storage organelle in plant and animal cells.

gravitation The tendency of objects in space to move towards each other.

gravity The force of attraction between two bodies. It is the force that causes objects to fall to earth.

Greenhouse Effect A warming of the earth caused by blankets of carbon dioxide and other gases that prevent sun rays that strike the surface from radiating back into space.

H

habitat The immediate surroundings or environment in which a particular species may live.

half-life The length of time required for the degradation to another substance of half the molecules in an amount of radioactive substance. The half-lives of radioactive ISOTOPES of elements can be used to date material containing radioactive substances. An example is the carbon-14 dating of living material.

Harvey, William An English physician and anatomist (1578–1657) who discovered how the blood moves through the body.

heat A form of energy.

heat shock proteins A protein that prevent the denaturation of other proteins when the temperature rises to abnormally high levels.

hemoglobin A type of protein molecule that is bright red in color and binds reversibly to oxygen. It is carried within ERYTHROCYTES, enabling them to transport oxygen.

hemophilia A GENETIC DISORDER caused by inheritance of a defective gene for one of the proteins that act as blood-clotting factors. The blood of affected persons fails to clot normally if an injury occurs, creating the danger that they might bleed to death from even minor wounds.

heredity The transmission of traits from generation to generation.

homeostasis The maintenance of internal balance by a living organism

hormone A chemical regulator of many bodily activities. A hormone is produced by an endocrine gland.

hydridoma Recombinant (mixed) cells produced by the fusion of plasma cells and cancer cells.

hydrogen The chemical element with the smallest atom. It exists as a gas and is common in nature. Hydrogen is important to living organisms because it is a constituent of water and most organic coinpounds.

hypha A mycelial thread; one of the "strands" making up a MYCELIUM, which is a fungus body.

hypothesis An unproven explanation of something that has happened or might happen.

I

immunity Resistance to a particular disease or condition. *See* ACTIVE IMMUNITY, ACQUIRED IMMUNITY. NATURAL IMMUNITY, PASSIVE IMMUNITY.

immunization The process of making one immune, usually by the giving of antigens to induce active immunity via the production of antibodies.

immuno-globulins Antibodies.

indicator A substance whose color is sensitive to the hydrogen-ion concentration of the solution to which it is added.

inorganic An adjective meaning "not organic" and applying to any atom other than carbon or to a molecule not containing carbon. *See* ORGANIC.

insecticides Chemical combinations used to destroy or control harmful insects.

interferon An antiviral agent secreted by cells under attack from viruses.

interstellar An adjective meaning "between stars."

ion An atom or radical that has acquired a positive charge by giving up or losing electron(s), or a negative charge by gaining electron(s).

ionic bond A type of chemical bond created by one atom giving up all electron or electrons to another atom to achieve the maximum number of electrons in the outer orbit of each atom. Ionic compounds will separate in water to yield IONS. This process is called *dissociation.*

isotopes Atoms that belong to the same chemical element but have a different atomic mass.

K

Kepler, Johannes A German astronomer (1571–1630) who made important discoveries about the orbits of planets.

kinetic energy Energy that is in motion. The energy of a boulder tumbling down a mountainside is an example of kinetic energy. *See* POTENTIAL ENERGY.

Koch, Robert A German doctor (1843–1910) who studied bacteria. He and LOUIS PASTEUR are considered the founders of the science of bacteriology.

Krebs Cycle The aerobic breakdown of glucose, forming carbon dioxide and water.

L

Lamarck, Chevalier de A French naturalist (1744–1829) who developed a theory of evolution. *See* DARWIN.

Lavoisier, Antoine A French chemist (1743–1794) who made important discoveries concerning combustion, the conservation of matter, and the role of oxygen in respiration.

leukocytes White corpuscles or blood cells.

lever system An assemblage of parts for moving weight with the least amount of applied force. A lever system consists of a rigid rod *(lever)* applied to the weight, a point of balance *(fulcrum)* for the lever, and mechanical force applied to the lever. These parts can be arranged in different ways to accommodate different amounts of weight, but a common principle of all lever systems is that the greatest amount of lifting force is achieved when the point at which the force is applied is farthest from the fulcrum.

light year The distance light travels in one year.

Linnaeus, Carolus A Swedish botanist (1707–1778) best known for developing a system of nomenclature for animals and plants.

lipopaly-saccharide A polymer of simple sugars linked with fragments of lipid molecules.

litmus An indicator used to test for pH, or hydrogen-ion concentration. Litmus is red in acid solutions and blue in basic solutions.

litmus paper A special paper containing LITMUS, used by chemists to test for acid and alkali.

lunar An adjective referring to the moon. A lunar eclipse is an eclipse of the moon. *See* SOLAR; ECLIPSE.

lymph A colorless fluid that has passed from the bloodstream through capillary walls into the intercellular spaces; lymph is collected by lymph ducts and returned to the bloodstream.

lysosomes Cellular organelles that contain powerful hydrolytic enzymes.

M

mandible The lower jaw bone of vertebrates; the mouth part of arthropods that resembles a jaw and functions in biting.

marine An adjective meaning "of or relating to the sea."

mechanics The study of the effects of force on moving or motionless bodies; a branch of PHYSICS.

meiosis A type of cellular division that results in gametes (sex cells) or gametic nuclei. It consists of two divisions resulting in four daughter cells, and the number of chromosomes in each daughter is reduced by half (haploid).

membrane A thin sheet forming a semipermeable boundary, as in (1) a thin layer of soft tissue; (2) the outer boundary of a cell (*see* PLASMA MEMBRANE); or (3) the enclosing boundary of an intracellular structure (for example, the nucleus).

Mendel, Gregor Johann An Austrian monk and botanist (1822–1884) who made important discoveries concerning HEREDITY.

metabolism A cellular process by which food is oxidized for the release of energy and utilized for synthesis of cellular materials.

meteorology A science that studies the weather and the atmosphere.

microscope An instrument that produces a magnified image of an object. Light microscopes use a set of glass lenses to focus and magnify rays of light that either pass through or bounce off the object. Electron microscopes use magnetic lenses and beams of electrons to produce more sharply focused and highly magnified images than can be produced with a light microscope.

mineral An INORGANIC substance that occurs naturally in rocks or soil. Minerals such as calcium, sodium, potassium, and zinc are used by living organisms in various metabolic processes.

mitochondrion The cellular organelle of EUKARYOTES in which cellular oxidation (*cellular respiration*) generates energy.

mitosis A type of cellular division that results in exact duplicates of the parent cell, as in asexual reproduction or growth. It consists of one division resulting in two daughter cells, and the number of chromosomes in each daughter is the same as in the parent (diploid).

molecule The smallest unit into which a compound can be divided and still retain its original properties. Molecules are made up of atoms.

mollusks Animals of the phylum *Mollusca*, characterized by a *mantle*, a *radula*, and a *muscular foot*. Some mollusks are aquatic, like the octopus, clam, and oyster. Others are terrestrial, like the snail and slug.

mutation A stable and abrupt change in a gene, and thus in the trait the gene determines, that is transmitted from generation to generation.

mutualism A symbiotic relationship of mutual benefit to its partners.

mycelium A mass of fungal threads or hyphae, composing the fungus body.

N

natural immunity Immunity or resistance to disease with which a person is born.

nebula A cloudy and gaseous mass found in INTERSTELLAR space.

nephron A functional unit of the kidney, consisting of Bowman's capsule with its glomerulus, and the associated ducts and convoluted tubules, with their capillaries.

neutron A small particle that is part of the atom and has no electrical charge. *See* ELECTRON and PROTON.

Newton, Isaac An English mathematician and natural philosopher (1642–1727) who made major discoveries in astronomy and PHYSICS. His most important work was his study of GRAVITATION and OPTICS.

nonpolar compound A substance in which the electromagnetic charge of each molecule is balanced so that there is no positively or negatively charged end to the molecule. Oils and fats are examples. *See* POLAR and SOLUBLE.

norepinephrine A biogenic amine derivative of tyrosine that serves as a neurotransmitter in central nervous system and the peripheral nervous system.

nuclear An adjective referring to the NUCLEUS of the atom or of a cell.

nuclear fission The splitting of an atom in order to produce energy.

nuclear fusion The joining together of lightweight atoms resulting in the release of energy.

nucleic acid DNA and RNA; the nucleic acids code and transcribe information about heredity.

nucleolus A separate area within the NUCLEUS in which RNA is synthesized.

nucleotide The "building unit" of NUCLEIC ACIDS, consisting of a sugar (ribose or deoxyribose), a phosphate, and a base (a purine or a pyrimidine).

nucleus The center core of an object, as (1) the center of an atom, containing protons and neutrons; or (2) the regulatory center of a cell of an organism.

O

observatory A specially constructed building containing one or more telescopes for observation of the heavens.

ohm A unit for measuring electric resistance.

oncogen specific genes that initiate malignancies.

optics The study of light and its effects, a branch of PHYSICS.

orbit The route that an object in space (such as the moon) takes around another body (such as the earth).

organ A structure consisting of several different types of TISSUE combined into a single unit. A single organ can perform one or more major functions and is usually linked with other organs to form a *system.*

organelle An intracellular structure that performs a major function for the cell; the cellular equivalent of an organ.

organic Characteristic of, pertaining to, or derived from organisms; an adjective referring to living things or organisms.

organism A living thing, such as a human, a plant, or an animal.

osmosis The movement of water across a semipermeable membrane.

oxidation Any chemical reaction that results in a molecule losing an electron, losing a hydrogen atom, or gaining an oxygen atom.

oxide A compound made of oxygen and another element.

P

parasitism A symbiotic relationship in which one organism (*parasite*) lives on and at the expense of another (*host*).

passive Immunity (usually temporary) imparted without the person's body acting in its immunity build-up; the immunity is imparted by the administration of foreign antibodies.

Pasteur, Louis A French chemist (1822–1895) who made major discoveries in chemistry and biology, especially in the control of many diseases. He and ROBERT KOCH were the founders of the science of bacteriology.

pasteurization The heating of milk, or some other beverage, to a certain temperature for a definite period of time to destroy certain pathogens without changing the flavor or quality of the beverage.

PCR Polymerase chain reaction is an invitro technique for the rapid reproduction of many copies of DNA segments.

peptide bond A chemical bond that joins two amino acid by connecting the carbohl group of one amino acid and the amino group of the other.

peptidoglycan A substance in bacterial cell walls made of polypeptide-linked carbohydrates.

pH A symbol used in expression of acidity or alkalinity. It denotes the negative logarithm of the concentration of hydrogen ions in gram atoms per liter.

phagotroph An organism that feeds on other organisms, usually while they are still alive, by engulfing them to allow digestion and absorption to take place within the body.

phenyike-tonuria (PKU) A GENETIC DISORDER caused by inheritance of a damaged gene for the enzyme that converts excess molecules of the AMINO ACID phenylalanine to the AMINO ACID tyrosine. High levels of phenylalanine and phenylketones, molecules intermediate between phenylalanine and tyrosine, accumulate in the blood of the affected person unless dietary intake of phenylalanine is severely restricted. Untreated PKU in infants results in severe brain damage and mental retardation.

physics The study of matter and energy, and their interactions.

phytogeo-graphic map A map showing plant life.

Planck, Max A German physicist (1858–1947) who did notable work in thermodynamics; the "father of quantum physics."

planet A large body that moves around the sun. The earth is a planet.

plankton A group of sea life—both plant and animal—that drifts with tides and currents.

plasma The liquid portion of the blood in which proteins and other substances are dissolved.

plasma membrane The cell membrane, the living covering of the cell.

plasmid Small circular DNA molecules in bacterial cells capable of self-duplication often different genes are inserted.

plastids Cellular organelles that are found in plant cells and may contain pigments. The types of plastids are: (1) *chloroplasts,* which contain the chlorophyll and carotenoid pigments and which are green; (2) *chromoplasts,* which contain carotenoid pigments and range in color from yellow to brown; and (3) *leucoplasts,* which are colorless.

polar compound A substance in which the electromagnetic charge of each molecule is unevenly distributed so that the molecule is positively charged on one end and negatively charged on the other end. Water is an example. *See* NONPOLAR COMPOUND and SOLUBLE.

potential energy Energy that is available for use. The energy of a boulder balanced on a mountainside is an example of potential energy. It becomes *kinetic energy* when the boulder begins to roll.

precipitation The settling out of particles suspended in liquid. Precipitation can be the result of a chemical reaction in which dissolved reactants form an insoluble product. Material that settles out of a suspension is a *precipitate.*

Priestley, Joseph The English chemist (1738–1804) who discovered oxygen, though the element was named and its importance first recognized by LAVOISIER.

primeval An adjective meaning "the first" or "early."

prokaryote An organism characterized by cells not containing a true or definite NUCLEUS surrounded by a nuclear membrane.

protein A complex organic compound consisting of AMINO ACIDS.

proton A positively charged particle found in the nucleus of atoms.

protoplasm An outdated term for the living substance within a cell. Current terminology divides cellular content into CYTOPLASM and *nucleoplasm* (material within the nuclear membrane).

protoplast The entire cellular contents, surrounded by and including the cell membrane. The cell wall and/or capsule are not a part of the protoplast.

R

radical A group of atoms that carries a charge and stays together as a unit during chemical reactions or in solutions, such as the nitrate ion and the sulfate ion.

radio astronomy The study of radio waves received from outer space.

reduction Any chemical reaction that results in a molecule gaining an electron, gaining a hydrogen atom, or losing an oxygen atom.

regeneration The ability of an organism to regrow pairs of itself after an injury.

replication The process by which DNA duplicates itself for distribution to daughter nuclei during mitosis and/or meiosis.

reproduction The process by which organisms create offspring of their own species.

respiration In cells, the oxidation of food for the release of energy; in aerobes, the intake of oxygen and the release of carbon dioxide.

restriction fragment A piece of DNA produced by breaking a large piece of DNA at specific points with restriction enzymes extracted from bacteria.

retrovirus An RNA virus that produces new DNA from its RNA, as catalized by the enzyme reverse transcriptase.

RFLP Restriction fragment length polymorphism; differences in the lengths of RESTRICTION FRAGMENTS seen when DNA from different individuals is exposed to the same set of restriction enzymes. Using RFLP's to determine the identity of a person with DNA obtained from blood or other bodily materials is often referred to as "DNA fingerprinting." RFLP's can also be used to diagnose the presence of genetic disorders resulting from damaged genes.

ribosome An intracellular structure consisting of RNA and protein whose function is to provide a site for the TRANSLATION phase of protein synthesis.

RNA Ribonucleic acid; a large, helical, single-stranded molecule whose different types perform various tasks in the process of protein synthesis.

S

salinity The degree of SALT present. Usually refers to the amount of salt in a fluid.

salt A substance formed when an acid is mixed with a base.

saprotroph An organism feeding on dead organic matter, usually digesting the food externally and absorbing the digested material into its body.

satellite An object that orbits around a planet, such as a moon. In recent years, the earth has had several man-made satellites.

serotonin A biogenic amine derivative of tryptophan that serves as a neurotransmitter in the central nervous system.

serum The fluid portion of blood plasma after clotting.

sickle cell anemia A GENETIC DISORDER caused by inheritance of a damaged gene for two of the four PROTEIN subunits of the HEMOGLOBIN molecule. The defective hemoglobin molecules stick to one another, forming clusters that distort the shape of the ERYTHROCYTES, reducing their ability to transport oxygen. Defective erythrocytes can also burst or clog capillaries.

slime mold Large amoeboid protozoans that form spores similar to those of fungi.

solar An adjective referring to the sun. A solar eclipse is an eclipse of the sun. See LUNAR; ECLIPSE.

solar system The sun, planets, satellites, and asteroids.

soluble The ability of a substance to mix completely with a liquid at the molecular level such that no particles of any kind are visible in the mixture. The substance must be compatible with the liquid; nonpolar substances will not dissolve in polar liquids or the reverse. Dissolved substances will often be able to pass through semipermeable membranes. *See* NONPOLAR COMPOUND, POLAR COMPOUND, SOLUTE, and SOLUTION.

solute The substance dissolved in a fluid to form a solution. *See* SOLUTION, SOLUBLE, and SOLVENT.

solution A solution is a type of mixture formed when one substance mixes completely with a liquid at the molecular level. For example, when sugar (POLAR COMPOUND) is mixed with hot water (also a POLAR COMPOUND), the result is a solution. *See* SOLUTE, SOLVENT, and SOLUBLE.

solvent The fluid in which a solute is dissolved to form a SOLUTION. *See* SOLUBLE.

sonic An adjective referring to sound.

spawn Eggs of certain aquatic animals. Also used as a verb meaning "to lay eggs." Both forms are usually used in connection with fish.

stimulus Any change in the external or internal environment of a living organism. Many stimuli cause a change in the organism's activity (response). For example, if a person has not eaten for some time, the smell of the food might make his mouth water. The stimulus is the sudden presence of food (detected by smell); the response is secretion of saliva.

sublimation The transformation of a substance from a solid directly to a gaseous state without passing through a liquid state when warmed.

substratum A layer lying beneath the top layer (geology); the surface of a medium on which microorganisms grow (biology); a material or compound on which enzymes act (biology). Also called the *substrate.*

supersonic An adjective meaning "faster than sound."

suspension A type of mixture in which large particles are mixed with a liquid and remain mixed only as long as they are agitated. The particles in a suspension will settle out if not continuously agitated. An example is the suspension of blood cells in the plasma of blood. Particles in suspension will not pass through a semipermeable membrane. *See* COLLOID and SOLUTION.

symbiosis A relationship between two different species living together. The relationship may be PARA SITISM, MUTUALISM, or COMMENSALISM.

synergism A phenomenon in which the total is greater than the sum of the individual parameters.

T

theory An explanation of natural events based on hypotheses confirmed by testing.

thermodynamics The study of heat and energy flow.

tissue A group of similar CELLS specialized to perform a single task. When different tissues are combined, they are arranged in sequential layers. *See* ORGAN.

transcription The formation of messenger RNA from the coded DNA.

transduction The passage of genetic material from one bacterial cell to another by means of viral parasites called *phages.*

transformation The passage of genetic material from one bacterium to another through the medium in which they are growing.

translation The formation of proteins from amino acids by the use of the coded information in the messenger RNA.

translocation The movement of materials throughout a plant.

U

unicellular An adjective meaning "one-celled." *See* CELL.

universe All things that exist in space, taken as a whole.

V

valence The number of electrons that can be accepted by, given up by, or shared by an atom or RADICAL. Positive valence numbers indicate electrons that can be given up to or shared with another atom or radical; negative valence numbers indicate electrons that can be accepted from another atom or radical. The positive and negative valences of reactants must balance for a chemical reaction to happen.

vapor The gaseous phase of a substance that is usually in a liquid state. Vaporization (*evaporation*) of water or another liquid is accomplished by heating the liquid.

vascular tissue Tissue used to transport materials in multicellular organisms. In higher animals, blood is vascular tissue; in higher plants, xylem and phloem are vascular tissues.

vector An organism, usually an arthropod, that carries and transmits pathogens from one animal to another.

velocity The rate of motion of one object relative to another object.

Vesalius, Andreas A Flemish anatomist (1514–1564) who studied the body. His discoveries were so important that he is often referred to as "the father of anatomy." *See* ANATOMY.

virus An obligate intracellular parasite consisting essentially of a nucleic acid surrounded by a protein coat.

vitamin An organic substance other than an ENZYME that is necessary for the proper maintenance of a metabolic process. A vitamin deficiency will cause metabolic dysfunction and an over all decline in health. Animals, including humans, must get their vitamins from the food they eat.

volt The practical unit of measurement of electric potential and electromotive force.

W/X/Y/Z

water table The level nearest to the surface of the ground where water is found.

work The result of energy expenditure. Common examples of work are movement, chemical reactions, and changes from one physical state to another.

yeast A unicellular nonmycelial fungus. Some yeasts are of commercial importance in brewing and baking industries.

zoology The study of animals. The science is a branch of BIOLOGY.

PHYSICAL SCIENCES TESTS ANSWER SHEET

TEST 1: PHYSICAL SCIENCES

1. Ⓐ Ⓑ Ⓒ Ⓓ
2. Ⓐ Ⓑ Ⓒ Ⓓ
3. Ⓐ Ⓑ Ⓒ Ⓓ
4. Ⓐ Ⓑ Ⓒ Ⓓ
5. Ⓐ Ⓑ Ⓒ Ⓓ
6. Ⓐ Ⓑ Ⓒ Ⓓ
7. Ⓐ Ⓑ Ⓒ Ⓓ
8. Ⓐ Ⓑ Ⓒ Ⓓ
9. Ⓐ Ⓑ Ⓒ Ⓓ
10. Ⓐ Ⓑ Ⓒ Ⓓ
11. Ⓐ Ⓑ Ⓒ Ⓓ
12. Ⓐ Ⓑ Ⓒ Ⓓ
13. Ⓐ Ⓑ Ⓒ Ⓓ
14. Ⓐ Ⓑ Ⓒ Ⓓ
15. Ⓐ Ⓑ Ⓒ Ⓓ
16. Ⓐ Ⓑ Ⓒ Ⓓ
17. Ⓐ Ⓑ Ⓒ Ⓓ
18. Ⓐ Ⓑ Ⓒ Ⓓ
19. Ⓐ Ⓑ Ⓒ Ⓓ
20. Ⓐ Ⓑ Ⓒ Ⓓ
21. Ⓐ Ⓑ Ⓒ Ⓓ
22. Ⓐ Ⓑ Ⓒ Ⓓ
23. Ⓐ Ⓑ Ⓒ Ⓓ
24. Ⓐ Ⓑ Ⓒ Ⓓ
25. Ⓐ Ⓑ Ⓒ Ⓓ
26. Ⓐ Ⓑ Ⓒ Ⓓ
27. Ⓐ Ⓑ Ⓒ Ⓓ
28. Ⓐ Ⓑ Ⓒ Ⓓ
29. Ⓐ Ⓑ Ⓒ Ⓓ
30. Ⓐ Ⓑ Ⓒ Ⓓ
31. Ⓐ Ⓑ Ⓒ Ⓓ
32. Ⓐ Ⓑ Ⓒ Ⓓ
33. Ⓐ Ⓑ Ⓒ Ⓓ
34. Ⓐ Ⓑ Ⓒ Ⓓ
35. Ⓐ Ⓑ Ⓒ Ⓓ
36. Ⓐ Ⓑ Ⓒ Ⓓ
37. Ⓐ Ⓑ Ⓒ Ⓓ
38. Ⓐ Ⓑ Ⓒ Ⓓ
39. Ⓐ Ⓑ Ⓒ Ⓓ
40. Ⓐ Ⓑ Ⓒ Ⓓ
41. Ⓐ Ⓑ Ⓒ Ⓓ
42. Ⓐ Ⓑ Ⓒ Ⓓ
43. Ⓐ Ⓑ Ⓒ Ⓓ
44. Ⓐ Ⓑ Ⓒ Ⓓ
45. Ⓐ Ⓑ Ⓒ Ⓓ
46. Ⓐ Ⓑ Ⓒ Ⓓ
47. Ⓐ Ⓑ Ⓒ Ⓓ
48. Ⓐ Ⓑ Ⓒ Ⓓ
49. Ⓐ Ⓑ Ⓒ Ⓓ
50. Ⓐ Ⓑ Ⓒ Ⓓ
51. Ⓐ Ⓑ Ⓒ Ⓓ
52. Ⓐ Ⓑ Ⓒ Ⓓ
53. Ⓐ Ⓑ Ⓒ Ⓓ
54. Ⓐ Ⓑ Ⓒ Ⓓ
55. Ⓐ Ⓑ Ⓒ Ⓓ
56. Ⓐ Ⓑ Ⓒ Ⓓ
57. Ⓐ Ⓑ Ⓒ Ⓓ
58. Ⓐ Ⓑ Ⓒ Ⓓ
59. Ⓐ Ⓑ Ⓒ Ⓓ
60. Ⓐ Ⓑ Ⓒ Ⓓ
61. Ⓐ Ⓑ Ⓒ Ⓓ
62. Ⓐ Ⓑ Ⓒ Ⓓ
63. Ⓐ Ⓑ Ⓒ Ⓓ
64. Ⓐ Ⓑ Ⓒ Ⓓ
65. Ⓐ Ⓑ Ⓒ Ⓓ

TEST 2: PHYSICAL SCIENCES

1. Ⓐ Ⓑ Ⓒ Ⓓ
2. Ⓐ Ⓑ Ⓒ Ⓓ
3. Ⓐ Ⓑ Ⓒ Ⓓ
4. Ⓐ Ⓑ Ⓒ Ⓓ
5. Ⓐ Ⓑ Ⓒ Ⓓ
6. Ⓐ Ⓑ Ⓒ Ⓓ
7. Ⓐ Ⓑ Ⓒ Ⓓ
8. Ⓐ Ⓑ Ⓒ Ⓓ
9. Ⓐ Ⓑ Ⓒ Ⓓ
10. Ⓐ Ⓑ Ⓒ Ⓓ
11. Ⓐ Ⓑ Ⓒ Ⓓ
12. Ⓐ Ⓑ Ⓒ Ⓓ
13. Ⓐ Ⓑ Ⓒ Ⓓ
14. Ⓐ Ⓑ Ⓒ Ⓓ
15. Ⓐ Ⓑ Ⓒ Ⓓ
16. Ⓐ Ⓑ Ⓒ Ⓓ
17. Ⓐ Ⓑ Ⓒ Ⓓ
18. Ⓐ Ⓑ Ⓒ Ⓓ
19. Ⓐ Ⓑ Ⓒ Ⓓ
20. Ⓐ Ⓑ Ⓒ Ⓓ
21. Ⓐ Ⓑ Ⓒ Ⓓ
22. Ⓐ Ⓑ Ⓒ Ⓓ
23. Ⓐ Ⓑ Ⓒ Ⓓ
24. Ⓐ Ⓑ Ⓒ Ⓓ
25. Ⓐ Ⓑ Ⓒ Ⓓ
26. Ⓐ Ⓑ Ⓒ Ⓓ
27. Ⓐ Ⓑ Ⓒ Ⓓ
28. Ⓐ Ⓑ Ⓒ Ⓓ
29. Ⓐ Ⓑ Ⓒ Ⓓ
30. Ⓐ Ⓑ Ⓒ Ⓓ
31. Ⓐ Ⓑ Ⓒ Ⓓ
32. Ⓐ Ⓑ Ⓒ Ⓓ
33. Ⓐ Ⓑ Ⓒ Ⓓ
34. Ⓐ Ⓑ Ⓒ Ⓓ
35. Ⓐ Ⓑ Ⓒ Ⓓ
36. Ⓐ Ⓑ Ⓒ Ⓓ
37. Ⓐ Ⓑ Ⓒ Ⓓ
38. Ⓐ Ⓑ Ⓒ Ⓓ
39. Ⓐ Ⓑ Ⓒ Ⓓ
40. Ⓐ Ⓑ Ⓒ Ⓓ

PHYSICAL SCIENCES TESTS

TEST 1: PHYSICAL SCIENCES

65 QUESTIONS • TIME—65 MINUTES

Directions: Read each question carefully and consider all possible answers. When you have decided which choice is best, blacken the corresponding space on your answer sheet. There is only one best answer for each question.

1. Oxygen gas can be obtained in appreciable quantities by heating all of the following *except*

   (A) H_2O
   (B) H_2O_2
   (C) HgO
   (D) PbO_2

2. All of the reactions between the following pairs will produce hydrogen *except*

   (A) copper and hydrochloric acid
   (B) iron and sulfuric acid
   (C) magnesium and steam
   (D) sodium and alcohol

3. When hydrochloric acid is added to sodium sulfite and the gas that is formed is bubbled through barium hydroxide, the salt formed is

   (A) $BaCl_2$
   (B) $BaSO_3$
   (C) NaCl
   (D) NaOH

4. If 3480 calories of heat are required to raise the temperature of 300 grams of a substance from 50°C to 70°C, the substance would be:

   Use the formula: c = Q/MDT

   c = specific heat

   Q = number of calories

   M = mass

   T = temperature

Substances	Specific Heat
(A) ethyl alcohol	0.581
(B) aluminum	0.214
(C) liquid ammonia	1.125
(D) water	1.0

5. Ozone is a molecular variety of

   (A) oxygen
   (B) chlorine
   (C) hydrogen
   (D) sulfur

6. If a eudiometer tube is filled with 26 milliliters of hydrogen and 24 milliliters of oxygen and the mixture exploded, which of the following would remain uncombined?

   (A) 2 milliliters hydrogen
   (B) 14 milliliters hydrogen
   (C) 23 milliliters hydrogen
   (D) 11 milliliters oxygen

7. The gas resulting when hydrochloric acid is added to a mixture of iron filings and sulfur is

   (A) H_2S
   (B) SO_2
   (C) SO_3
   (D) H_2

8. Calculate the time required for 100 milligrams of I^{131} (dissociation constant, K = 0.086625) to decay to 50 milligrams. Use the formular K = $0.693/t\frac{1}{2}$

   (A) 0.5 days
   (B) 0.4 days
   (C) 64 days
   (D) 8 days

9. What is the percentage composition of oxygen in a mole of glucose ($C_6H_{12}O_6$)?

   (C = 12, H = 1, O = 16)

   (A) 53
   (B) 35
   (C) 6
   (D) 20

10. In sulfuric acid the valence number of sulfur is

    (A) plus 2
    (B) minus 2
    (C) minus 4
    (D) plus 6

11. The boiling points of the following gases are as follows: argon, –185.7°C; helium, –268.9°C; nitrogen, –195.8°C; oxygen, –183°C. In the fractional distillation of liquid air, the gas that boils off last is

    (A) argon
    (B) helium
    (C) nitrogen
    (D) oxygen

12. The chemical reaction: $2Zn + 2HCl = 2ZnCl + H_2$ is an example of

    (A) double displacement
    (B) synthesis
    (C) analysis
    (D) single displacement

13. When carbon dioxide gas is bubbled through water in a test tube, the product is

    (A) ozone
    (B) methane
    (C) hydrogen peroxide
    (D) carbonic acid

14. Bronze is an alloy of copper and

    (A) iron
    (B) lead
    (C) zinc
    (D) tin

15. Which of the following substances will raise the pH of a solution of hydrochloric acid?

    (A) NaCl
    (B) H_2CO_3
    (C) $NaHCO_3$
    (D) HNO_3

16. An oxide whose water solution will turn litmus red is

    (A) BaO
    (B) Na_2O
    (C) P_2O_3
    (D) CaO

17. A compound that has a high heat for formation is normally

    (A) easy to form from its elements and easy to decompose
    (B) easy to form from its elements and difficult to decompose
    (C) difficult to form from its elements and easy to decompose
    (D) difficult to form from its elements and difficult to decompose

18. A solution of zinc chloride should *not* be stored in a tank made of aluminum because

    (A) aluminum will displace the zinc in the zinc chloride solution
    (B) the zinc would become contaminated
    (C) the chloride ion will react with impurities in the solution
    (D) the two metals will react to produce an undesirable compound

19. The valence number of sulfur in the ion SO_4^{-2} is

    (A) –2
    (B) +2
    (C) +6
    (D) +10

20. The chemical name for sulfuric acid is

    (A) hydrogen sulfate
    (B) hydrogen sulfite
    (C) sulfur trioxide
    (D) hydrogen sulfide

21. The number of grams of hydrogen formed by the action of 6 grams of magnesium (atomic weight = 24) on an appropriate quantity of acid is

    (A) 0.5
    (B) 8
    (C) 22.4
    (D) 72

22. The symbol for two molecules of hydrogen is

    (A) H_2
    (B) 2H
    (C) 2H+
    (D) $2H_2$

23. The formula for sodium bisulfate is

    (A) $NaBiSO_4$
    (B) $NaHSO_4$
    (C) NaH_2SO_4
    (D) Na_2SO_4

24. The law of multiple proportions was first proposed by

    (A) Dalton
    (B) Davy
    (C) Priestley
    (D) Williams

25. One liter of a certain gas, under standard conditions, weighs 1.16 grams. A possible formula for the gas is

    (A) C_2H_2
    (B) CO
    (C) NH_3
    (D) O_2

26. Which of the following compounds would be classified as a salt?

    (A) Na_2CO_3
    (B) $Ca(OH)_2$
    (C) H_2CO_3
    (D) CH_3OH

27. Of the following, which is an aromatic compound?

    (A) benzene
    (B) ethyl alcohol
    (C) iodoform
    (D) methane

28. Of the following, which is a monosaccharide?

    (A) dextrose
    (B) glycogen
    (C) lactose
    (D) sucrose

29. Fats belong to the class of organic compounds represented by the general formula, RCOOR', where R and R' represent hydrocarbon groups; therefore, fats are

    (A) ethers
    (B) soaps
    (C) esters
    (D) lipases

30. Oil and water are immiscible (do not mix) because

    (A) oil is polar and water is polar
    (B) oil is nonpolar and water is polar
    (C) water is nonpolar and oil is polar
    (D) water is nonpolar and oil is nonpolar

31. The chemical bond that forms between the carboxyl (RCOOH) group of one amino acid and the amino (RC-NH2) of another is a/an

    (A) peptide bond
    (B) coordinate covalent
    (C) ionic bond
    (D) high energy bond

32. Two atoms have the same atomic number but different atomic weights (masses); therefore, these atoms are

    (A) compounds
    (B) isotopes
    (C) neutrons
    (D) different elements

33. Commercial bleach has the formula

    (A) $CaCl_2$
    (B) CaOCL
    (C) $CaOCl_2$
    (D) $Ca(ClO_3)_2$

34. In forming an ionic bond with an atom of chlorine, a sodium atom will

    (A) receive one electron from the chlorine atom
    (B) receive two electrons from the chlorine atom
    (C) give up one electron to the chlorine atom
    (D) give up two electrons to the chlorine atom

35. Which of the following is an example of a transition element? (Refer to the periodic table on page 201.)

    (A) aluminum
    (B) astatine
    (C) nickel
    (D) rubidium

36. A gas lighter than air is

    (A) CH_4
    (B) C_6H_6
    (C) HCl
    (D) N_2O

37. Of the following gases, which is odorless and heavier than air?

    (A) CO
    (B) CO_2
    (C) H_2S
    (D) N_2

38. In a volume of air at a pressure of one atmosphere at sea level, the partial pressure of oxygen is equal to

(A) 593 mm of mercury
(B) 494 mm of mercury
(C) 380 mm of mercury
(D) 160 mm of mercury

39. The complete combustion of carbon disulfide would yield carbon dioxide and

(A) sulfur
(B) sulfur dioxide
(C) sulfuric acid
(D) water

40. Alcoholic beverages contain

(A) wood alcohol
(B) isopropyl alcohol
(C) glyceryl alcohol
(D) ethyl alcohol

41. Of the following compounds, which is more difficult to decompose than lithium fluoride?

(A) lithium bromide
(B) lithium chloride
(C) lithium iodide
(D) none of the above

42. Which of the following molecules would be classified as a ketone?

(A)
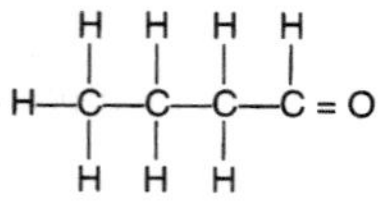

(B)
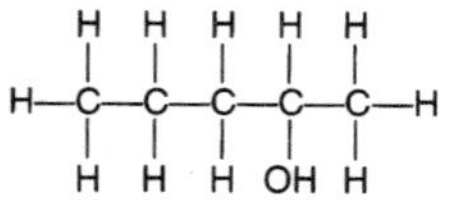

(C)
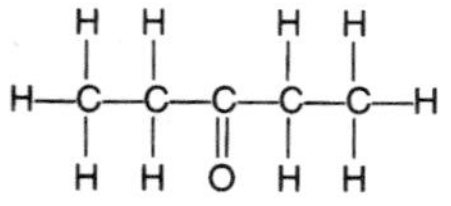

(D)
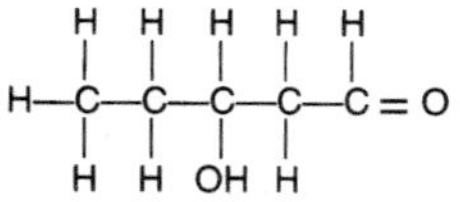

43. The periodic table (page 201) shows that the atomic number of fluorine is 9; this indicates that the fluoride atom contains

(A) nine neutrons in its nucleus
(B) nine protons in its nucleus and nine electrons in orbit around the nucleus
(C) a total of nine protons and neutrons
(D) a total of nine protons and electrons

44. The elements in group Zero of the periodic table (page 201) are considered inert gases because each has electrons in its outer-most energy level

(A) 8
(B) 7
(C) 4
(D) 2

45. Of four copper wires with the following dimensions, which one would have the greatest resistance to electrical current?

(A) length of one meter and diameter of 4 millimeters
(B) length of two meters and diameter of 8 millimeters
(C) length of one meter and diameter of 8 millimeters
(D) length of two meters and diameter of 2 millimeters

46. The general formula for an organic acid is

(A) RCOOR
(B) ROH
(C) ROR
(D) RCOOH

47. An example of a strong electrolyte is

(A) sugar
(B) calcium chloride
(C) glycerin
(D) boric acid

48. A lead ball, a wooden ball, and a styrofoam ball, all with a mass of one kilogram, are thrown at a wall 16 meters away, and all of them hit the wall in two seconds. Which ball will strike the wall with the greatest force?

(A) lead ball
(B) wooden ball
(C) styrofoam ball
(D) all strike with the same force

49. Identify the two atoms with the same number of electrons in their outer-most energy level (use the periodic table on page 201)

(A) Na/K
(B) K/Ca
(C) Na/Mg
(D) Ca/Na

50. When copper oxide is heated with charcoal, the reaction that occurs is an example of

(A) reduction only
(B) oxidation only
(C) both oxidation and reduction
(D) neither oxidation nor reduction

51. Nonmetal oxides, when dissolved in water, tend to form

(A) acids
(B) bases
(C) salts
(D) hydrides

52. The most important of the greenhouse gases contributing to global warning and altering the marine carbon cycle is

(A) SO_2
(B) CO
(C) NH_3
(D) CO_2

53. The best reducing agent is

(A) mercury
(B) hydrogen
(C) copper
(D) carbon dioxide

54. For a solution of H_2SO_4, the equivalency between molarity and normality would be (H = I, S = 32, O = 16)

(A) IM = IN
(B) IM = 2N
(C) IN = 2M
(D) IM = 0.5N

55. The test for a nitrate results in

(A) a precipitate
(B) a red flame
(C) a brown ring
(D) litmus turning blue

56. A solution that contains all the solute it can normally dissolve at a given temperature must be

(A) concentrated
(B) supersaturated
(C) saturated
(D) unsaturated

57. The oxides of barium and sulfur combine to form

(A) a salt
(B) a base
(C) an acid
(D) an anhydride

58. A pencil is dropped into a glass half filled with water. It looks as if the end that is underwater does not match up with the end that is in the air. This optical illusion is the result of

(A) diffraction of light
(B) convection of light
(C) diffusion of light
(D) refraction of light

59. The reason why concentrated H_2SO_4 is used extensively to prepare other acids is that concentrated sulfuric acid

(A) is highly ionized
(B) is an excellent dehydrating agent
(C) has a high specific gravity
(D) has a high boiling point

60. In a 0.001 M solution of HCI, the pH is:

(A) 2
(B) –3
(C) 1
(D) 3

61. By use of the periodic table on page 201, it can be determined that the atoms with the greatest affinity would be

(A) Na and Cl
(B) K and F
(C) Na and F
(D) K and Cl

62. Using the periodic table on page 201, determine if the valence of a sodium ion is:

(A) +1
(B) 0
(C) -1
(D) +12

63. The portion of an atom directly involved in the ionic bonding is/are

(A) protons in the nucleus
(B) neutrons in the nucleus
(C) electrons in the outer energy level
(D) electrons in the inner-most energy level

64. If the toxicity of a pesticide or a herbicide is in the range that a few drops could be fatal, the label should read

(A) Warning
(B) Caution
(C) Avoid
(D) Danger

65. A tornado passed over a house and destroyed it, primarily because

(A) the air pressure over the roof was lower than the pressure in the attic
(B) the air pressure over the roof was equal to the pressure in the attic
(C) the air pressure over the roof was higher than the pressure in the attic
(D) none of the above

TEST 1: PHYSICAL SCIENCES ANSWER KEY

1. **A**
2. **A**
3. **B**
4. **A**
5. **A**
6. **D**
7. **D**
8. **D**
9. **A**
10. **D**
11. **D**
12. **D**
13. **D**
14. **D**
15. **C**
16. **C**
17. **B**
18. **A**
19. **C**
20. **A**
21. **A**
22. **D**
23. **B**
24. **A**
25. **A**
26. **A**
27. **A**
28. **A**
29. **C**
30. **B**
31. **A**
32. **B**
33. **C**
34. **C**
35. **C**
36. **A**
37. **B**
38. **D**
39. **B**
40. **D**
41. **D**
42. **C**
43. **B**
44. **A**
45. **D**
46. **D**
47. **B**
48. **D**
49. **A**
50. **C**
51. **A**
52. **D**
53. **B**
54. **B**
55. **C**
56. **C**
57. **A**
58. **D**
59. **D**
60. **B**
61. **B**
62. **A**
63. **C**
64. **D**
65. **A**

TEST 1: PHYSICAL SCIENCES EXPLANATORY ANSWERS

1. **(A)** Heating water to a very high temperature (about 2000°C) will cause only about two percent of the water to dissociate into hydrogen and oxygen—a not very economical or efficient way of obtaining oxygen. Electrolysis will decompose water at a much lower temperature. Hydrogen peroxide and many oxides or metals can be decomposed more easily by heating alone.

2. **(A)** All acids contain hydrogen, which may be displaced by certain metals. However, copper ranks below hydrogen in the *electromotive* or *activity series. Activity* refers to the activity of a metal in displacing hydrogen in acids and in water. Metals ranked below hydrogen in the series do not displace hydrogen from acids.

3. **(B)** Hydrochloric acid can react with sodium hydrogen sulfite to produce sodium chloride, water, and sulfur dioxide. Sulfur dioxide can react with barium hydroxide to form barium sulfite and water.

4. **(A)** The problem can be solved by using the formula: $c = Q/MDT$. Inasmuch as Q, M, D, and T are given, no algebraic rearrangement is necessary to solve for c (specific heat).

5. **(A)** Ozone is a molecule variety of oxygen in which three oxygen atoms bond to make one molecule of O_3. Ozone is easily formed by the action of electricity or ultraviolet radiation on the normal diatomic form (O_2) of oxygen.

6. **(D)** Since there is twice as much hydrogen as there is oxygen in a molecule of water (H_2O), the 26 milliliters of hydrogen could combine with only 13 milliliters of oxygen. This would leave 11 of the 24 milliliters of oxygen uncombined.

7. **(D)** Hydrochloric acid reacts with active metals, forming the chloride of that metal and releasing hydrogen.

8. **(D)** Inasmuch as 100 milligrams will decay to 50.0 milligrams, the formula: $K = 0.693/t_{\frac{1}{2}}$ should algebraically rearranged to solve for $t_{\frac{1}{2}}$ (half-life). To do this, multiple both sides by $t_{\frac{1}{2}}$ and divide both sides by K.

9. **(A)** The percentage composition of oxygen in 1 mole of glucose (180 grams) is calculated as follows

Atomic Mass		# Atoms
Carbon 12 ×	6	= 72
Hydrogen 1 ×	12	= 12
Oxygen 16 ×	6	= 96
		180

% Comp. $O_2 = 96/180 \times 100$

10. **(D)** Sulfuric acid (H_2SO_4) contains four oxygens, each with a valence of minus 2; the total negative valence is 8. Each of the two hydrogens has a valence of plus 1; the total hydrogen valence equals plus 2. Therefore, sulfur would need a valence of plus 6 to equalize the positive and negative valences in the molecule.

11. **(D)** Fractional distillation can be used to separate the components of a mixture; the mixture is heated to boiling and the temperature is constantly raised. The component with the lowest boiling point vaporizes first; the component with the highest boiling point will vaporize last. Liquid oxygen has a boiling point of −183°C, which is higher than the boiling point of the other components. So oxygen will boil off last.

12. **(D)** Only one substance (HCl) is dissociated. Therefore, the reaction is a single displacement.

13. **(D)** Free carbon dioxide and water will combine to produce carbonic acid (H_2CO_3). Different reactants would be needed to produce ozone (O_3), methane (CH_4), or hydrogen peroxide (H_2O_2).

14. **(D)** Bronze is an alloy of copper and tin. An alloy is made by mixing two or more different metals while they are in molten condition and then allowing the mixture to cool and solidify. The metals remain completely dissolved in one another after solidification, forming a homogenous substance with properties different from any of the constituent metals in their pure forms. For example, bronze is both harder and more resistant to corrosion than pure copper.

15. **(C)** $NaHCO_3$ will combine with HCl (hydrochloric acid) to form NaCL and H_2CO_3. H_2CO_3 is a weaker acid than HCl; therefore the net effect of replacing HCl molecules with H_2CO_3 molecules is to raise the pH of the solution. In causing this reaction, $NaHCO_3$ is acting as a *buffer*. NaCl is a salt that will have no effect on the pH of an HCl solution. The other two compounds are acids that would lower the pH of the solution further if added.

16. **(C)** Litmus turns red in acid solution. When phosphorus trioxide dissolves in water, phosphorus acid is formed. The other compounds named form alkaline solutions.

17. **(B)** The amount of heat absorbed or lost in a chemical reaction is the heat of reaction. It equals the heat content of the product(s) minus the heat content of the reactants. Heat is absorbed if more energy is stored in the products than in the reactants, and released if more energy is stored in the reactants than in the product(s). In the formation of a compound, the heat of reaction is called the heat of formation for that compound. A compound with more energy stored in it than is in the reactants (a compound with a high heat of formation) can be formed but is difficult to decompose.

18. **(A)** Zinc is ranked above the others but below aluminum in the activity series of metals. The higher the metal is ranked, the more energetic it is in its displacement ability. Therefore, aluminum could displace zinc in the zinc chloride solution, forming aluminum chloride. So one should not store zinc chloride in a tank made of aluminum because aluminum will displace the zinc in the zinc chloride.

19. **(C)** The four oxygen ions would have a total *valence* of negative 8 (each oxygen, minus 2); if the valence of the SO_4 ion is minus 2, the remaining valence of 6 would be matched to a positive valence. Therefore, sulfur must have a valence of plus 6.

20. **(A)** Sulfuric acid is composed of two hydrogen ions and one sulfate ion. The chemical formula is H_2SO_4; thus, its chemical name is hydrogen sulfate.

21. **(A)** Magnesium has an atomic weight of 24; hydrogen's atomic weight is approximately 1. As is true with many metals, magnesium can react with an acid, such as hydrochloric acid, to produce hydrogen ($Mg + 2HC1 \rightarrow MgCl_2 + H_2$). The amount of hydrogen produced can be calculated by using the following equation:

$$\frac{\text{amount Mg}}{\text{atomic weight}} = \frac{\text{amount } H_2 0}{\text{atomic weight}}$$

Substituting in the equation, we get the following:

$$\frac{6 \text{ grams}}{24} = \frac{x \text{ grams}}{2} = 0.5 \text{ grams}$$

In working out problems in which one must determine the amount of a substance derived from a given reaction, the chemical equation must be balanced and molecular weight must be used. Thus, for diatomic gases, use twice the atomic weight.

22. **(D)** Hydrogen in molecular form is composed of two atoms; the formula for one molecule of hydrogen is H_2. Therefore, two molecules of hydrogen is $2H_2$.

23. **(B)** Sodium bisulfate differs from sodium sulfate in having hydrogen as a part of the molecule. Since the sulfate ion has a valence of minus 2, and hydrogen and sodium each have a valence of plus 1, then one sodium and one hydrogen must be in combination with the sulfate ion. ($NaHSO_4$)

24. **(A)** John Dalton discovered the facts concerning chemical combinations and suggested that materials are composed of atoms. He first proposed the law of multiple proportions in 1804. The law states that in a series of compounds formed by the same two or more elements, given a definite weight for one element, the different weights of the second element are in the ratio of small whole numbers to the weight of the first. For example, in sulfur dioxide (SO_2), the weight of oxygen is 32 (atomic weight = 16); in sulfur trioxide (SO_3), the weight of oxygen is 48. Therefore, the ratio is 2:3.

25. **(A)** One mole *(gram molecular weight)* of a gas occupies 22.4 liters under standard conditions. Since one liter of the gas in question is $\frac{1}{22.4}$ of one mole, it is $\frac{1}{22.4}$ of its gram molecular weight. Knowing this, the molecular weight of the gas can be determined. We can set up the equation as follows:

$$\frac{x \text{ unknown gram mol. wt.}}{22.4 \text{ liters}} = \frac{1.16 \text{ grams}}{1 \text{ liter}}$$

Solving the equation, we get 26 as one gram molecular weight. C_2H_2 (ethane) fits this weight. ($C = 12 \times 2$, $H = 1 \times 2$)

26. **(A)** A salt is an ionic compound that yields ions other than hydrogen ions (H^+) or hydroxide ions (OH^-) when it dissociates. Na_2CO_3 will yield neither when it dissociates into 2 Na^+ + $CO_3{}^{2-}$. $Ca(OH)_2$ will yield hydroxide ions when it dissociates, and H_2CO_3 will yield hydrogen ions. CH_3OH is a covalent compound and will not dissociate.

27. **(A)** *Aromatic* compounds are so named because of their odors; they occur in ring structure (molecular structure) and include such compounds as benzene, tolulene, and xylene.

28. **(A)** Dextrose is a *monosaccharide,* in that its molecule is composed of one "sugar unit" and cannot be hydrolyzed into simpler sugars. Lactose and sucrose are *disaccharides,* each yielding two monosaccharides by hydrolysis. Glycogen is a *polysaccharide* composed of a large number of monosaccharide units.

29. **(C)** Fats are glyceryl esters that, when hydrolized, yield glycerol and fatty acids. The cleavage of the ester linkage upon hydrolysis can be achieved by saponification, acids, superheated steam, or lipase, which is an enzyme that hydrolyzes fats. This may be represented as follows:

$$RCOOR' + H_2O \rightarrow RCOOH + R'OH$$

30. **(B)** As a rule, polar liquids dissolve in polar liquids and non-polar liquids dissolve in non-polar liquids. Water is polar and oil is non-polar. Therefore, oil and water are immiscible.

31. **(A)** The bond formed between the carboxy (RCOOH) and the amino ($R - (NH_2)$) of two amino acid is a peptide bond, and the resulting compound is a depeptide.

32. **(B)** The *atomic number* represents the number of protons within the nucleus of an atom; since an atom is electrically neutral, the atomic number also equals the number of electrons of the atom. The atomic weight (*mass number*) represents the total number of nuclear particles (protons plus neutrons). All atoms of the same element have the same number of protons and, thus, the same atomic number. If the number of neutrons differ, the mass number is different; these atoms, then, are *isotopes.*

33. **(C)** Calcium hypochlorite ($CaOCl_2$) is effective as a bleach due to the oxidizing activity of hypochlorous acid (HClO), which is produced from calcium hypochloride and from which chlorine gas can also be liberated.

34. **(C)** An ionic bond will form between two atoms if the loss of electrons from one to the other will result in both atoms having a completely filled outer electron orbit. A sodium atom has 11 electrons, two in its first electron orbit, eight in its second electron orbit, and one in its outer electron orbit. The loss of one electron from the sodium atom will eliminate its outer electron orbit, making the next orbit in toward the nucleus the new outer orbit with a full complement of eight electrons. A chlorine atom has 17 electrons, two in its first electron orbit, eight in its second, and seven in its outer electron orbit. The acceptance of one electron by the chlorine atom will fill its outer electron orbit with the full complement of eight electrons.

35. **(C)** Transition elements are characterized by atoms in which the two highest energy levels are incompletely filled. Consulting the periodic table indicates that of those listed, only nickel is a transition element (see the periodic table on page 201).

36. **(A)** Air is a mixture of gases; the gases present in greatest quantity are nitrogen and oxygen. The quantity of nitrogen in the air is almost four times that of oxygen. Of the compounds listed, methane (CH_4), with a molecular weight of 16, is lighter than air.

37. **(B)** Carbon dioxide is an odorless gas that is heavier than air. It is colorless, soluble in water, and about one and one-half times as heavy as air. It is a component of air, but comprises less than 0.05 percent of it.

38. **(D)** The pressure of a gas is measured by the distance in millimeters that it will lift a column of mercury in a barometer. The pressure of air is 760 mm of mercury at sea level. Air is a mixture of gases, and the pressure of each gas in such a mixture, referred to as its *partial pressure,* is equal to its concentration in the mixture. Oxygen constitutes 21% of air; therefore, its partial pressure at sea level would be 21% of 760 mm of mercury of pressure, or 160 mm of mercury.

39. **(B)** Carbon disulfide is highly inflammable; its complete combustion yields carbon dioxide and sulfur dioxide.

$CS_2 + 3O_2 \rightarrow CO_2 + 2SO_2$

40. **(D)** The ethyl alcohol of alcoholic beverages is produced by fermentation of monosaccharides; usually yeast is used to supply the enzymes needed, and the fermentation process supplies the energy needed by the yeast.

$C_6H_{12}O_6 \rightarrow 2C_2H_5OH + 2CO_2$

41. **(D)** Because fluorine is extremely active, it does not occur freely in nature but combines naturally with all elements except the inert gases, forming very stable compounds. Because it is a vigorous oxidizing agent, it cannot be oxidized by other oxidizing agents. For these reasons, fluorides are more difficult to decompose than are compounds of the other halogens.

42. **(C)** A *ketone* is an organic molecule that contains a carbon atom double-bonded to an oxygen atom located between two other carbon atoms 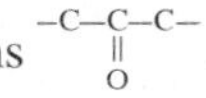. The compound shown in choice (A) is an aldehyde because it contains a terminal CHO 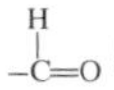 group. The compound shown in choice (B) is an alcohol because it contains an OH group bonded to a carbon. The compound shown in choice (D) is both an alcohol and an aldehyde.

43. **(B)** The atomic number indicates the number of *protons* (positively charged particles) within the nucleus of an atom. Since an atom is electrically neutral, the number of protons is equal to the number of *electrons* (negatively charged particles) of the atom. Thus, the atomic number can indicate the number of electrons as well as the number of protons.

44. **(A)** The atoms of each element in group Zero have 8 electrons in the outer-most energy level. The elements have atoms with complete octets of electrons, producing stable energy levels.

45. **(D)** The resistance of a metal wire is directly proportional to its length and inversely proportional to its cross-sectional area. The longest wire with the smallest diameter will therefore have the greatest resistance.

46. **(D)** An *organic* acid is characterized by the presence of a carboxyl group (—COOH), or

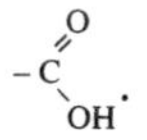

R represents a hydrocarbon group or a radical derived from a hydrocarbon.

47. **(B)** An *electrolyte* is a substance that forms an electrically conducting solution when dissolved in water. This is caused by the dissociation of the compound into ions, or *ionization*. The greater the ionization, the stronger the electrolyte. Calcium chloride ionizes to a much greater degree than the others and is a strong electrolyte.

48. **(D)** Force is a function of mass, distance, and acceleration. Since all of these factors are equal in this example, all of the balls strike the wall with the same force. The force is calculated as $1 \text{ kg} \times 16 \text{ m}/(2 \text{ sec})^2 = 4$ newtons.

49. **(A)** Sodium (Na) and potassium (K) are both in group IA, with one electron in the outer energy level. Sodium and potassium have three and four energy levels, respectively.

50. **(C)** Charcoal is an amorphous form of carbon, and carbon can react with oxides of many metals and other substances to form CO, CO_2, and the carbides of the metals. Thus, the oxides would be reduced by the removal of oxygen, and carbon would be oxidized to carbon monoxide or carbon dioxide. So oxidation and reduction occur.

51. **(A)** Nonmetal oxides, such as oxides of sulfur, carbon, and nitrogen, can react with water to form acids. The equations below are examples:

$CO_2 + H_2O \rightarrow H_2CO_3$

$SO_2 + H_2O \rightarrow H_2SO_3$

52. **(D)** Carbon dioxide (CO^2) comprises only approximately 0.04 percent of the earth's atmospheric gases. When this percentage increases, it prevents sun rays that strike the earth from radiating back into space. This produces warning of the atmosphere and the earth's surface to cause the greenhouse effect.

53. **(B)** Although hydrogen is relatively inert at ordinary temperatures, it can combine with free oxygen, with oxygen that is in chemical

combination, with some metallic elements, and with many nonmetallic elements. The addition of hydrogen reduces a substance.

54. **(B)** A 1.0 Molar solution of a substance is prepared by dissolving 1 gram-molecular weight of solution in enough solvent to equal 1 liter of solution. A 1 normal solution is prepared by dissolving an amount of solute (gram – molecular weight/total positive valence) in enough solvent to equal 1 liter of solution. (Atomic weights H = 1.0; S = 32; O = 16). mol. wt. = 98, 98g/L = 1M 98/2 = 49g/L = 1N.

55. **(C)** The nitrate test involves the use of a sulfate, such as iron sulfate, and sulfuric acid. The nitrate and sulfate ions react, forming nitric oxide. Nitric oxide then combines with the ferrous ion to form a ferrous-nitrogen-oxygen complex, which produces a brown color.

56. **(C)** A *saturated* solution is one that is in equilibrium; a condition of equilibrium exists between the solvent and the solute, and no more of the solute can dissolve.

57. **(A)** Oxides of barium and sulfur can combine to produce barium sulfate, a salt.

$BaO + SO_3 \rightarrow BaSO_4$

58. **(D)** The optical illusion described is the result of refraction, the abrupt bending of a ray of light when it passes at an angle from a medium of one density to a medium of a different density. Air and water have very different densities, resulting in the refraction of light. Diffraction is the separation of light into bands of different wavelength, as in a rainbow. Diffusion is the scattering of light, such as the effect produced when light passes through frosted glass. Convection does not apply to light; it is the transfer of heat by circulation of air or water.

59. **(D)** Sulfuric acid has a high boiling point: 317°C. Because of this, it is not very volatile and can be used to prepare more volatile acids, such as hydrochloric and nitric acids.

$NaCl + H_2SO_4 \rightarrow NaHSO_4 + HCl$

60. **(B)** The pH of a solution is a measure of the negative logarithm of the hydrogen ion concentration (e.g. pH = $-\log[H^+]$). The H+ in question is 1×10^{-3}. Therefore, the pH = $^+3$.

61. **(B)** Reactivity of elements in group IA increases from top-to-bottom because valence electrons are progressively further from the positive charges in the nucleus of atoms. Reactivity of elements in group VIIA increases from bottom-to-top because valence electrons are progressively closer the positive charges of the nucleus.

62. **(A)** Sodium (Na) is a metal in group IA, with 1.0 electron in its outer-most shell. Its most stable configuration is achieved by donating 1.0 electron, resulting in a +1 valence.

63. **(C)** The portion of an atom directly involved in ionic bonding are the electrons in the outer energy level. The outer energy level will either gain or loose electrons in order to achieve a complete octet (eight electrons).

64. **(D)** The Federal Government requires that all pesticides have a label with a signal word. The pesticide will read DANGER (highly toxic) if only a few drops could be fatal.

65. **(A)** The circular winds that form a tornado create an area of extremely low pressure in the center. When rotating areas of low pressure move over most structures that have areas of higher air pressure, the structure explodes outward, as air is forced down a pressure gradient.

TEST 2: PHYSICAL SCIENCES

40 QUESTIONS • TIME—40 MINUTES

Directions: Read each question carefully and consider all possible answers. When you have decided which choice is best, blacken the corresponding space on your answer sheet. There is only one best answer for each question.

1. Which of the following properties is considered a physical property?

(A) flammability
(B) boiling point
(C) reactivity
(D) osmolarity

2. Which one of the following substances is a chemical compound?

(A) blood
(B) water
(C) oxygen
(D) air

3. What are the differentiating factors for potential and kinetic energy?

(A) properties—physical or chemical
(B) state—solid or liquid
(C) temperature—high or low
(D) activity—in motion or in storage

4. How many calories are required to change the temperature of 2000 grams of H_2O from 20°C to 38°C?

(A) 36 calories
(B) 24 calories
(C) 18 calories
(D) 12 calories

5. The oxidation of one gram of CHO produces four calories. How much CHO must be oxidized in the body to produce 36 calories? (CHO is a carbohydrate.)

(A) 4 grams
(B) 7 grams
(C) 9 grams
(D) 12 grams

6. What is the atomic weight of the element in the figure below?

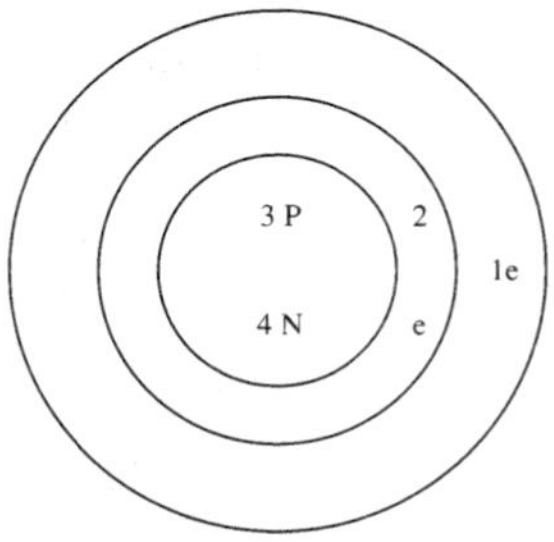

(A) 2
(B) 3
(C) 4
(D) 7

7. Which of the following kinds of radiation is most penetrating?

(A) alpha
(B) beta
(C) gamma
(D) X rays

8. I^{131} has a half-life of eight days. A 100-milligram sample of this radioactive element would decay to what amount after eight days?

(A) 50 milligrams
(B) 40 milligrams
(C) 30 milligrams
(D) 20 milligrams

9. A direct physiological effect of radiation on human tissues is

(A) impairment of cellular metabolism
(B) proliferation of white blood cells
(C) formation of scar tissue
(D) reduction of body fluids

10. What is the gram molecular weight of $C_6H_{12}O_6$? (C = 12, H = 1, O = 16)

    (A) 29 grams
    (B) 174 grams
    (C) 180 grams
    (D) 696 grams

11. Which one of the following equations is balanced?

    (A) $H_2O \rightarrow H_2 \uparrow + O_2 \uparrow$
    (B) $Al + H_2SO_4 \rightarrow Al_2(SO_4)_3 + H_2 \uparrow$
    (C) $S + O_2 \rightarrow SO_3$
    (D) $2HgO \rightarrow 2Hg + O_2 \uparrow$

12. A person with a fever would be expected to have

    (A) an increase in pulse rate
    (B) a decrease in pulse rate
    (C) no change in pulse rate
    (D) any one of the above

13. Which of the following bodily substances is a catalyst?

    (A) bile
    (B) hemoglobin
    (C) enzyme
    (D) mucus

14. In order to increase the temperature of a gas in a closed unit, it would be necessary to

    (A) increase the pressure
    (B) decrease the density
    (C) decrease the volume
    (D) increase the space

15. Which of the following equations represents an oxidation-reduction reaction?

    (A) $2Na + Cl_2 \rightarrow NaCl$
    (B) $CO_2 + H_2O \rightarrow H_2CO_3$
    (C) $HNO_3 + KOH \rightarrow KNO_3 + H_2O$
    (D) $CaO + H_2O \rightarrow Ca(OH)_2$

16. Which one of the following equations represents neutralization?

    (A) $2Na + Cl_2 \rightarrow 2NaCl$
    (B) $CO_2 + H_2O \rightarrow H_2CO_3$
    (C) $HNO_3 + KOH \rightarrow KNO_3 + H_2O$
    (D) $CaO + H_2O \rightarrow Ca(OH)_2$

17. What happens when a small amount of soap is added to hard water?

    (A) Copious suds are formed.
    (B) A scum is formed.
    (C) All sediments filter out.
    (D) Sediments diffuse equally throughout the solution.

18. A ten-percent solution of glucose will contain

    (A) 1 gram of glucose per 1000 milliliters of solution
    (B) 1 gram of glucose per 100 milliliters of solution
    (C) 1 gram of glucose per 10 microliters of solution
    (D) 10 grams of glucose per 100 milliliters of solution

Questions 19–22 refer to the diagrams below.

Each diagram represents one solution: One gram molecular weight of NaOH, one of KOH, and one of HCl, each dissolved in enough H_2O to make one liter.

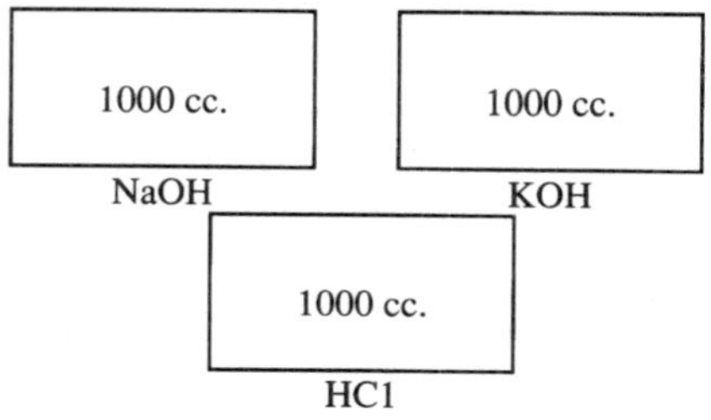

19. What is the molecular weight of NaOH? (Atomic weights: Na = 23; 0 = 16; H = 1)

    (A) 40×1
    (B) 40×10
    (C) 40×100
    (D) 40×1000

20. These are molar quantities because

    (A) their molecular weights are equal to each other
    (B) the volume for each solution is the same
    (C) each solution contains one gram molecular weight
    (D) the percentage of solute to solvent is equal in each solution

21. Identify the products of the chemical reaction between 1 cubic centimeter of KOH and 1 cubic centimeter of HCl

    (A) $K^+ + Cl_2 + 2H + OH$
    (B) $KCl + H_2 + O_2$
    (C) $K + Cl + HOH$
    (D) $KCl + H_2O$

22. CA^{++} (atomic weight 40) is bivalent; hence, one gram equivalent weighs

    (A) 40 grams
    (B) 30 grams
    (C) 20 grams
    (D) 10 grams

23. A covalent bond between two amino acid molecules can be created by

    (A) inserting a water molecule between them
    (B) removing a water molecule from them
    (C) inserting a carbon atom between them
    (D) removing a carbon atom from one of them

24. Identify those elements in the periodic table at the bottom of the page that are inert gases (refer to columns).

    (A) IA
    (B) Zero
    (C) IIIB-VIIB
    (D) VIII

25. The basic inorganic raw materials for photosynthesis are

    (A) water and oxygen
    (B) water and carbon dioxide
    (C) oxygen and carbon dioxide
    (D) sugar and carbon dioxide

26. Production of Salk vaccine against polio depended upon discovery of a method for

    (A) growing the polio virus outside the human body
    (B) killing the polio virus
    (C) observing the polio virus in the human body
    (D) producing a polio antitoxin

27. Ringworm is caused by a(n)

    (A) alga
    (B) bacterium
    (C) fungus
    (D) protozoan

28. The process responsible for the continuous removal of carbon dioxide from the atmosphere is

    (A) respiration
    (B) metabolism
    (C) oxidation
    (D) photosynthesis

IA	IIA	IIIB	IVB	VB	VIB	VIIB	VIII			IB	IIB	IIIA	IVA	VA	VIA	VIIA	Zero
H 1																H 1	He 2
Li 3	Be 4											B 5	C 6	N 7	O 8	F 9	Ne 10
Na 11	Mg 12											Al 13	Si 14	P 15	S 16	Cl 17	Ar 18
K 19	Ca 20	Sc 21	Ti 22	V 23	Cr 24	Mn 25	Fe 26	Co 27	Ni 28	Cu 29	Zn 30	Ga 31	Ge 32	As 33	Se 34	Br 35	Kr 36
Rb 37	Sr 38	Y 39	Zr 40	Nb 41	Mo 42	Tc 43	Ru 44	Rh 45	Pd 46	Ag 47	Cd 48	In 49	Sn 50	Sb 51	Te 52	I 53	Xe 54
Cs 55	Ba 56	*La 57	Hf 72	Ta 73	W 74	Re 75	Os 76	Ir 77	Pt 78	Au 79	Hg 80	Tl 81	Pb 82	Bi 83	Po 84	At 85	Rn 86
Fr 87	Ra 88	**Ac 89															

*LANTHANIDE SERIES	Ce 58	Pr 59	Nd 60	Pm 61	Sm 62	Eu 63	Gd 64	Tb 65	Dy 66	Ho 67	Fr 68	Tm 69	Yb 70	Lu 71
**ACTINIDE SERIES	Th 90	Pa 91	U 92	Np 93	Pu 94	Am 95	Cm 96	Bk 97	Cf 98	Es 99	Fm 100	Md 101	No 102	Lr 103

29. All of the following concepts in genetics were first clearly stated by Gregor Mendel *except*

(A) dominance
(B) independent assortment
(C) segregation
(D) hybrid vigor

30. The relation between termites and their intestinal protozoa is an example of

(A) trophism
(B) parasitism
(C) mutualism
(D) commensalism

31. When completed, the number of DNA base pairs comprising the human genome is expected to be approximately

(A) 10 thousand
(B) 10 million
(C) 3 billion
(D) 3 trillion

32. A completed human genomic map identifies the nucleotide sequences on the following chromosomal pairs

(A) 22 autosomes + 1 sex chromosome
(B) 48 autosomes + 1 sex chromosome
(C) 23 autosomes + 1 sex chromosome
(D) 92 autosomes + 2 sex chromosomes

33. A technique (in which a catheter is inserted into the uterus to retrieve tissue samples) for the prenatal diagnosis of genetic diseases is called

(A) amniocentesis
(B) positional cloning
(C) chorionic villus sampling (CVS)
(D) none of the above

34. Identify the correct statement about DNA fingerprinting analysis of human tissues

(A) It is effective with small samples (e.g. less than 100 microliters of blood)
(B) It produces identical bond patterns from all tissues in an individual
(C) It is effective on tissues more than 1,000 years old
(D) All of the above

35. In a DNA fingerprinting analysis of blood samples from a mother (M), a child (C), and an alleged father (F), the banding pattern in the child's blood was: 50 percent (F), 27.3 percent (M), and 22.3 percent (FM). The statistical probability that the accused man is the child's father is

(A) 50 percent
(B) greater than 50 percent
(C) less than 50 percent
(D) zero

36. Glycogenesis occurs primarily in the

(A) blood cells and spleen
(B) pancreas and gallbladder
(C) small intestines and stomach
(D) liver and muscles

37. The end-products of the Krebs Cycle are

(A) carbon dioxide and water
(B) urea and bile pigments
(C) lactic acid and pyruvic acid
(D) ketones and acetones

38. The functional unit (or nephron) of the human kidney consists of

(A) Bowman's capsule and veins
(B) Bowman's capsule, the glomerulus, and renal tubule
(C) the ureter and renal tubule
(D) the ureter, urethra, and renal tubule

39. An organ that functions both as an endocrine and an exocrine gland is the

(A) salivary gland
(B) gall bladder
(C) thyroid gland
(D) pancreas

40. Aerobic oxidation of glucose occurs in two major stages; these are

(A) glycolysis and reduction
(B) synthesis and the Krebs Cycle
(C) glycolysis and the Krebs Cycle
(D) degradation and hydrolysis

TEST 2: PHYSICAL SCIENCES ANSWER KEY

1. **B**
2. **B**
3. **D**
4. **A**
5. **C**
6. **D**
7. **C**
8. **A**
9. **A**
10. **C**
11. **D**
12. **A**
13. **C**
14. **A**
15. **A**
16. **C**
17. **B**
18. **D**
19. **A**
20. **C**
21. **D**
22. **C**
23. **B**
24. **B**
25. **B**
26. **A**
27. **C**
28. **D**
29. **D**
30. **C**
31. **C**
32. **A**
33. **C**
34. **D**
35. **B**
36. **D**
37. **A**
38. **B**
39. **D**
40. **C**

TEST 2: PHYSICAL SCIENCES EXPLANATORY ANSWERS

1. **(B)** Physical properties are those that do not involve any change in the nature or chemical composition of the substance. Heating a substance to the temperature at which it boils (its *boiling point*) will change its physical state but will not alter its chemical state.

2. **(B)** Water is a compound formed by oxygen and hydrogen in chemical combination. Blood and air are mixtures, and oxygen is an element.

3. **(D)** *Potential energy* is, in effect, energy in storage, as energy that can be released when conditions are conducive. *Kinetic energy* is energy of activity; the energy is released as the activity occurs.

4. **(A)** One calorie (kilocalorie) will raise one kilogram (1000 grams) of water one degree Celsius. It would take 18 calories to raise 1000 grams of water 18 degrees (38° – 20°), or 36 calories to raise 2000 grams of water 18 degrees Celsius.

5. **(C)** If one gram of carbohydrate produces four calories, nine grams are required to produce 36 calories. 36 calories ÷ 4 calories/ gram = 9 grams.

6. **(D)** The atomic weight (or mass number of an atom) equals the total of the number of protons and neutrons in the nucleus of the atom, or the total number of particles in the nucleus.

7. **(C)** Nearly every unstable nucleus of an atom gives off one or more of the three kinds of radiation: alpha, beta, and gamma. *Alpha* and *beta* radiation are particle emission; *gamma* rays are shortwave energy rays similar to X rays, but stronger and more penetrating. Both gamma rays and X rays are more penetrating than alpha and beta radiation.

8. **(A)** The *half-life period* can be defined as the time needed for half of a given amount of a substance to undergo spontaneous decomposition. This varies with different radioactive elements. There would be 50 milligrams left of a 100 milligram sample of material with a half-life of eight days after the eight days pass.

9. **(A)** Radiation can cause *mutations,* or genetic change. Any change in the genetic code would alter or destroy the trait associated with that particular gene. This could involve changes in enzyme produced and other factors associated with cellular metabolism.

10. **(C)** Gram molecular weight may be defined as the weight of the molecule expressed in grams. The molecular weight of glucose ($C_6H_{12}O_6$) is 180, as the following indicates: The weight of the six atoms of carbon equals 72 (6×12); twelve hydrogens weigh 12 (12×1); the weight of the six oxygens equals 96 (6×16). The total is 180; thus, the gram molecular weight of glucose is 180 grams.

11. **(D)** Equation (D) is balanced, because the amount of each substance is equal on both sides of the equation. There are two mercury atoms and two oxygen atoms on each side.

12. **(A)** A person with a fever has a higher temperature than normal. This reflects an increase in metabolic activities, since heat is given off as a waste product when energy in the form of ATP is used for metabolic purposes. Consequently, the pulse rate of a person with a fever is higher than normal because the heart is pumping blood at a greater rate so that the transport of materials like oxygen and glucose in the blood can accommodate this increased metabolic activity. Also, the circulatory system has to work harder to carry the greater amount of heat generated away from the tissues to be radiated from the surface of the body.

13. **(C)** Enzymes are called *organic catalysts,* in that they are produced by the organisms and catalyze reactions that occur within that organism. The other substances named do not function as catalysts.

14. **(A)** Gases are affected by temperature and pressure. If the gas is in a closed system, it cannot change its volume if temperature or pressure changes. Therefore, in a closed system, increasing the pressure would increase the temperature.

15. **(A)** For every oxidation, there must be a reduction. Oxidation can involve the removal of electrons, the removal of hydrogen, or the addition of oxygen; reduction, the opposite. In equation (A) metallic sodium loses an electron to become a positively charged ion; chlorine gains an electron to become a negatively charged chloride ion. Thus, sodium is oxidized and chlorine is reduced.

16. **(C)** Nitric acid reacts with the base potassium hydroxide to form potassium nitrate and water. For each hydrogen ion of the acid, there is a hydroxyl ion of the base to combine with it to form water. Therefore, neutralization occurs.

17. **(B)** Hard water contains calcium sulfate, calcium bicarbonate, or magnesium compounds. Soap is a mixture of sodium salts of organic acids that will react with these dissolved minerals. The insoluble calcium salt of the organic acid is precipitated out. This is the *scum,* or insoluble curdy material, that forms first. If enough soap is added, the soap acts as a cleansing agent after the first portion has precipitated the calcium ion.

18. **(D)** The concentration of a solution, on a percentage basis, contains a specific amount of solute in grams per 100 milliliters of solution. Thus, a ten-percent solution would have ten grams of solute per 100 milliliters of solution.

19. **(A)** The molecular weight of sodium hydroxide (NaOH) is 40×1 or 40. This can be calculated by adding the atomic weights of the atoms composing the molecule.

20. **(C)** A molar solution contains one gram molecular weight (the molecular weight of the molecule expressed in grams), or one mole per liter of solution. Therefore, each is a one-molar solution.

21. **(D)** Potassium hydroxide (KOH) and hydrochloric acid (HCl) react to form potassium chloride (KCl) and water. This is a double displacement.

$$KOH + HCl \rightarrow K^+ Cl^- + H_2O$$

22. **(C)** An *equivalent weight* of an element is that weight of the element that combines with or displaces one atomic weight of hydrogen. Since calcium has a valence of plus 2 while hydrogen has a valence of plus 1, one-half of the atomic weight of calcium will displace one atomic weight of hydrogen. Calcium has an atomic weight of 40; therefore, its equivalent weight is 20, or, expressed as grams, 20 grams. The following equation can apply:

equivalent weight = [atomic weight/valence]

23. **(B)** Two amino acid molecules can be bonded together by removing a hydrogen atom from the amino group (NH_2) of one amino acid molecule and removing a hydroxyl ion (OH^-) from the carboxyl group (COOH) of the other. The result is a molecule of water removed from the two amino acids and a covalent bond between the nitrogen atom in the amino group of one amino acid and the carbon atom in the carboxyl group of the other. This type of reaction is called *dehydration synthesis* and results in the production of water within cells that is called *metabolic water*. Creation of a bond between two amino acids can be illustrated as follows (R represents any of the 20 different side chains that can be included in amino acids):

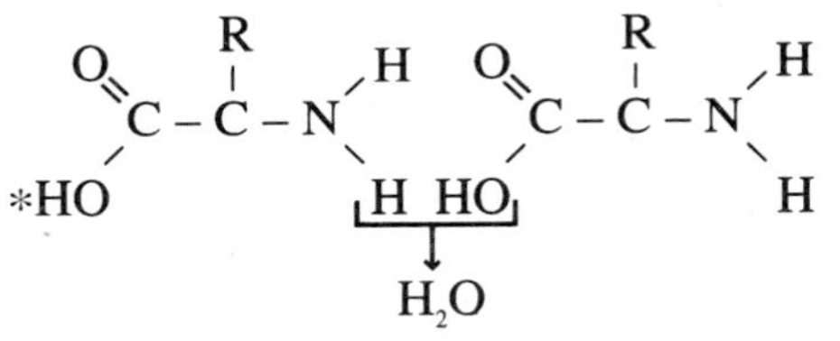

Removing this water molecule will create a bond between the nitrogen and carbon.

24. **(B)** The periodic table places elements according to similarities in properties due to the number and arrangement of electrons in the atom. Group Zero is the inert gases. Metals and nonmetals are included in the remaining groups.

25. **(B)** Carbon dioxide and water, in the presence of light and the chlorophylls, yield glucose and oxygen. The water is absorbed by the root system of green plants and translocated through xylem to the leaves and other parts, which are the photosynthetic organs. Carbon dioxide enters the plants through epidermal stomates.

26. **(A)** Salk vaccine is prepared from inactivated polio virus. Viruses are obligate intracellular parasites; therefore, a method for growing viruses outside the human body had to be discovered and refined. Viruses typically are cultured in chick embryos.

27. **(C)** Ringworm is caused by fungi known as dermatophytes. These are sometimes known as the *Tineas*.

28. **(D)** *Photosynthesis* is the process characteristic of green plants by which carbon dioxide and water react to produce glucose and oxygen. The carbon dioxide used in the process enters the tissue from the air, passing in through stomata of the epidermis; oxygen produced by the reaction passes through the stomata into the air. This process occurs only in the presence of light, and therefore continuous carbon dioxide removal occurs only in the presence of light.

29. **(D)** Mendel's Laws clearly stated the concepts of dominance and segregation (first law—Law of Segregation) and of independent assortment (second law—Law of Independent Assortment), but did not deal with the concept of hybrid vigor.

30. **(C)** Any relationship between two individual species is *symbiosis*. The word *symbiosis* means "life together." There are several kinds of symbiotic relationships, including commensalism, parasitism, and mutualism. A *mutualistic* relationship is one in which strong bonds exist between the two species, and each member benefits from the relationship. This kind of symbiotic relationship exists between termites and the protozoans (flagellates) of their intestinal tract. There is evidence that some bacteria in the termite's intestinal tract also play a role in the relationship. The flagellates and bacteria digest the cellulose that the termites consume.

31. **(C)** The Human Genome Project, which is funded by the National Institutes of Health and the Department of Energy, was initiated in 1990 and is expected to be completed (identify about 3 billion base pairs) by the beginning of the next millenium.

32. **(A)** The human genomic contains 22 pairs of autosomes and 1 pair of sex chromosomes in each somatic cell.

33. **(C)** Chorionic villus sampling (CVS) involves inserting a catheter into the uterus to take samples of the fetal chorion.

34. **(D)** DNA fingerprinting analyses produce identical band patterns from all tissues of an individual and can be done with less than 100 microliters of tissue. These techniques have been done on samples from Egyptian mummies, over 2,000 years old.

35. **(B)** All bands in the child's blood were inherited from either the father or the mother. Inasmuch as the father, in this case, produced half of the bands and contributed to an additional one-quarter of them, paternity can be assigned with high statistical confidence.

36. **(D)** *Glycogenesis* is the formation of glycogen from glucose; glycogen is the form in which carbohydrates are stored in animals. Glycogen is stored in larger quantities and more permanently in the liver; some is produced and stored temporarily in muscle.

37. **(A)** Carbon dioxide and water are the end-products of the Krebs Cycle, which is the second phase of aerobic cellular oxidation of glucose for the release of energy.

38. **(B)** The kidney has the function of filtering wastes from the blood. Each nephron performs this function; thus, it is the functional unit. Wastes and water are filtered out from the blood in the glomerulus, a mass of capillaries lying in Bowman's capsule; the water and wastes pass through the capsule wall into the renal tubule. Much of the water is reabsorbed into the bloodstream through the walls of the capillaries surrounding the loop of Henle of the renal tubule. The remaining liquid, or urine, passes into the renal pelvis, to the ureter and bladder, and is eventually eliminated through the urethra.

39. **(D)** An endocrine (or ductless) gland secretes hormone(s) directly into the bloodstream. The hormone is transported by the blood and will affect only the target tissue. An exocrine gland passes its secretion through a duct to a specific site. The pancreatic islet cells secrete the hormone, insulin; other cells of the pancreas secrete pancreatic juice, containing enzymes, through the pancreatic duct into the duodenum.

40. **(C)** In the first stage of aerobic oxidation, glucose is oxidized to pyruvic acid; this is known as glycolysis. The two pyruvates resulting from glycolysis of a molecule of glucose enter into the Krebs Cycle (Citric Acid Cycle) and are oxidized to carbon dioxide and water.

LIFE SCIENCES TESTS ANSWER SHEET

TEST 3: LIFE SCIENCES

1. Ⓐ Ⓑ Ⓒ Ⓓ	19. Ⓐ Ⓑ Ⓒ Ⓓ	37. Ⓐ Ⓑ Ⓒ Ⓓ	55. Ⓐ Ⓑ Ⓒ Ⓓ
2. Ⓐ Ⓑ Ⓒ Ⓓ	20. Ⓐ Ⓑ Ⓒ Ⓓ	38. Ⓐ Ⓑ Ⓒ Ⓓ	56. Ⓐ Ⓑ Ⓒ Ⓓ
3. Ⓐ Ⓑ Ⓒ Ⓓ	21. Ⓐ Ⓑ Ⓒ Ⓓ	39. Ⓐ Ⓑ Ⓒ Ⓓ	57. Ⓐ Ⓑ Ⓒ Ⓓ
4. Ⓐ Ⓑ Ⓒ Ⓓ	22. Ⓐ Ⓑ Ⓒ Ⓓ	40. Ⓐ Ⓑ Ⓒ Ⓓ	58. Ⓐ Ⓑ Ⓒ Ⓓ
5. Ⓐ Ⓑ Ⓒ Ⓓ	23. Ⓐ Ⓑ Ⓒ Ⓓ	41. Ⓐ Ⓑ Ⓒ Ⓓ	59. Ⓐ Ⓑ Ⓒ Ⓓ
6. Ⓐ Ⓑ Ⓒ Ⓓ	24. Ⓐ Ⓑ Ⓒ Ⓓ	42. Ⓐ Ⓑ Ⓒ Ⓓ	60. Ⓐ Ⓑ Ⓒ Ⓓ
7. Ⓐ Ⓑ Ⓒ Ⓓ	25. Ⓐ Ⓑ Ⓒ Ⓓ	43. Ⓐ Ⓑ Ⓒ Ⓓ	61. Ⓐ Ⓑ Ⓒ Ⓓ
8. Ⓐ Ⓑ Ⓒ Ⓓ	26. Ⓐ Ⓑ Ⓒ Ⓓ	44. Ⓐ Ⓑ Ⓒ Ⓓ	62. Ⓐ Ⓑ Ⓒ Ⓓ
9. Ⓐ Ⓑ Ⓒ Ⓓ	27. Ⓐ Ⓑ Ⓒ Ⓓ	45. Ⓐ Ⓑ Ⓒ Ⓓ	63. Ⓐ Ⓑ Ⓒ Ⓓ
10. Ⓐ Ⓑ Ⓒ Ⓓ	28. Ⓐ Ⓑ Ⓒ Ⓓ	46. Ⓐ Ⓑ Ⓒ Ⓓ	64. Ⓐ Ⓑ Ⓒ Ⓓ
11. Ⓐ Ⓑ Ⓒ Ⓓ	29. Ⓐ Ⓑ Ⓒ Ⓓ	47. Ⓐ Ⓑ Ⓒ Ⓓ	65. Ⓐ Ⓑ Ⓒ Ⓓ
12. Ⓐ Ⓑ Ⓒ Ⓓ	30. Ⓐ Ⓑ Ⓒ Ⓓ	48. Ⓐ Ⓑ Ⓒ Ⓓ	66. Ⓐ Ⓑ Ⓒ Ⓓ
13. Ⓐ Ⓑ Ⓒ Ⓓ	31. Ⓐ Ⓑ Ⓒ Ⓓ	49. Ⓐ Ⓑ Ⓒ Ⓓ	67. Ⓐ Ⓑ Ⓒ Ⓓ
14. Ⓐ Ⓑ Ⓒ Ⓓ	32. Ⓐ Ⓑ Ⓒ Ⓓ	50. Ⓐ Ⓑ Ⓒ Ⓓ	68. Ⓐ Ⓑ Ⓒ Ⓓ
15. Ⓐ Ⓑ Ⓒ Ⓓ	33. Ⓐ Ⓑ Ⓒ Ⓓ	51. Ⓐ Ⓑ Ⓒ Ⓓ	69. Ⓐ Ⓑ Ⓒ Ⓓ
16. Ⓐ Ⓑ Ⓒ Ⓓ	34. Ⓐ Ⓑ Ⓒ Ⓓ	52. Ⓐ Ⓑ Ⓒ Ⓓ	70. Ⓐ Ⓑ Ⓒ Ⓓ
17. Ⓐ Ⓑ Ⓒ Ⓓ	35. Ⓐ Ⓑ Ⓒ Ⓓ	53. Ⓐ Ⓑ Ⓒ Ⓓ	
18. Ⓐ Ⓑ Ⓒ Ⓓ	36. Ⓐ Ⓑ Ⓒ Ⓓ	54. Ⓐ Ⓑ Ⓒ Ⓓ	

TEST 4: LIFE SCIENCES

1. Ⓐ Ⓑ Ⓒ Ⓓ	16. Ⓐ Ⓑ Ⓒ Ⓓ	31. Ⓐ Ⓑ Ⓒ Ⓓ	46. Ⓐ Ⓑ Ⓒ Ⓓ
2. Ⓐ Ⓑ Ⓒ Ⓓ	17. Ⓐ Ⓑ Ⓒ Ⓓ	32. Ⓐ Ⓑ Ⓒ Ⓓ	47. Ⓐ Ⓑ Ⓒ Ⓓ
3. Ⓐ Ⓑ Ⓒ Ⓓ	18. Ⓐ Ⓑ Ⓒ Ⓓ	33. Ⓐ Ⓑ Ⓒ Ⓓ	48. Ⓐ Ⓑ Ⓒ Ⓓ
4. Ⓐ Ⓑ Ⓒ Ⓓ	19. Ⓐ Ⓑ Ⓒ Ⓓ	34. Ⓐ Ⓑ Ⓒ Ⓓ	49. Ⓐ Ⓑ Ⓒ Ⓓ
5. Ⓐ Ⓑ Ⓒ Ⓓ	20. Ⓐ Ⓑ Ⓒ Ⓓ	35. Ⓐ Ⓑ Ⓒ Ⓓ	50. Ⓐ Ⓑ Ⓒ Ⓓ
6. Ⓐ Ⓑ Ⓒ Ⓓ	21. Ⓐ Ⓑ Ⓒ Ⓓ	36. Ⓐ Ⓑ Ⓒ Ⓓ	51. Ⓐ Ⓑ Ⓒ Ⓓ
7. Ⓐ Ⓑ Ⓒ Ⓓ	22. Ⓐ Ⓑ Ⓒ Ⓓ	37. Ⓐ Ⓑ Ⓒ Ⓓ	52. Ⓐ Ⓑ Ⓒ Ⓓ
8. Ⓐ Ⓑ Ⓒ Ⓓ	23. Ⓐ Ⓑ Ⓒ Ⓓ	38. Ⓐ Ⓑ Ⓒ Ⓓ	53. Ⓐ Ⓑ Ⓒ Ⓓ
9. Ⓐ Ⓑ Ⓒ Ⓓ	24. Ⓐ Ⓑ Ⓒ Ⓓ	39. Ⓐ Ⓑ Ⓒ Ⓓ	54. Ⓐ Ⓑ Ⓒ Ⓓ
10. Ⓐ Ⓑ Ⓒ Ⓓ	25. Ⓐ Ⓑ Ⓒ Ⓓ	40. Ⓐ Ⓑ Ⓒ Ⓓ	55. Ⓐ Ⓑ Ⓒ Ⓓ
11. Ⓐ Ⓑ Ⓒ Ⓓ	26. Ⓐ Ⓑ Ⓒ Ⓓ	41. Ⓐ Ⓑ Ⓒ Ⓓ	56. Ⓐ Ⓑ Ⓒ Ⓓ
12. Ⓐ Ⓑ Ⓒ Ⓓ	27. Ⓐ Ⓑ Ⓒ Ⓓ	42. Ⓐ Ⓑ Ⓒ Ⓓ	57. Ⓐ Ⓑ Ⓒ Ⓓ
13. Ⓐ Ⓑ Ⓒ Ⓓ	28. Ⓐ Ⓑ Ⓒ Ⓓ	43. Ⓐ Ⓑ Ⓒ Ⓓ	58. Ⓐ Ⓑ Ⓒ Ⓓ
14. Ⓐ Ⓑ Ⓒ Ⓓ	29. Ⓐ Ⓑ Ⓒ Ⓓ	44. Ⓐ Ⓑ Ⓒ Ⓓ	59. Ⓐ Ⓑ Ⓒ Ⓓ
15. Ⓐ Ⓑ Ⓒ Ⓓ	30. Ⓐ Ⓑ Ⓒ Ⓓ	45. Ⓐ Ⓑ Ⓒ Ⓓ	60. Ⓐ Ⓑ Ⓒ Ⓓ

LIFE SCIENCES TESTS

TEST 3: LIFE SCIENCES

70 QUESTIONS • TIME—70 MINUTES

Directions: Read each question carefully and consider all possible answers. When you have decided which choice is best, blacken the corresponding space on your answer sheet. There is only one best answer for each question.

1. Diabetes mellitus initially results from

   (A) oversecretion of pancreatin
   (B) undersecretion of insulin
   (C) excessive intake of sugar
   (D) inadequate intake of fats

2. The so-called "bag of water," which breaks during labor in the pregnant female, is the

   (A) amniotic sac
   (B) yolk sac
   (C) placenta
   (D) chorionic membrane

3. Sebaceous glands are most numerous in areas where

   (A) there are small amounts of hair
   (B) there are large amounts of hair
   (C) the skin is thin
   (D) sweat glands are located

4. Hereditary determiners are found in

   (A) PKU
   (B) RNA
   (C) DNA
   (D) SMA

5. Skin color varies with the amount of

   (A) melanin
   (B) matrix
   (C) hair
   (D) keratin

6. The deciduous teeth contain no

   (A) cuspids
   (B) bicuspids
   (C) canines
   (D) incisors

7. The material covering the surface of the tooth below the gum line is

   (A) cementum
   (B) dentine
   (C) enamel
   (D) pulp

8. Hemoglobin is a molecule composed principally of

   (A) ferritin
   (B) amino acids
   (C) iron
   (D) myosin

9. The sex of the new individual is determined by

   (A) the female
   (B) the male
   (C) either the female or the male
   (D) neither the female nor the male

10. The umbilical cord is cut immediately after a baby is born because

    (A) of the need to stop circulation between the fetus and the placenta
    (B) the mother's blood will contaminate the baby's blood
    (C) the baby has less need for blood
    (D) the mother will hemorrhage

11. The major difference between plasma and blood is

    (A) cellular content
    (B) acid-base balance
    (C) anion-cation placement
    (D) solute-solvent concentrations

12. The blood cells that cause blood clotting are called

    (A) leucocytes
    (B) erythrocytes
    (C) thrombocytes
    (D) lymphocytes

13. The longest, strongest, and heaviest bone in the body is the

    (A) tibia
    (B) spinal column
    (C) femur
    (D) radius

14. Iron is needed for

    (A) development of nervous tissue
    (B) formation of red blood cells
    (C) growth of hair and nails
    (D) utilization of vitamins

15. Which of the following is necessary for digestion?

    (A) transamination
    (B) glucogenolysis
    (C) Krebs cycle
    (D) peristalsis

16. Which of the following organs is vital to life?

    (A) adrenal glands
    (B) thymus
    (C) liver
    (D) spleen

17. Gram-negative bacterial pathogens are generally more difficult to treat clinically than gram-positive due to differences in

    (A) cell wall compositions
    (B) ribosomes
    (C) nucleon regions
    (D) mesosomes

18. Three-dimensional vision is related to which of the following structures?

    (A) iris
    (B) pupil
    (C) optic chiasma
    (D) retina

19. Urea formation is the human body's method of eliminating excess

    (A) carbon
    (B) hydrogen
    (C) nitrogen
    (D) phosphorus

20. Which of the following hormones is predominant in females?

    (A) androgen
    (B) testosterone
    (C) gonadotrophin
    (D) estrogen

21. Proteins are polymers of

    (A) hydrocarbons
    (B) amino acids
    (C) heterocyclics
    (D) alcohols

22. Which one of the following statements is true?

    (A) Bone marrow produces red blood cells in the adult.
    (B) The spleen synthesizes vitamins in the child.
    (C) The liver manufactures glucose and stores bile.
    (D) The lymphatic system refines fats and stores water.

23. The most widely distributed of all tissues is

    (A) epithelial
    (B) muscle
    (C) connective
    (D) nervous

24. The chemical reaction that supplies immediate energy for muscular contractions can be summarized as

    (A) $ATP \rightarrow ADP + P$
    (B) lactic acid $\rightarrow CO_2 + H_2O$
    (C) lactic acid $\rightarrow$ glycogen
    (D) glycogen $\rightarrow$ ATP

25. The body's reaction to stress includes which of the following mechanisms?

    (A) conversion of carbohydrates into glycogen
    (B) decreased pumping action of the heart
    (C) secretion of adrenalin
    (D) pooling of blood in the veins

26. After rigorous exercise, the body is depleted of

    (A) Na and H_2O
    (B) Glucose and H_2O
    (C) H_2O and K
    (D) H_2O and colloids

27. Which of the following is related to the cause of heart disease?

    (A) absence of serum transaminase
    (B) accumulation of urea nitrogen
    (C) decreased levels of bilirubin
    (D) increased levels of blood cholesterol

28. The endocrine glands in the body have the function of

    (A) purifying the blood
    (B) regulating bodily activities
    (C) controlling the blood distribution
    (D) preventing antigenic action

29. Persons with overactive thyroids have which of the following changes in body functions?

    (A) decrease in metabolic rate
    (B) increase in metabolic rate
    (C) loss of appetite
    (D) gain in weight

30. The basic unit of the lung tissue is

    (A) lacuna
    (B) nephron
    (C) alveolus
    (D) cyton

31. Hemorrhoids, commonly called piles, affect which of the following structures?

    (A) pyloric sphincter
    (B) rectal sphincter
    (C) urethral orifice
    (D) mitral orifice

32. Before amino acids can be metabolized to release energy, which of the following must occur?

    (A) fermentation
    (B) hydrolysis
    (C) deamination
    (D) anabolism

33. A biochemical reaction, common to the digestion of carbohydrates, lipids, and proteins, is enzymatic

    (A) fermentation
    (B) deamination
    (C) glycogenolysis
    (D) hydrolysis

34. Fats yield more calories per gram and oxidize slower than carbohydrates, proteins, and nucleic acids due to excess atoms of

    (A) hydrogen
    (B) oxygen
    (C) nitrogen
    (D) phosphorus

35. In the circulatory system, oxygenated blood is pumped out of the heart from the

    (A) right ventricle
    (B) left ventricle
    (C) right atrium
    (D) left atrium

36. A person who escapes major infections and accidental death, has an enhanced probability of living to age 100 if his/her apolipoprotein (E) allelic gene combination is

    (A) E-2/E-4
    (B) E-3/E-4
    (C) E-2/E-2
    (D) E-4/E-4

37. Smooth muscle tissue is found in the

    (A) heart
    (B) kidneys
    (C) intestines
    (D) skeletal muscles

38. The exchange of gases between the respiratory system and the circulatory system is by means of the pulmonary

    (A) arteries
    (B) veins
    (C) capillaries
    (D) venules

39. In the production of monoclonal antibodies, antigens and lymphocytes from an experimental animal are fused with malignant cells to form an internseleate cell known as

    (A) hydroma
    (B) polycloma
    (C) hybridoma
    (D) none of the above

40. In systemic circulation, venous blood is different from arterial blood in that the

    (A) CO_2 concentration is lower than the O_2 concentration
    (B) CO_2 concentration is higher than the O_2 concentration
    (C) overall concentration is high and the rate of flow is low
    (D) overall concentration is low and the rate of flow is high

41. Sperm and egg cells have the haploid number of chromosomes as a result of

    (A) meiosis
    (B) cleavage
    (C) mitosis
    (D) fertilization

42. Fraternal twins develop from

    (A) one fertilized egg
    (B) two fertilized eggs
    (C) one egg fertilized by two sperms
    (D) two eggs fertilized by the same sperm

43. The term *restriction fragment length polymorphism (RFLP)* refers to differences in length between

    (A) chromosome fragments
    (B) fragments of DNA
    (C) ribosomal fragments
    (D) fragments of protein molecules

44. The "pacemaker" of the heart is located in the

    (A) left atrium
    (B) left ventricle
    (C) right atrium
    (D) right ventricle

45. Which generalization concerning sex determination is true?

    (A) The female determines the sex of the offspring
    (B) The XY chromosomes are found in the male
    (C) The sex of the offspring is first determined during maturation
    (D) There is a greater chance of getting female offspring than male offspring

46. A decrease in the number of red corpuscles would result in a corresponding decrease in the blood's ability to

    (A) transport oxygen
    (B) destroy disease germs
    (C) form fibrinogen
    (D) absorb glucose

47. Heat shock proteins (HSPs) may enable structural and functional proteins, under conditions of elevated temperatures to

    (A) expand their active sites
    (B) re-establish their molecular geometry
    (C) lower their optimal temperature
    (D) crystallize

48. In a normal person the largest part of the central nervous system is the

    (A) cerebrum
    (B) cerebellum
    (C) medulla
    (D) spinal cord

49. Which one of the following terms is *not* directly associated with the same sense organ as the three others?

    (A) stapes
    (B) cochlea
    (C) tympanic membrane
    (D) cornea

50. The effect of human activity on the earth's biodiversity has been that

    (A) more species have occupied the total available space
    (B) a decrease in biodiversity
    (C) no change in overall space-species relationship
    (D) an increase in biodiversity

51. If the order of strength of the following bases is: $HCO_3 > C_2H_3O_2 > HSO_4 > Cl$, the weakest acid is

    (A) $HCl\ (H^+ + Cl^-)$
    (B) $HC_2H_3O_2\ (H^+ + C_2H_3O_2^-)$
    (C) $H_2SO_4\ (H^+ + HSO_4^-)$
    (D) $H_2CO_3\ (H^+ + HCO_3^-)$

52. In a chemical reaction [A] and [B] combine to form [C] and [D], as expressed by the reaction [A][B] = [C][D]. Select the statement which best describes the equilibrium condition.

 (A) Reaction is shifted to the right.
 (B) Concentrations of reactants and products are constant.
 (C) Reaction is shifted to the left.
 (D) Concentration of products is greater than the concentration reactants.

53. Down syndrome is a genetic disorder caused by

 (A) an extra copy of chromosome 21
 (B) a defective gene on chromosome 21
 (C) fragmentation of one copy of chromosome 23
 (D) a missing copy of chromosome 23

54. In cellular metabolism, glycolysis

 (A) requires O_2
 (B) does not require O_2
 (C) occurs only in animal cells
 (D) produces $CO_2 + H_2O$

55. If 5×10^5 lbs of NaCl were dumped into a 0.5 acre pond, what would happen to the water concentration inside the frog's body cells?

 (A) no change
 (B) It would increase.
 (C) It would decrease.
 (D) It would approach boiling.

56. An astronaut, without a pressurized suit and with a blood pressure of 120/70, is accidentally sucked out of a spacecraft, halfway between earth and the moon. He/she would

 (A) experience a collapse of his blood vessels
 (B) rapidly develop cancer
 (C) experience an expansion of blood vessels
 (D) experience no adverse medical effect

57. Which of the following viruses have been associated with cancer in animals?

 (A) adenovirus
 (B) retrovirus
 (C) papovavirus
 (D) all of the above

58. The major contributions of whole wheat or enriched bread or cereal to the diet are

 (A) carbohydrate and vitamin B complex
 (B) protein and iron
 (C) calcium and riboflavin
 (D) protein and vitamin B complex

59. A good label for canned goods always includes

 (A) picture of product to give idea of color, size, and appearance
 (B) net contents, number of portions, and quality of product
 (C) brief but specific instructions or directions for use
 (D) brand name

60. Caloric needs are highest during

 (A) infancy
 (B) childhood
 (C) adulthood
 (D) middle age

61. Isolated genes shown to initiate malignancies are known as

 (A) carcinogens
 (B) oncogenes
 (C) prions
 (D) none of the above

62. One of the most contentious current problems relative to science ethics involves

 (A) organ transplants
 (B) blood transfusion
 (C) human embryonic stem cell research
 (D) hospitalization time

63. In the life cycle of the AIDS-causing virus (HIV), the pathogens bind to lymphocyte membrane receptors by their surface

 (A) glycoproteins
 (B) capsids
 (C) reverse transcriptase molecules
 (D) prions

64. After an AIDS virus enters a lymphocyte, it synthesizes viral DNA from a template composed of

(A) double stranded DNA
(B) double stranded RNA
(C) single stranded DNA
(D) single stranded RNA

65. In patients with cystic fibrosis, the accumulation of mucus around the membranes of cells in the lungs, liver, and pancreas has been shown to be caused by the blockage of ionic channels for

(A) CA^{++}
(B) Cl^{-}
(C) K^{+}
(D) Na^{+}

66. Choose the correct statement, relative to the distribution of sodium (Na^{+}) and potassium (K^{+}) on opposites of cell membranes.

(A) high Na^{+} outside
(B) high K^{+} outside
(C) low Na^{+} outside
(D) low K^{+} inside

67. Which of the following are requirements for cloning a gene?

(A) an enzyme to fragment DNA
(B) a vector (a bacterial plasmid or a virus)
(C) a host cell or organism
(D) all of the above

68. Small circular self-duplicating DNA molecule s found in bacterial cells are

(A) microbodies
(B) oligaproteins
(C) plasmids
(D) none of the above

69. Enzymes necessary for fragmenting genes to be cloned are

(A) restriction enzymes
(B) splicing enzymes
(C) recombinases
(D) polymerases

70. In the formation of recombinant DNA, the DNA from two different sources is spliced by an enzyme

(A) polymerase
(B) DNA ligase
(C) recombinant dehydrogenase
(D) none of the above

TEST 3: LIFE SCIENCES ANSWER KEY

1. **B**
2. **A**
3. **B**
4. **C**
5. **A**
6. **B**
7. **A**
8. **B**
9. **B**
10. **A**
11. **A**
12. **C**
13. **C**
14. **B**
15. **D**
16. **C**
17. **A**
18. **C**
19. **C**
20. **D**
21. **B**
22. **A**
23. **C**
24. **A**
25. **C**
26. **A**
27. **D**
28. **B**
29. **B**
30. **C**
31. **B**
32. **C**
33. **D**
34. **A**
35. **B**
36. **C**
37. **C**
38. **C**
39. **C**
40. **B**
41. **A**
42. **B**
43. **B**
44. **C**
45. **B**
46. **A**
47. **B**
48. **A**
49. **D**
50. **B**
51. **D**
52. **B**
53. **A**
54. **B**
55. **C**
56. **C**
57. **D**
58. **A**
59. **B**
60. **A**
61. **B**
62. **C**
63. **A**
64. **D**
65. **B**
66. **A**
67. **D**
68. **C**
69. **A**
70. **B**

TEST 3: LIFE SCIENCES EXPLANATORY ANSWERS

1. **(B)** Insulin increases the permeability of the cell membrane to glucose, thus enhancing the uptake of glucose from the blood by the cells. If insulin is deficient, glucose is not removed from the blood and utilized by the cells, resulting in an excess of glucose in the blood and leading to other symptoms of diabetes.

2. **(A)** The amnion is one of the extraembryonic structures formed during embryonic development. It surrounds the embryo and becomes filled with fluid in which the embryo floats. The amniotic fluid probably provides protection from mechanical shock for the embryo.

3. **(B)** Sebaceous glands are associated with hair follicles: the cells lining the glands form the secretion, and the entire cellular lining, plus the fatty secretion, form sebum, which is expelled into the hair follicle. Sebum serves to keep the hair and skin pliable.

4. **(C)** DNA (deoxyribonucleic acid) is found in the nucleus of each cell and "stores" genetic information, or the genetic code. DNA replicates itself before mitosis or meiosis begins, and genetic information is distributed equally to the daughter nuclei. RNA (ribonucleic acid), transcribed on DNA, translates the genetic or hereditary information.

5. **(A)** Melanin is a dark pigment found in the cells of the basal layers of the skin. Skin color varies with the size and density of the melanin particles: the more melanin present, the darker the skin.

6. **(B)** Each person has a set of 20 deciduous teeth, as contrasted to 32 permanent or nondeciduous teeth, The set of deciduous teeth contains no bicuspids, and only two molars per quadrant rather than three molars. A set per quadrant of deciduous teeth includes two incisors, one canine, and two molars; a set per quadrant of nondeciduous teeth includes two incisors, one canine, two premolars (bicuspids), and three molars.

7. **(A)** Cementum covers the surface of roots of teeth; enamel covers the surface of the crowns of teeth.

8. **(B)** The bulk of a hemoglobin molecule consists of 4 subunits, each one of which is a chain of amino acids. Iron is also present in hemoglobin but does not comprise as large a part of the entire molecule as the 4 chains of amino acids. Ferritin is an iron-containing molecule stored in the liver. Myosin is a major component of muscle cells.

9. **(B)** The XY chromosomes are found in the male, while the female carries XX. As a result of meiosis, a sperm will carry either an X or Y chromosome; all eggs will carry one X. Fertilization of an X-bearing egg by a Y-bearing sperm produces an XY zygote, which develops into a male. Fertilization of an X-bearing egg by an X-bearing sperm produces an XX zygote, which develops into a female.

10. **(A)** The fetus and the mother have independent circulatory systems, Fetal blood passing to and from the placenta by way of the umbilical blood vessels is separated from the mother's blood in the placenta by thin tissues; food, gases, and metabolic wastes can diffuse through these tissues between the two bloodstreams. After birth, the placenta's function has ended and as the baby's systems become "active," there is no longer an exchange of materials between the two blood-streams.

11. **(A)** *Plasma* is the liquid portion of the blood. *Whole blood* consists of plasma with its dissolved materials, and the blood cells.

12. **(C)** Thrombocytes disintegrate when blood flows from a blood vessel, releasing a phospholipid, thrombokinase, that acts to convert prothrombin in the plasma to thrombin. Thrombin acts enzymatically on fibrinogen in the plasma, converting it to fibrin, which is insoluble and forms a mesh trapping blood cells. This mesh is the blood clot.

13. **(C)** The femur is the thigh bone of the leg. It is the longest, strongest, and heaviest bone of the body.

14. **(B)** Iron is a part of the hemoglobin molecule, the red, oxygen-carrying pigment of red blood cells. If iron is deficient, hemoglobin cannot be produced, and the formation of red blood cells is inhibited.

15. **(D)** *Peristalsis* is the wave of muscular contractions that pushes food through the esophagus into the stomach and through the intestine. Food must reach the digestive sites, the stomach and small intestine, for digestion to occur. The other possible answers are involved in metabolic processes, not in digestion.

16. **(C)** The liver is the largest glandular organ of vertebrates and has the important function of regulating organic materials such as wastes, glucose, and proteins in the blood. It can also perform other essential functions, such as detoxifying blood by converting toxic substances into harmless wastes, fat digestion and storage functions, immune responses, and protein metabolism. It is essential for life.

17. **(A)** The cell walls of gram-negative bacteria are more complex than gram-positives—with less peptidoglycan and more lipopalysaccharides, which renders them more difficult for drugs to cross.

18. **(C)** Nerve fibers from the retina of the eye form the optic nerve of the eye; at the crossover point (*optic chiasma*), fibers from the nasal halves (inner halves) of each retina cross to the opposite side of the brain, while fibers of the temporal halves (outer halves) of each retina remain uncrossed. Thus, each optic nerve, after the chiasma, contains fibers from both retinas. This means that objects in one field of vision (either left or right) produce effects in two eyes that are transmitted to one side of the brain. In other words, the two halves of the retina of each eye are represented on opposite sides of the brain, producing a stereoscopic effect and permitting perception of depth.

19. **(C)** Many aquatic animals excrete ammonia as their nitrogenous waste, egg-laying animals excrete uric acid, and intra-uterine animals excrete urea.

20. **(D)** *Estrogen* is a complex of female sex hormones that is responsible for the appearance of secondary sex characteristics, such as widening of the pelvis, breasts, etc. Estrogen also functions in the menstrual cycle, preparing the uterus for implantation of the embryo.

21. **(B)** A *polymer* is a large, chain-like organic molecule that is formed by bonding together many smaller organic molecules of the same kind. A protein is a chain of many amino acid molecules joined to one another by peptide bonds. The amino acid molecules present and the sequence in which they are joined is considered the *primary structure* of the protein and determines its physical or chemical properties.

22. **(A)** Red blood cells are produced in the bone marrow in the adult. The other statements are incorrect as follows: vitamins typically are consumed with food (two possible exceptions); glucose is a product of digestion, and bile is stored in the gallbladder; water is a part of almost all tissues, and fats are refined by the bile from the liver.

23. **(C)** *Connective tissues* are those whose cells are not contiguous but scattered throughout a noncellular matrix. Connective tissues can bind and support other tissues; therefore, they are widely distributed. Some examples of connective tissues are blood, bone, cartilage, adipose, and tissues composing tendons or ligaments.

24. **(A)** The limited amount of ATP stored in muscle tissue supplies immediate energy for contraction when the ATP is converted to ADP. When the ATP is used up, it is recreated by energy from a reserve, creatine phosphate. When the creatine phosphate is consumed, oxidation of glucose to CO2 and water provides energy for muscle contraction and for the resynthesis of creatine phosphate. Lactic acid can form anaerobically during severe muscle exertion, and its accumulation is partly responsible for the feeling of fatigue. Lactic acid diffuses out of the muscle tissue into the bloodstream and thus to the liver, where some of it is oxidized to produce further energy, and some can be converted to glycogen for carbohydrate storage.

25. **(C)** Adrenalin, or epinephrine, secreted by the adrenal medulla, is normally released in small quantities and helps to regulate blood circulation and carbohydrate metabolism. Under stressful conditions, the adrenal medulla is stimulated to release larger amounts of adrenalin, which increases blood pressure, heart rate, carbohydrate metabolism, and conversion of glycogen to sugar, thus raising the blood sugar level, etc. This prepares the body to cope with the stressful situation. Hence, the "flight or fight" response.

26. **(A)** Exercise will cause perspiration, which evaporates from the skin. *Perspiration* is a liquid composed of water, salt, and a small amount of urea and is drawn from the bloodstream (from capillaries in the sweat glands) and released to the body surface through pores. Thus, rigorous exercise will cause the body to lose sodium (salt) and water.

27. **(D)** Cholesterol is a lipid that is insoluble in fluids such as blood; therefore, it is bound to proteinaceous carriers for transport. Evidence indicates that cholesterol is involved in the fatty deposits in arteries, even infiltrating cells and the intercellular spaces of arterial walls, if carried by certain carriers. This can lead to plaque and clot formation, blocking off the arteries and interfering with blood circulation. This same plaque and clot formation can occur in the coronary artery supplying heart muscle, causing a heart attack.

28. **(B)** The endocrine glands secrete hormones directly into the bloodstream; the hormones are transported throughout the body, but only specific "target" cells or tissues can pick up a specific hormone. Thus, the hormone may regulate cellular activities in tissues some distance from the cells that secreted it. By regulating cellular activities of tissues, hormones regulate body activities.

29. **(B)** The thyroid hormone controls the rate of cellular metabolism for the release of energy. An overactive gland secretes an excess of hormone, which will increase the metabolic rate. A deficiency of thyroid hormone causes the rate of metabolism to be lowered.

30. **(C)** The *alveolus* is a small, thin-walled sac of the lung; it is the blind end of the smallest bronchioles. Each alveolus (approximately 300 million are present in human lungs) is surrounded by, or adjacent to, small capillaries. It is here that gaseous exchange between the blood and lungs occur. Carbon dioxide passes into the alveolus from the blood, and oxygen passes from the alveolus into the bloodstream through the capillary walls.

31. **(B)** A *hemorrhoid* is a dilation of veins in the anal region. This can lead to a enlargement of tissue, especially the rectal sphincter, which is a ring-shaped muscle controlling the anal opening.

32. **(C)** The amino nitrogen must be removed from amino acids in order to give them the basic hydrocarbon skeleton similar to carbohydrates. After the amino group is removed, the resulting compounds may enter the same metabolic pathways used by carbohydrates.

33. **(D)** The chemistry of life is closely dependent upon the chemistry of water. Water, in the presence of the proper enzymes, must be added to the bonds that bind monosaccharides in carbohydrates, amino acids in proteins, and fatty acids and glycerol in fats to degrade these polymers to their subunits.

34. **(A)** Energy production, in the degradation of foods, is associated with the release of hydrogen (oxidation). The ratio of hydrogen to oxygen is significantly greater in fats than in carbohydrates and proteins.

35. **(B)** Oxygenated blood passes from the lungs to the left atrium of the heart by way of the pulmonary veins. From the left atrium blood moves to the left ventricle, from which it is pumped through the aorta to the arterial system of the body, and thus throughout the body, where oxygen is diffused into the cells and carbon dioxide is picked up by the blood. The carbon dioxide-laden blood is returned to the heart, entering the right atrium, and passing to the right ventricle. From the right ventricle, it is pumped to the lungs through the pulmonary arteries, where it becomes oxygenated again.

36. **(C)** Studies conducted by Dr. Allan Roses and D. Warren Stuttmatter at the Duke University Medical Center and reported in the Wall Street Journal (October 19, 1995) indicated that the apoliprotein (E) gene occurs as E-2, E-3, and E-4 subtypes. The potential of gene E for promoting cell maintenance and protection against Alzheimer's, heart disease, and diabetes is in order of potency of E-2 > E-3 > E-4. Therefore, E-2 is the good gene and E-4 is the bad form.

37. **(C)** The three basic kinds of muscle tissue are *smooth, skeletal*, and *cardiac*. Smooth muscle is characteristic of the digestive tract and arteries, organs not under voluntary control. Cardiac muscle is found in the heart. Skeletal muscle (striated) makes up the muscles associated with voluntary movement. The kidney is nonmuscular.

38. **(C)** Gaseous exchange between the respiratory system and the circulatory system occurs by means of the capillaries present in the lungs surrounding alveoli. These are referred to as the *pulmonary capillaries.*

39. **(C)** Thy hybridoma, formed by fusing lymphocytes with cancer cells, produces a single type of antibody. The hybridoma can be injected into a mouse or cultured, in vitro, to increase production of the single antibody type.

40. **(B)** Blood in systemic veins is returning to the right atrium of the heart from the cells of the body. Therefore, it is high in concentrations of carbon dioxide and metabolic wastes that were received from the cells as a result of cellular metabolism. Venous blood of the pulmonary system is returning to the left atrium of the heart from the lungs, where it gave up carbon dioxide to be expelled from body and acquired oxygen. Therefore, it has a higher concentration of oxygen.

41. **(A)** The first division of *meiosis* results in a reduction of the number of chromosomes because the members of each pair of chromosomes are separated from one another. Each daughter nucleus resulting from meiosis receives only one chromosome of each pair present in the parent nucleus, or one-half the number of chromosomes of the parent nucleus. Nuclei resulting from meiosis are *haploid,* as contrasted to the *diploid* condition of the parent nucleus.

42. **(B)** *Fraternal,* or nonidentical, twins result from two fertilized eggs, or *zygotes.* If two eggs are released during ovulation and both are fertilized (one sperm per egg), fraternal twins result. These twins are like ordinary siblings, whereas identical twins resulting from a single *zygote* are genetically identical.

43. **(B)** *Restriction fragment length polymorphisms* are differences in the lengths of fragments of DNA produced by exposing DNA from genetically different individuals to a bacterial restriction enzyme that cuts DNA at specific points.

44. **(C)** Specialized muscle cells, known as the "pacemaker" of the heart, make up a region of the right atrium. When these cells are excited, the atria are stimulated to contract, emptying the blood into the ventricles. Certain muscle fibers then carry the excitation stimulus, by way of the atrio-ventricular node, to muscles of the ventricles, stimulating them to contract and force blood from the heart.

45. **(B)** The XY chromosomes are found in the male, while the female carries XX. As a result of meiosis, a sperm will carry either an X or a Y chromosome; all eggs will carry an X. Fertilization of an X-bearing egg by a Y-bearing sperm produces an XY zygote, which develops into a male. Fertilization of an X-bearing egg by an X-bearing sperm produces an XX zygote, which develops into a female.

46. **(A)** Red blood cells contain the pigment hemoglobin, which has as its function the transport of oxygen. If the number of red blood cells is decreased, the ability of the blood to transport oxygen is decreased.

47. **(B)** Temperatures greater than 40°C will denature (destroy) the molecular geometry of most proteins. In many plant and animal cells, special proteins (heat shock proteins) are synthesized to prevent denaturation at these temperatures.

48. **(A)** The cerebrum is the largest division of the central nervous system of man. It originates thinking and controls learning, memory, thought, some voluntary movements, and the senses. In the animal kingdom, observations indicate that intelligence increases with cerebrum size. Man has the largest cerebrum, in proportion to body size, in the animal kingdom.

49. **(D)** The stapes, cochlea, and tympanic membrane are all parts of the ear: The *stapes* is one of the vibrating bones of the middle ear, the *cochlea* is the receptor portion of the inner ear from which electrical impulses ("messages") are transmitted to the brain through the auditory nerve, and the *tympanic membrane* is the eardrum. The *cornea,* on the other hand, is the transparent covering over the front of the lens of the eye.

50. **(B)** Human activities (e.g. agricultural and industrial) generally destroy food and alter physical conditions required to complete the life cycle in some species. The overall effect is a reduction in the total number of species that occupy a habitat.

51. **(D)** Acidity is determined by the concentration of hydrogen ion H^+s per unit of volume. Strong bases allow fewer H^+s to escape in aqueous solution than weak bases, producing weaker acids (e.g. Cl^- is a weak base, making HCl and strong acid, whereas HCO_3 is a strong base making H_2CO_3 a weak acid).

52. **(B)** The arrows directed to the right in chemical equations represent products generated from the forward reaction and those directed to the left represent reactants produced by the reverse reaction. The arrow length symbolizes the concentration of the substances on both sides of the equation.

53. **(A)** In humans and other animals, it is normal for an individual to have two copies of each type of chromosome in the nucleus of any body cell except an egg or a sperm. There are 23 different types of chromosomes in humans; therefore, the normal complement of chromosomes in human cells is 46. Individuals with Down syndrome receive an extra copy of chromosome 21 from one of their parents. They have three copies of chromosome 21 and a total of 47 chromosomes in the nuclei of their cells.

54. **(B)** In cellular metabolism, glycolysis is an anaerobic process (requires no O_2), produces reduced nicotinamide adeninedinucleotide ($NADH_2$) and small amounts of ATP, and occurs in all types of cells.

55. **(C)** Osmosis is the movement of water across cell membranes from solutions of low solute concentration to solutions with higher concentrations of solute. The salt gives the water a higher solute concentration than the frog's intracellular fluids. Therefore, the water concentration inside the cells would decrease as water flowed to the outside.

56. **(C)** The air (atmosphere) around the earth exerts a normal pressure of 760 mmHg (1.0 atmosphere). The pressure in interplanetary space is zero (a vacuum). Since the pressure inside the astronaut's blood vessels is greater than zero, the vessels would push outward.

57. **(D)** All of these viruses have been associated with cancer: adenoviruses (respiratory tract tumors), retroviruses (leukemia and AIDS), and papovaviruses (cervical cancer).

58. **(A)** Cereals (grains) are rich in certain members of the vitamin B complex; because of the starchy endosperm in seeds, cereals also are high in carbohydrates.

59. **(B)** Labels on canned goods may include a variety of information about the product, but the net contents by weight or volume and the quality should always be included. The number of portions may vary per net contents, according to the nature of the product; so knowledge of the number of servings is useful information. Other information may also be included on the label.

60. **(A)** Caloric needs vary with age as well as with physiological state, activity, and the size of the individual. Both physical and mental growth and development are more rapid during infancy and early childhood than at any other time in one's life. Therefore, more food is needed in proportion to size to provide the needed calories of energy and to provide the materials for growth. A proper diet is essential for normal development.

61. **(B)** Genes shown to cause cancerous growths are called oncogenes.

62. **(C)** Many individuals believe that the use of tissues from aborted fetuses in ethically unacceptable.

63. **(A)** The AIDS virus uses its surface glycoproteins to bind to membrane receptors of host cells, to initiate the infection by infusing viral RNA into the host cell.

64. **(D)** The AIDS virus uses an enzyme, reverse transcriptase, as the normal pattern of synthesis (using DNA as a template to produce RNA) to a reverse method (using RNA as a template to form DNA).

65. **(B)** The inability to pass Cl^- to the outside of cells in cystic fibrosis patients causes water to enter the cells by osmosis, making the intercellular mucus thicker than normal.

66. **(A)** Cell membranes maintain their high external Na^+ and high internal K^+ concentrations by using ATP to energize membrane carrier proteins that form the sodium-potassium pump. This is an active transport mechanism, which moves both ions against concentration gradients.

67. **(D)** The general procedure for cloning includes: isolating DNA plasmid from a bacterium, isolating the DNA comprising the gene of interest from a different cell type, mixing the gene of interest with the plasmid to form a hybrid type of DNA called recombinant DNA, infecting a vector (bacteria or virus) with the recombinant DNA, culturing the vector (containing the recombinant DNA) to produce many identical copies of itself (a clone)

68. **(C)** Plasmids, small, circular self-duplicating DNA molecules isolated from bacteria, are major requirements for recombinant DNA technology.

69. **(A)** The restriction enzymes recognize and fragment the DNA (at the proper location) of the genes to be cloned.

70. **(B)** The splicing of DNA from two different sources is accomplished by the enzyme, DNA ligase, which catalyzed bonding by the complementarity of base pairing.

TEST 4: LIFE SCIENCES

60 QUESTIONS • TIME—60 MINUTES

Directions: For each of the following items, select the choice which best answers the question or completes the statement. Blacken the corresponding space on your answer sheet.

1. Passage of water through the membrane of a cell is called

(A) assimilation
(B) osmosis
(C) circulation
(D) transpiration

2. The largest portion of the iron supplied to the body by foods is used by the body for the

(A) growth of hard bones and teeth
(B) manufacture of insulin
(C) development of respiratory enzymes
(D) formation of hemoglobin

3. Phenylketonuria is a genetic disorder which involves an inability of

(A) blood to clot properly
(B) one amino acid to be convened to another
(C) blood cells to carry a sufficient load of oxygen
(D) lung alveoli to stay open

4. A new drug for treatment of tuberculosis was being tested in a hospital. Patients in group A actually received doses of the new drug; those in group B were given only sugar pills. Group B represents a(n)

(A) scientific experiment
(B) scientific method
(C) experimental error
(D) experimental control

5. Which is most closely associated with the process of transpiration?

(A) spiracles of a grasshopper
(B) root of a geranium
(C) leaf of a maple
(D) gills of a fish

6. Which term includes all the others?

(A) organ
(B) tissue
(C) system
(D) organism

7. When several drops of pasteurized milk were placed in a petri dish containing sterilized nutrient agar, many colonies developed. This experiment shows the milk

(A) contained some bacteria
(B) contained harmful bacteria
(C) should have been sterilized
(D) was incorrectly stamped "pasteurized"

8. The growth of green plants toward light is related most specifically to the distribution in the plant of

(A) minerals
(B) enzymes
(C) auxins
(D) amino acids

9. In humans, the digestion of carbohydrates begins in the

(A) stomach
(B) small intestine
(C) mouth
(D) liver

10. To determine whether an unknown black guinea pig is pure or hybrid black, it should be crossed with

(A) a white
(B) a hybrid black
(C) a pure black
(D) another unknown

11. In a series of rock layers arranged one on top of another, fossils found in the lowest layers are
    (A) completely different from fossils found in the upper layers
    (B) older than the fossils found in the upper layers
    (C) of organisms simpler than organisms fossilized in the upper layers
    (D) of organisms more complex than organisms fossilized in the upper layers

12. The principal way in which forests help to prevent soil erosion is that the
    (A) trees provide homes for wildlife
    (B) leaves of the trees manufacture food
    (C) forest floors absorb water
    (D) forest shields the soil from the sun's heat

13. Which factor in the environment of an organism causes it to react?
    (A) a stimulus
    (B) a response
    (C) a reflex
    (D) an impulse

14. A breeder wanted to develop a strain of beef cattle with good meat and the ability to thrive in a hot, dry climate. How can she best accomplish this?
    (A) continued selection among the members of a prize herd
    (B) crossbreeding followed by selection
    (C) inbreeding to bring out desirable hidden traits
    (D) inbreeding followed by selection

15. The inhaling and the exhaling of air by the human lungs is mainly an application of
    (A) Boyl's Law—the inverse relationship between the pressure and the volume of a gas
    (B) the volume of a gas at standard temperature and pressure (STP)
    (C) Charles' Law—the direct relationship between the temperature and the volume of a gas
    (D) the number of O_2 and CO_2 particles per mole

16. Which plant tissues are mostly concerned with storage?
    (A) phloem and xylem
    (B) phloem and cambium
    (C) palisade cells and epidermis
    (D) pith and spongy cells

17. The Hubble Telescope is able to produce images of very distant celestial objects more clearly than other telescopes because
    (A) its reflector is able to concentrate more light on the lens
    (B) its images are enhanced by computer
    (C) its view is not obstructed by atmosphere
    (D) it has a larger lens

18. Which reagent should be used in the urine test for diabetes?
    (A) iodine
    (B) nitric acid
    (C) ammonia
    (D) Benedict's solution

19. The major benefit of buffer systems is that they
    (A) increase pH significantly
    (B) resist significant changes in pH
    (C) decrease pH significantly
    (D) none of the above

20. The Kreb cycle produces
    (A) H_2O and NADH
    (B) CO_2 and H_2
    (C) pyruvic acid and lactic acid
    (D) amino acids

21. The removal for microscopic examination of a small bit of living tissue from a patient is called
    (A) biopsy
    (B) surgery
    (C) dissection
    (D) therapy

22. The presence of which substance is most important for all cell activity?
    (A) light
    (B) carbon dioxide
    (C) water
    (D) chlorophyll

23. The end-products of digestion that enter the lacteals are
    (A) glucose
    (B) amino acids
    (C) minerals
    (D) fatty acids

24. A student in the laboratory tossed two pennies from a container one hundred times and recorded these results: both heads, 25; one head and one tail, 47; both tails, 28. Which cross between plants would result in approximately the same ratio?

(A) Aa × AA
(B) Aa × Aa
(C) AA × aa
(D) Aa × aa

25. In the equation below for photosynthesis, the oxygen comes

$$CO_2 + H_2O \rightarrow C_6H_{12}O_6 + O_2$$

(A) entirely from CO_2
(B) from a simple sugar molecule
(C) partially from CO_2 and H_2O
(D) entirely from H_2O

26. Tissue culture has been extensively used as a research method in all of the following fields of biological investigation *except*

(A) photosynthesis
(B) virology
(C) development of nerve cells
(D) experimental embryology

27. After each transfer of a culture of bacteria, the wire loop should be

(A) dipped into alcohol
(B) held in a flame
(C) dipped into liquid soap
(D) washed repeatedly in water

28. Identify the statement which is **not** true of cellular respiration.

(A) Is a down-hill process
(B) Occurs in both plant and animal cells
(C) Uses CO_2 and H_2O for reactants
(D) Is an exergonic process

29. In which one of the following ways does combustion differ from cellular respiration?

(A) More heat is produced.
(B) More energy is wasted.
(C) It is less rapid.
(D) It occurs at a higher temperature.

30. Of the following, an enzyme responsible for the digestion of proteins is

(A) maltase
(B) trypsin
(C) ptyalin
(D) steapsin

31. Failure of blood to clot readily when exposed to air may be due to a(n)

(A) oversupply of erythrocytes
(B) deficiency of leucocytes
(C) overabundance of fibrin
(D) inadequacy of thrombokinase

32. Cone cells are most closely associated with the function of

(A) digestion
(B) absorption
(C) vision
(D) secretion

33. The part of the vertebrate eye that controls the amount of light entering the eye is the

(A) cornea
(B) ciliary body
(C) iris
(D) conjunctiva

34. Most of the carbon dioxide in the blood is carried in the

(A) liquid portion
(B) leucocytes
(C) erythrocytes
(D) platelets

35. Increased blood pressure may be brought about by excess secretion of

(A) thyroxin
(B) insulin
(C) ACTH
(D) adrenalin

36. Of the following, the plant hormone concerned with growth is

(A) auxin
(B) estrogen
(C) testosterone
(D) ATP

37. Bread mold resembles ferns in that both develop

(A) mycelia
(B) hyphae
(C) pinnules
(D) spores

38. Sap rises in woody stems because of root pressure and

(A) transpiration pull
(B) enzyme action
(C) molecular adhesion
(D) photosynthesis

39. Vascular tissues present in the body of a flowering plant are xylem and

(A) cambium
(B) phloem
(C) meristem
(D) lenticels

40. Stored food for the embryo of a bean seed is found in the

(A) plumule
(B) hypocotyl
(C) cotyledons
(D) testa

41. Which of the following is not a characteristic of cancer cells?

(A) high power for self-affinity
(B) altered genetic material
(C) uncontrolled division
(D) loss of normal functions

42. In the structure of a flower, the stigma is most closely positioned to the

(A) style
(B) ovary
(C) sepal
(D) ovule

43. The basic structure of cell membranes is a

(A) protein bilayer
(B) protein-impregnated phospholipid bilayer
(C) carbohydrate bilayer
(D) phospholipid bilayer

44. When catalyzed by sucrase, sucrose decomposes to yield glucose + fructose. The reaction is

(A) fermentation
(B) hydrolysis
(C) denaturation
(D) condensation

45. Continental drift is caused by

(A) fluctuations in Earth's magnetic field
(B) extrusion of molten rock through cracks is sea floors
(C) fragmentation of larger land masses into smaller ones
(D) Coriolis force generated by the rotation of the earth

46. Carbohydrates are a combination of carbon, hydrogen, and oxygen in an approximate ratio of

(A) 2:1:2
(B) 3:2:1
(C) 1:2:1
(D) 1:1:1

47. Rod-shaped bacteria are classified as

(A) bacilli
(B) cocci
(C) vibrios
(D) spirilla

48. A stain used in classifying bacteria is

(A) Gram's
(B) Wright's
(C) Loeffler's
(D) Giemsa

49. A bacteriophage is a kind of

(A) enzyme
(B) toxin
(C) bacterium
(D) virus

50. Of the following, the marsupial native to the United States is the

(A) raccoon
(B) wombat
(C) opossum
(D) armadillo

51. The first fully terrestrial vertebrates were the

(A) amphibians
(B) reptiles
(C) birds
(D) mammals

52. Enzyme molecules are all of the following, except

(A) lipids
(B) proteins
(C) macromolecules
(D) biological catalysts

53. The size of most eukaryotic cells is

(A) 0.1–1.0 microns
(B) 10–100 microns
(C) 1.0–10 microns
(D) greater than 100 microns

54. Sickle cell anemia is a genetic disorder that involves an inability of

(A) erythrocytes to contain a sufficient amount of hemoglobin
(B) bone marrow to produce a sufficient number of erythrocytes
(C) bone marrow to produce erythrocytes of normal size
(D) erythrocytes to carry a sufficient lead of oxygen

55. Of the following, a crustacean that lives on land is the

(A) centipede
(B) millipede
(C) sow bug
(D) tick

56. Where would you find a leucoplast?

(A) in a liver cell
(B) in white blood cell
(C) in a white potato
(D) in a bacterium

57. Of the following, the hydra is most closely related to

(A) coral
(B) flatworm
(C) sponge
(D) roundworm

58. An unforeseen result of the widespread use of DDT is the

(A) control of mosquitoes
(B) development of insects immune to DDT
(C) development of fishes immune to DDT
(D) destruction of harmful birds

59. Cytoplasmic structures that contain powerful hydrolysis enzymes which could lead to cell destruction in the absence of surrounding membranes are

(A) lysosomes
(B) golgi
(C) ribosomes
(D) none of the above

60. If the carrying capacity (k-value) represents the maximum number of individuals of a species that a habitat can support, it suggests that the population

(A) is regulated by density-dependent factors
(B) will ultimately become extinct
(C) is regulated by density-independent factors
(D) can increase at an exponential rate, indefinitely

TEST 4: LIFE SCIENCES ANSWER KEY

1. **B**
2. **D**
3. **B**
4. **D**
5. **C**
6. **D**
7. **A**
8. **C**
9. **A**
10. **A**
11. **B**
12. **C**
13. **A**
14. **B**
15. **A**
16. **D**
17. **C**
18. **D**
19. **B**
20. **B**
21. **A**
22. **C**
23. **D**
24. **B**
25. **D**
26. **A**
27. **B**
28. **C**
29. **D**
30. **B**
31. **D**
32. **C**
33. **C**
34. **A**
35. **D**
36. **A**
37. **D**
38. **A**
39. **B**
40. **C**
41. **A**
42. **A**
43. **B**
44. **B**
45. **B**
46. **C**
47. **A**
48. **A**
49. **D**
50. **C**
51. **B**
52. **A**
53. **B**
54. **D**
55. **C**
56. **C**
57. **A**
58. **B**
59. **A**
60. **A**

TEST 4: LIFE SCIENCES EXPLANATORY ANSWERS

1. **(B)** Although other mechanisms may be involved in passage of materials through a cell membrane, the passage of some materials, especially water, occurs by diffusion; *diffusion* occurs from regions of higher concentrations of the substance to regions of lower concentration. Diffusion through a membrane, such as the cell membrane, is known as *osmosis.*

2. **(D)** Iron is a part of the hemoglobin molecule, and, as such, is essential for its formation. Hemoglobin is the oxygen-carrying pigment found in red corpuscles.

3. **(B)** *Phenylketonuria (PKU)* is a genetic disorder characterized by the inability of the affected person to convert excess molecules of the amino acid phenylalanine to molecules of the amino acid tyrosine. It is caused by inheriting a defect in the gene for the enzyme that catalyzes the conversion.

4. **(D)** A *control* is used with experiments for comparison. The control is treated in the same manner as is the experimental group except for one variable. In this case, the variable would be the administering of the drug or sugar pills. Thus, any differences between the groups in experimental results could be attributed to this one variable.

5. **(C)** *Transpiration* is the loss of water in a gaseous state, through epidermal stomata, from the aerial parts of a plant. Most transpiration occurs through the leaf epidermis. Stomata are not found in root epidermis.

6. **(D)** An organism is a living thing or individual. An organism consists of "systems," which consist of organs, which consist of tissues, especially in the case of higher organisms. This statement would not apply to lower organisms that have not reached the system level of phylogenetic development.

7. **(A)** Milk is not sterile; it contains numerous bacteria. Pasteurization does not sterilize milk, but does destroy certain harmful bacteria that can be carried in milk.

8. **(C)** *Auxins* are growth hormones found in plants; in stems, auxins stimulate growth. If a plant is unevenly illuminated, auxins are more concentrated on the side of the stem that is more poorly illuminated, stimulating growth on that side. This will cause the stem to bend toward the light.

9. **(A)** In the humans, carbohydrate digestion begins in the mouth with the enzyme ptyalin produced by the salivary glands.

10. **(A)** Black is dominant over white in this case; therefore, the white guinea pig carries only white genes and is *homozygous* or pure recessive. When such a test backcross is made, the offspring will indicate the genotype of the black guinea pig. If the black guinea pig is hybrid or *heterozygous* black (carrying one white gene), black and white offspring will result in a theoretical ratio of 1:1; if the black guinea pig is pure or homozygous black, all offspring will be black because of dominance, although all of the offspring will be hybrid because they carry a white gene.

11. **(B)** Fossils found in the lowest rock layers are the oldest because these layers were deposited before the ones that lie above them. Fossils in upper layers are not always different from the lower layers. Some species have very long histories and leave fossils in more than one layer. Conversely, fossils in upper layers are never completely the same as fossils in lower layers. At least some species of organisms whose fossils lie in lower layers would have become extinct and been replaced by fossils of different organisms by the time upper layers were deposited. Older organisms were not always simpler than modern organisms and were certainly not more complex.

12. **(C)** The roots of plants help to hold the soil in place and prevent soil erosion; the ground can absorb water. Eroded lands do not absorb water readily. Water may run off, carrying with it some of the topsoil; and this reduces the quality of the land. Where plants are present, the run-off is reduced or diminished, and the ground absorbs water.

13. **(A)** A *stimulus* is anything that can cause a *reaction* or response by the organism. The reaction may be involuntary, such as batting the eye when an object approaches, or voluntary, such as moving from an area of discomfort.

14. **(B)** Crossbreeding between strains with the desired traits, followed by selection of the offspring for future breeding and establishing the herd, is the best way to accomplish the breeder's goal. Inbreeding is just as likely to bring out undesirable hidden traits.

15. **(A)** The inhaling and the exhaling of air by the human lungs demonstrates Boyle's Law. Inhaling results from the expansion of the chest cavity (increase in volume and decrease in air pressure) and exhaling results from compression of the chest cavity (decrease in volume and increase in air pressure). These changes accomplished by movement of the ribs and diaphragm.

16. **(D)** Pith typically consists of *parenchyma* cells, which store starch in typical green plants. Spongy cells, characteristic of dicot leaves, also store starch, but temporarily.

17. **(C)** The Hubble Telescope is able to produce sharper images of objects than other telescopes because it is in orbit around Earth and does not have its view obstructed by atmosphere. Images seen through telescopes on Earth's surface are always obscured to some degree by the scattering of light as it passes through the atmosphere and by the passage of air currents created by heating of the atmosphere.

18. **(D)** A symptom of diabetes is sugar (glucose) in the urine. *Benedict's solution* is a reagent used to test for the presence of reducing sugars such as glucose.

19. **(B)** Buffer Systems resist significant changes in pH. When a strong acid or a strong base is added to a buffer system they produce a weak acid and a salt or a weak base and water, respectively. In each case the pH would change only slightly.

20. **(B)** Each turn of the Kreb cycle generates 2 moles of CO_2 and four pairs of H_2.

21. **(A)** A small amount of living tissue can be removed from a specific organ of a patient and examined by a pathologist to give the attending physician information needed for diagnosis. This excision and diagnostic study of living tissue is a *biopsy,* a useful diagnostic tool—specially for diseases of a cancerous nature.

22. **(C)** Water constitutes about 75–85 percent of the typical living cell. No activities associated with life can occur without water.

23. **(D)** Fats are *emulsified,* or broken up into small droplets, by bile secreted from the liver into the small intestine. The enzyme lipase then digests the fat droplets into fatty acids and glycerin. These products are not absorbed through capillary walls directly into the bloodstream, but enter the small lymph vessels, or *lacteals,* located in the villi of the intestine.

24. **(B)** The results of the penny toss approximate a 1:2:1 ratio, which is the same ratio that is obtained from a monohybrid cross:

    $Aa \times Aa \rightarrow 1AA{:}2Aa{:}1aa.$

25. **(D)** In the light phase of photosynthesis, H_2O is dissociated into $H_2 + O_2$. The O_2 comes entirely from the water molecules. The resulting H_2 is then used to reduce CO_2 to simple sugar.

26. **(A)** Tissue culture is the technique of growing tissues or cells in solutions of water and nutrients. This technique is especially useful in studying growth, differentiation, and morphology.

27. **(B)** Incineration is an effective method of sterilization; holding a loop in a flame sterilizes the loop, preventing contamination of surfaces on work areas, etc., and the possible spread of infectious bacteria.

28. **(C)** Cellular respiration oxidizes digested food molecules and produces CO_2 and H_2O as end products. It is a down-hill reaction and occurs in both plant and animal cells.

29. **(D)** *Combustion,* or burning, is a rapid reaction giving off much heat and light in a short period of time. The energy is expended more rapidly; thus, the reaction occurs at a higher temperature since the temperature of the combustible material must be raised to a combustion point. Cellular respiration occurs more slowly, at lower temperatures, and is controlled by enzymes. If cellular respiration occurred at combustion temperatures, cells would be destroyed.

30. **(B)** *Trypsin,* an enzyme found in pancreatic juice, digests proteins, peptones, and proteoses to peptides. The digestion of peptides to amino acids also occurs in the small intestine under the control of the enzyme erepsin. Some protein digestion (to peptones and proteoses) occurs in the stomach, under the control of the enzyme pepsin. Ptyalin and maltase act on carbohydrates; steapsin, on fats.

31. **(D)** Thrombocytes disintegrate when ruptured, as when blood flows from an injured blood vessel, releasing thrombokinase (thromboplastin), which acts to convert prothrombin to thrombin. Thrombin acts on fibrinogen in the plasma, converting it to insoluble fibrin, the material that forms the clot. Inadequacy of thrombokinase would prevent the first step of clotting, the formation of thrombin from prothrombin.

32. **(C)** *Cone cells* are photoreceptor cells found in the retina of the eye. They are responsible for color vision. Cone cells are functional only in bright light; therefore, color is not perceived in dim light.

33. **(C)** The *iris* is a circular muscle that regulates the diameter of the *pupil,* the aperture that allows light to enter the posterior chamber of the eye where the light-sensitive retina is located. The *cornea* allows light to enter the eye but does not regulate the amount of light entering. The *ciliary body* is a muscle that changes either position or shape of the lens to focus the light coming through the pupil. The *conjunctiva* is a thin, protective layer of epithelium that covers the exposed surface of the eyeball.

34. **(A)** Most of the carbon dioxide is transported in the blood plasma in the form of sodium bicarbonate ($NaHCO_3$). *Erythrocytes, leucocytes,* and *platelets* (thrombocytes) are blood cells suspended in the plasma.

35. **(D)** *Adrenalin,* a hormone secreted by the adrenal glands, causes increases in blood pressure, heart rate, breathing, glucose blood levels, etc., preparing the body for stressful situations.

36. **(A)** *Auxins* are plant growth hormones; *testosterone* and *estrogen* are animal sex hormones. *ATP* (adenosine triphosphate) is an energy-transport compound found in cells.

37. **(D)** Bread mold is a fungus, while ferns are vascular plants. Both bread mold and ferns, however, produce spores as asexual reproductive cells. A *mycelium* is a mass of fungal hyphae and is not a part of the fern-plant body. *Pinnules* are the "leaflets" of a fern frond and are not part of a fungus.

38. **(A)** *Transpiration* is the loss of gaseous water from a plant through epidermal stomata of the aerial parts of the plant, especially the leaves. Water forms a continuous column in the xylem tissue. The pull of water effected by transpiration is a factor in the rise of *sap* (water plus dissolved materials). The process is much the same as drinking liquid through a straw.

39. **(B)** Xylem and phloem serve the purpose of transporting materials in vascular tissues. Upward translocation of plant sap is accomplished mainly through vessels (in angiosperms) and tracheids of xylem. Downward translocation is accomplished through the sieve tubes of phloem.

40. **(C)** The cotyledons of dicotyledonous plants (such as beans) store food for use by the plant embryo as it develops into a seedling that can carry on photosynthesis. The *plumule* is composed of the embryonic or first leaves of the embryo; the *hypocotyl* is the lower embryonic stem, and the *testa* is the seed coat.

41. **(A)** Normal cells have high power of self-affinity (tendency to adhere to their own bind). Cancer cells loose their ability, as demonstrated by the spreading of cancer from one organ to another (malignancy).

42. **(A)** The *stigma* is the top portion of the pistil on which pollen lands in pollination. The *style* is the neck-like portion of the pistil, located between the stigma and the ovary, the basal part. *Ovules* are potential seeds.

43. **(B)** Intensive research has demonstrated the basic structure of cell membranes is a mosaic of proteins in an outer and inner layer of phospholipids.

44. **(B)** The enzyme sucrase adds a molecule of water (hydrolysis to the band that binds the monosaccharides forming sucrose) to decompose the dissaccharide to simple sugars.

45. **(B)** The movement of continents relative to one another is mostly the result of the spreading apart of sea floor between continental masses caused by the extrusion of molten rock through cracks in the sea floor. Fluctuations in Earth's magnetic field and Coriolis force are real events, but neither has any effect on continental drift. Fragmentation of large land masses to make smaller ones has sometimes been a part of continental drift, but it qualifies as a result rather than a cause.

46. **(C)** The generic formular for carbohydrates is $(CH_2O)^n$ = 1C:2H:1O (1:2:1)

47. **(A)** There are three morphological types, or shapes, of bacteria: spherical-shaped bacteria are called *cocci;* rod-shaped bacteria are called *bacilli;* curved or spiral-shaped bacteria are usually known as *spirilla.*

48. **(A)** Bacteria are classified as gram positive or gram negative; this depends on their ability to retain crystal violet, the primary stain of the gram stain. Those bacteria that cannot be decolorized with ethanol but retain crystal violet are classified as gram positive. Those that can be decolorized are gram negative. The difference is due to the chemical composition of the cell wall.

49. **(D)** A *bacteriophage* is a kind of virus that attacks and destroys the bacterial cell. The viruses can pass their DNA into the bacterial cells and cause the cells to manufacture vital DNA and viral protein.

50. **(C)** A *marsupial* is a viviparous mammal that gives birth to immature embryos; the development of the young is completed in the female's pouch, located on her ventral side. Nourishment for the embryo is from the mammary glands, the nipples of which are located in the pouch.

51. **(B)** Reptiles are the first vertebrates in evolutionary development that spend the early or developmental part of their lives, as well as adult stages, on land. They do not possess gills for breathing in water as do the larval stages of amphibians.

52. **(A)** Enzymes are macromolecular proteins that serve as biological catalysts that lower activation energy requirements in cellular reactions.

53. **(B)** Most eukaryotic cells are in the range of 10 microns to 100 microns.

54. **(D)** *Sickle cell anemia* is caused by inheriting the defective form of a gene that codes for part of the protein portion of the hemoglobin molecule. The number of erythrocytes produced and the amount of hemoglobin in each erythrocyte are normal, but the altered structure of the hemoglobin molecules causes them to stick together in a manner that distorts erythrocytes into an abnormal crescent shape, making them less able to carry oxygen. Other types of anemia are due to insufficient hemoglobin within erythrocytes, too few erythrocytes, or erythrocytes that are abnormally small.

55. **(C)** All named are members of the phylum Arthropoda, but only the sowbug is a crustacean. The characteristics of the class Crustacea are two pairs of antennae, three pairs of mouth parts, and a three-part body. Most crustaceans are aquatic, gilled animals, but a few live on land. The sowbug is one of these.

56. **(C)** Leucoplasts are cellular plastids that store starches and are found only in plant cells.

57. **(A)** The hydra and corals are coelenterates, diploblastic animals characterized by a gastrovascular cavity.

58. **(B)** Many insects have developed an immunity to or tolerance of DDT, so it does not kill them. However, DDT can accumulate in the bodies of insects and then be transferred to the tissues of birds, fishes, and other insect predators. These predators can accumulate DDT and, when consumed by their predators, pass on the DDT. Thus, this harmful insecticide can be passed up the food chain with the concentration in animal tissues increasing at each level, and it can have harmful effects on higher animals that consume the lower DDT-containing animals.

59. **(A)** Lysosomes store powerful hydrolysis enzymes.

60. **(A)** All environments have limited amounts of food and space, that allow animal populations to increase up to these limits, and regulate the populations by the number of individual per unit of space (density-dependent).

GENERAL SCIENCE TEST ANSWER SHEET

1. Ⓐ Ⓑ Ⓒ Ⓓ	18. Ⓐ Ⓑ Ⓒ Ⓓ	35. Ⓐ Ⓑ Ⓒ Ⓓ	52. Ⓐ Ⓑ Ⓒ Ⓓ
2. Ⓐ Ⓑ Ⓒ Ⓓ	19. Ⓐ Ⓑ Ⓒ Ⓓ	36. Ⓐ Ⓑ Ⓒ Ⓓ	53. Ⓐ Ⓑ Ⓒ Ⓓ
3. Ⓐ Ⓑ Ⓒ Ⓓ	20. Ⓐ Ⓑ Ⓒ Ⓓ	37. Ⓐ Ⓑ Ⓒ Ⓓ	54. Ⓐ Ⓑ Ⓒ Ⓓ
4. Ⓐ Ⓑ Ⓒ Ⓓ	21. Ⓐ Ⓑ Ⓒ Ⓓ	38. Ⓐ Ⓑ Ⓒ Ⓓ	55. Ⓐ Ⓑ Ⓒ Ⓓ
5. Ⓐ Ⓑ Ⓒ Ⓓ	22. Ⓐ Ⓑ Ⓒ Ⓓ	39. Ⓐ Ⓑ Ⓒ Ⓓ	56. Ⓐ Ⓑ Ⓒ Ⓓ
6. Ⓐ Ⓑ Ⓒ Ⓓ	23. Ⓐ Ⓑ Ⓒ Ⓓ	40. Ⓐ Ⓑ Ⓒ Ⓓ	57. Ⓐ Ⓑ Ⓒ Ⓓ
7. Ⓐ Ⓑ Ⓒ Ⓓ	24. Ⓐ Ⓑ Ⓒ Ⓓ	41. Ⓐ Ⓑ Ⓒ Ⓓ	58. Ⓐ Ⓑ Ⓒ Ⓓ
8. Ⓐ Ⓑ Ⓒ Ⓓ	25. Ⓐ Ⓑ Ⓒ Ⓓ	42. Ⓐ Ⓑ Ⓒ Ⓓ	59. Ⓐ Ⓑ Ⓒ Ⓓ
9. Ⓐ Ⓑ Ⓒ Ⓓ	26. Ⓐ Ⓑ Ⓒ Ⓓ	43. Ⓐ Ⓑ Ⓒ Ⓓ	60. Ⓐ Ⓑ Ⓒ Ⓓ
10. Ⓐ Ⓑ Ⓒ Ⓓ	27. Ⓐ Ⓑ Ⓒ Ⓓ	44. Ⓐ Ⓑ Ⓒ Ⓓ	61. Ⓐ Ⓑ Ⓒ Ⓓ
11. Ⓐ Ⓑ Ⓒ Ⓓ	28. Ⓐ Ⓑ Ⓒ Ⓓ	45. Ⓐ Ⓑ Ⓒ Ⓓ	62. Ⓐ Ⓑ Ⓒ Ⓓ
12. Ⓐ Ⓑ Ⓒ Ⓓ	29. Ⓐ Ⓑ Ⓒ Ⓓ	46. Ⓐ Ⓑ Ⓒ Ⓓ	63. Ⓐ Ⓑ Ⓒ Ⓓ
13. Ⓐ Ⓑ Ⓒ Ⓓ	30. Ⓐ Ⓑ Ⓒ Ⓓ	47. Ⓐ Ⓑ Ⓒ Ⓓ	64. Ⓐ Ⓑ Ⓒ Ⓓ
14. Ⓐ Ⓑ Ⓒ Ⓓ	31. Ⓐ Ⓑ Ⓒ Ⓓ	48. Ⓐ Ⓑ Ⓒ Ⓓ	65. Ⓐ Ⓑ Ⓒ Ⓓ
15. Ⓐ Ⓑ Ⓒ Ⓓ	32. Ⓐ Ⓑ Ⓒ Ⓓ	49. Ⓐ Ⓑ Ⓒ Ⓓ	66. Ⓐ Ⓑ Ⓒ Ⓓ
16. Ⓐ Ⓑ Ⓒ Ⓓ	33. Ⓐ Ⓑ Ⓒ Ⓓ	50. Ⓐ Ⓑ Ⓒ Ⓓ	67. Ⓐ Ⓑ Ⓒ Ⓓ
17. Ⓐ Ⓑ Ⓒ Ⓓ	34. Ⓐ Ⓑ Ⓒ Ⓓ	51. Ⓐ Ⓑ Ⓒ Ⓓ	68. Ⓐ Ⓑ Ⓒ Ⓓ

GENERAL SCIENCE TEST

68 QUESTIONS • TIME—68 MINUTES

Directions: For each of the following items, select the choice that best answers the question or completes the statement. Blacken the corresponding space on your answer sheet.

1. A tree native to China and **not** to the United States is the
   (A) silvery maple
   (B) chestnut
   (C) gingko
   (D) tulip tree

2. Mammals are believed to have evolved directly from
   (A) fish
   (B) amphibians
   (C) reptiles
   (D) birds

3. The biochemical technique that would be used to separate differently sized pieces of DNA created by digesting a sample of DNA with a restriction enzyme is
   (A) diapedesis
   (B) liquid scintillation
   (C) electrophoresis
   (D) kinesthesia

4. Which of the following groups, in primate phylogeny, includes the primate most closely related to man?
   (A) Old World monkeys
   (B) great apes
   (C) New World monkeys
   (D) lemurs

5. Stanley Miller recently obtained evidence supporting the possibility of spontaneous generation by achieving laboratory synthesis of
   (A) amino acids
   (B) DNA
   (C) RNA
   (D) glucose

6. The part of a compound light microscope that focuses light before it passes through the specimen is the
   (A) objective
   (B) micrometer
   (C) ocular
   (D) condenser

7. During what season is hail most likely to occur during thunderstorms?
   (A) fall
   (B) winter
   (C) spring
   (D) summer

8. We can see only one side of the moon because the
   (A) earth rotates on its own axis
   (B) moon makes one rotation as it makes one revolution around the earth
   (C) moon has no refractive atmosphere
   (D) sun does not shine on the moon's unseen side

9. Which of the following is not an essential biotic element of all ecosystems?
   (A) producers
   (B) water
   (C) consumers
   (D) decomposers

10. The deadly property of carbon monoxide, if inhaled, is due to its
    (A) high affinity for O_2
    (B) low affinity for hemoglobin
    (C) high affinity for hemoglobin
    (D) conversion to cyanide gas

11. Of the following, vitamin B_{12} is most useful in combating
    (A) pernicious anemia
    (B) night blindness
    (C) rickets
    (D) goiter

12. Both malaria and yellow fever are
    (A) caused by protistans
    (B) cured with antibiotics
    (C) prevented by vaccination
    (D) controllable by swamp drainage or hormonal insecticides

13. An emission device in modern cars that uses platinum beads to oxides carbon monoxide and hydrocarbons to carbon dioxide and water is the
    (A) carburetor
    (B) catalytic converter
    (C) PCV valve
    (D) air filter

14. Of the following electrical devices found in the home, the one that develops the highest voltage is the
    (A) electric broiler
    (B) radio tube
    (C) television picture tube
    (D) electric steam-iron

15. Most soluble food substances enter the blood stream through the
    (A) small intestine
    (B) duodenum
    (C) capillaries in the stomach
    (D) hepatic vein

16. Air-polluting sulfa dioxide (SO_2) results primarily from
    (A) natural gas furnaces
    (B) leaded gasoline
    (C) paper waste
    (D) coal burning power plants

17. The "dark" side of the moon refers to the
    (A) craters, into which no sunlight has ever reached
    (B) south pole of the moon's axis
    (C) hemisphere that has never reflected the sun's rays on the earth
    (D) moon itself in the early phases of the month

18. Of the following, the one **not** characteristic of poison ivy is
    (A) milky juice
    (B) shiny leaves
    (C) three-leaflet clusters
    (D) white berries

19. Cholesterol is
    (A) a basic part of bone structure
    (B) an alcohol formed in the body
    (C) a substance found in blood
    (D) the cause of colitis

20. The diameter of the moon is approximately
    (A) 2,000 miles
    (B) 8,000 miles
    (C) 186,000 miles
    (D) 240,000 miles

21. Of the following, the one present in greatest amounts in dry air is
    (A) carbon dioxide
    (B) oxygen
    (C) water vapor
    (D) nitrogen

22. Which is **not** a characteristic of enzymes?
    (A) They are proteins.
    (B) They catalize metabolics reactions.
    (C) They act on substances.
    (D) They are phopholipids.

23. A ventral nerve cord is found in which of the following?
    (A) earthworm
    (B) frog
    (C) amphioxus
    (D) lamprey eel

24. Identify the statement which is **not** characteristic of exergonic reactions.
    (A) They are downhill reactions.
    (B) They have a negative energy change (–H).
    (C) They are uphill reactions.
    (D) The products have less energy than the reactants.

25. It is believed by scientists that worker bees indicate to their hive-mates the direction and distance of a supply of food by
    (A) strokes of their antennae
    (B) buzzing of sounds
    (C) an oriented dance in front of the hive
    (D) none of the above

26. The normal height of a mercury barometer at sea level is
    (A) 15 inches
    (B) 30 inches
    (C) 32 feet
    (D) 34 feet

27. Of the following phases of the moon, the invisible one is called
    (A) crescent
    (B) full moon
    (C) new moon
    (D) waxing and waning

28. Of the following, the statement that best describes a "high" on a weather map is that the air
    (A) extends farther up than normal
    (B) pressure is greater than normal
    (C) temperature is higher than normal
    (D) moves faster than normal

29. The nerve endings for the sense of sight are located in the part of the eye called the
    (A) cornea
    (B) sclera
    (C) iris
    (D) retina

30. Malaria is caused by
    (A) bacteria
    (B) mosquitoes
    (C) protistans
    (D) bad air

31. A 1000-ton ship must displace a weight of water equal to
    (A) 500 tons
    (B) 1000 tons
    (C) 1500 tons
    (D) 2000 tons

32. Of the following instruments, the one that can convert light into an electric current is the
    (A) radiometer
    (B) dry cell
    (C) electrolysis apparatus
    (D) photoelectric cell

33. On the film in a camera, the lens forms an image that by comparison with the original subject, is
    (A) right side up and reversed from left to right
    (B) upside down and reversed from left to right
    (C) right side up and not reversed from left to right
    (D) upside down and not reversed from left to right

34. Of the following, the plant whose seeds are *not* spread by wind is the
    (A) cocklebur
    (B) maple
    (C) dandelion
    (D) milkweed

35. Which of the following insects belongs to the order of insects containing the largest number of species?
    (A) housefly
    (B) flour beetle
    (C) grasshopper
    (D) cockroach

36. The part of a tomato plant that contains structures that correspond to the lungs of land animals is
    (A) roots
    (B) flowers
    (C) stems
    (D) leaves

37. Photosynthesis is a cellular process which
    (A) is an exergonic reaction
    (B) produces simple sugar and O_2
    (C) is initiated by chemical energy
    (D) produces CO_2 and H_2O

38. One-celled eukaryotes belong to the group of living things known as

(A) protistans
(B) poriferans
(C) annelids
(D) arthropods

39. Spiders can be distinguished from insects because spiders have

(A) hard outer coverings
(B) large abdomens
(C) four pairs of legs
(D) biting mouth parts

40. An important ore of uranium is called

(A) hematite
(B) bauxite
(C) chalcopyrite
(D) pitchblende

41. The lightest element known on earth is

(A) hydrogen
(B) helium
(C) oxygen
(D) air

42. Of the following gases in the air, the most plentiful is

(A) argon
(B) nitrogen
(C) oxygen
(D) carbon dioxide

43. The time it takes for light from the sun to reach the earth is approximately

(A) four years
(B) four months
(C) eight minutes
(D) sixteen years

44. Of the following kinds of clouds, the kind that occurs at the greatest height is called

(A) cirrus
(B) cumulus
(C) nimbus
(D) stratus

45. The time it takes for the earth to rotate 45 degrees is

(A) one hour
(B) three hours
(C) four hours
(D) ten hours

46. Of the following glands, the one that regulates the metabolic rate is the

(A) adrenal
(B) salivary
(C) thyroid
(D) thymus

47. In the small intestine, a digestive enzyme can break the peptide bond between two amino acids in a protein molecule by

(A) removing a water molecule from them
(B) inserting a water molecule between them
(C) removing a carbon atom from one of them
(D) inserting a carbon atom between them

48. The usual vector in the transmission to humans of rickettsial diseases is

(A) birds
(B) rodents
(C) arthropods
(D) snails

49. Passive immunity to diphtheria may be achieved by taking an injection of a(n)

(A) vaccine
(B) toxin
(C) toxoid
(D) antitoxin

50. Of the following, the only safe blood transfusion would be

(A) group A blood into a group O person
(B) group B blood into a group A person
(C) group O blood into a group AB person
(D) group AB blood into a group B person

51. If the effect of two or more factors is greater than the sum of the individual effects (e.g. $2 + 2 > 4$), the phenomenon is called

(A) synergism
(B) coopeativity
(C) antagonism
(D) none of the above

52. The water-conducting tissue in an angiosperm is

(A) phloem
(B) xylem
(C) pith
(D) cambium

53. The time that it takes the earth to complete a 60-degree rotation is

(A) 1 hour
(B) 4 hours
(C) 6 hours
(D) 24 hours

54. Of the following, the most common metal found in the earth's crust is

(A) iron
(B) copper
(C) aluminum
(D) tin

55. Of the following, the gas needed for burning is

(A) carbon dioxide
(B) oxygen
(C) nitrogen
(D) argon

56. Of the following, the process that will result in water most nearly chemically pure is

(A) aeration
(B) chlorination
(C) distillation
(D) filtration

57. The number of degrees on the Fahrenheit thermometer between the freezing point and the boiling point of water is

(A) 100 degrees
(B) 180 degrees
(C) 212 degrees
(D) 273 degrees

58. One is most likely to feel the effects of static electricity on a

(A) cold, damp day
(B) cold, dry day
(C) warm, humid day
(D) warm, dry day

59. Of the following planets, the one that has the largest number of satellites is

(A) Jupiter
(B) Mercury
(C) Neptune
(D) Pluto

60. The deserts of the earth generally occur on the __ side of the continents.

(A) west
(B) north
(C) east
(D) south

61. Atmospheric moisture (H_2O) combines with oxides of carbon, nitrogen and sulfur (CO_2, NO_3 and SO_2) to produce

(A) alkaline precipitation
(B) acid rain
(C) alcohol
(D) none of the above

62. As water is warmed, its solubility of oxygen (O_2)

(A) increases
(B) decreases
(C) remains constant
(D) fluctuates randomly

63. The chlorinated hydrocarbon pesticide, DDT, was banned from use in the United States during the 1970s because it

(A) has high affinity for milk and adipose tissues
(B) is deliterious to eggs of several species of birds
(C) is a biological concentration in ecosystem food chains
(D) all of the above

64. Of the 92 naturally occurring elements, the number found in the human body is closer to

(A) 50
(B) 10
(C) 25
(D) 75

65. Inasmuch as the molecular formular for glucose is $C_6H_{12}O_6$ and the molecular formular for fructose is $C_6H_{12}O_6$, the two substances are

(A) hextomers
(B) isomers
(C) heteromers
(D) anomers

66. Which of the following elements is the most abundant in the human body?

(A) carbon
(B) potassium
(C) nitrogen
(D) oxygen

67. The density of gold (Au) is $19.3 g/cm^3$ and that of iron (Fe) is $7.9 g/com^3$. A comparison of the volumes (V) of 50 gram samples of each metal would show that

    (A) $V_{Au} = V_{Fe}$
    (B) $V_{Au} < V_{Fe}$
    (C) $V_{Au} > V_{Fe}$
    (D) No predictable relationship between volumes

68. Among the tickborne diseases in the United States, the one usually identified by bull's eye rash near the bite site is

    (A) Rocky Mountain Spotted Fever
    (B) Tularema
    (C) Typhus
    (D) Lyme diseases

GENERAL SCIENCE TEST ANSWER KEY

1. **C**
2. **C**
3. **C**
4. **B**
5. **A**
6. **D**
7. **D**
8. **B**
9. **B**
10. **C**
11. **A**
12. **D**
13. **B**
14. **C**
15. **A**
16. **D**
17. **C**
18. **A**
19. **C**
20. **A**
21. **D**
22. **D**
23. **A**
24. **C**
25. **C**
26. **B**
27. **C**
28. **B**
29. **D**
30. **C**
31. **B**
32. **D**
33. **B**
34. **A**
35. **B**
36. **D**
37. **B**
38. **A**
39. **C**
40. **D**
41. **A**
42. **B**
43. **C**
44. **A**
45. **B**
46. **C**
47. **B**
48. **C**
49. **D**
50. **C**
51. **A**
52. **B**
53. **B**
54. **C**
55. **B**
56. **C**
57. **B**
58. **B**
59. **A**
60. **A**
61. **B**
62. **B**
63. **D**
64. **C**
65. **B**
66. **D**
67. **B**
68. **D**

GENERAL SCIENCE TEST EXPLANATORY ANSWERS

1. **(C)** The gingko is native to the Orient but has been imported into the United States and now is in widespread use as an ornamental tree.

2. **(C)** Evidence indicates that a primitive reptile known as a therapsid is the ancestor of mammals. These early reptiles of the Triassic period had acquired some mammalian characteristics such as warm bloodedness, hair, and mammary glands. They are sometimes referred to as "premammals."

3. **(C)** *Electrophoresis* is a technique that takes advantage of the fact that molecules in solution will migrate through a porous gel when an electrical current is passed through it. A mixture of differently sized molecules is placed into a depression at one end of the gel, and the current is turned on. Smaller molecules will travel farther through the gel than larger molecules, with the result that bands of molecules will accumulate at various distances from the starting point according to their size. These bands can be made visible by staining, allowing the results of one electrophoretic separation to be compared to another.

4. **(B)** Fossil evidence indicates that there was an isolation of ape-like forms, including hominids (man-like creatures), during the Pliocene period. These seemingly originated from the same "branch" of the evolutionary "tree." Lemurs, New World monkeys, and Old World monkeys apparently evolved earlier.

5. **(A)** It was found that if a mixture of methane, ammonia, and hydrogen is continuously bombarded with spark discharges as an energy source, amino acids are formed. If inorganic phosphate is added to the mixture, ATP, the energy compound of cells, is formed also. The earth, at its very early age, had the inorganic substances, and the sun could have provided the energy source.

6. **(D)** The *condenser* is an adjustable lens that focuses light before it reaches the specimen. This enhances the sharpness of the image produced by the magnifying lenses of the microscope. The *objective* and the *ocular* are the lenses used to create a magnified image of the light after it has passed through the specimen. A *micrometer* is a device used to measure objects viewed through the microscope.

7. **(D)** Thunderstorms, caused by a clash between warm and cold air masses, are more common in the summer because the reflection of heat from the earth warms the air of the lower atmosphere. The air of the upper atmosphere is much colder. Hail consists of pellets of ice and snow combined in alternating layers. Raindrops formed in the warm portions of the clouds are swept upward by air currents into the colder air masses, where the drops freeze into ice and collect a layer of snow. As they descend, they are coated with moisture and swept upward to freeze again. This up and down movement continues until the pellets are too heavy to be supported by the air. They then fall to earth as hail.

8. **(B)** As the moon revolves around the earth, it rotates on its axis so that only one side of the moon faces earth. Because the moon makes one rotation with one revolution around the earth, one side of the moon never faces the earth.

9. **(B)** In all ecosystems, producers (green plants or algae) convert CO_2 an H_2O into sugars which serve as food for consumers (animals), whose bodies are ultimately degraded by decomposers (bacteria and fungi). Water, although vital, is an inorganic substance.

10. **(C)** Carbon monoxide has a greater affinity than oxygen for hemoglobin. This binding blocks hemoglobin from binding oxygen for transport to body cells for metabolic needs.

11. **(A)** A deficiency of vitamin B_{12} leads to *pernicious anemia*, a condition in which red blood cells fail to mature. Vitamin B_{12} is essential for the formation of red blood cells.

12. **(D)** Both the virus that causes yellow fever and the protistan that causes malaria are transmitted by mosquitoes. Since mosquito eggs are laid and larvae develop in water, swamp drainage would reduce the breeding areas, thereby reducing mosquito populations and hence the incidence of the diseases. However, swamp drainage destroys the ecosystem of an area and is, therefore, undesirable. A juvenile hormone has been discovered in larvae that promotes the retention of larval characteristics and inhibits the molting hormone. Chemical analogs of the molting hormone have been used as insecticides; these produce abnormal final molts of the larva or block larval development, thus preventing the

larva from becoming an adult. These insecticides are very promising, and they are highly specific; they act only on the targeted insect and do not cause great changes in the environment.

13. **(B)** The catalytic converts use platinum to convert carbon monoxide and hydrocarbons to carbon dioxide and water, resulting in reduced air pollution.

14. **(C)** In a cathode-ray tube, such as is found in television sets (picture tube), a *cathode* (negative terminal) and an *anode* (positive terminal) are present. There is no material between the two through which electricity (electrons) can flow from one terminal to another: a vacuum exists in the tube. A heated cathode generates electrons, which become excited by heat and can acquire enough energy to leave the cathode. Once they do, they are attracted to the anode because of the difference in charges (electrons have a negative charge) and flow across the gap toward the anode. In other appliances, the material through which the electricity flows may produce some resistance; in a picture tube, the electrons are flowing across a space in a vacuum and encounter no resistance.

15. **(A)** The small-intestine lining is characterized by millions of *villi,* small, thin-walled projections into the lumen. Each villus is supplied with capillaries and a lacteal. The large number of villi greatly increase the absorptive area of the small intestine, and the blood vessels and lacteal are close to the food supply. Thus, digested foods are absorbed with ease through the thin-walled villus and thin capillary walls into the bloodstream or, in the case of fats, into the opened ends of the lacteals.

16. **(D)** Coal is the major source of SO_2 because gasoline, natural gas, and paper waste contain only small amounts of sulfur.

17. **(C)** The moon shines by the reflected light of the sun. Because the moon rotates on its axis as it revolves around the earth, one side of the moon never faces the earth. This side, the dark side of the moon, can never reflect the sun's light onto the earth.

18. **(A)** Poison ivy has a clear juice rather than a milky sap. Three-leaflet clusters, white berries, and shiny leaves are all characteristic of poison ivy.

19. **(C)** *Cholesterol* is a fatty substance found in animal fats. It can enter the bloodstream and become involved in the buildup of fatty deposits on the walls of capillaries and other blood vessels.

20. **(A)** The moon is a spherical body with a diameter of about 2,000 miles, revolving around the earth in an orbit approximately 240,000 miles distant from the earth.

21. **(D)** Air is a mixture of gases; dry air consists of about 78 percent nitrogen and 21 percent oxygen. The remaining one percent consists of other gases, including carbon dioxide.

22. **(D)** Enzymes are proteins that catalize reactions of substances known as substrates.

23. **(A)** The earthworm (and any other annelids) is characterized by a ventral nerve cord; this is true of arthropods as well. Members of the phylum *Chordata,* to which the lancelet amphioxus, the eel, and the frog belong, have a dorsal nerve cord.

24. **(C)** Exergonic reactions are downhill reactions.

25. **(C)** Bee behavior has been studied, and scientists can interpret some of the movements of the worker bees' dance. The movements are known to give information as to the location of the pollen or nectar they have discovered. The angle of the tail-wag, direction and pattern of movement, sound and duration of sound, and the duration of the dance are ways of giving information as to distance and direction to the food supply. Floral odors on the dancers' bodies indicate the correct flowers in the area.

26. **(B)** Air pressure at sea level is 14.7 pounds/square inch. This pressure, at 0 degrees C supports a barometer mercury column of 76 centimeters, or 30 inches. This is equivalent to one atmosphere of pressure.

27. **(C)** The moon phases occur because the moon shines only by the reflected light of the sun and because only one hemisphere is seen from the earth. The four phases, as seen from the northern hemisphere, are (1) the new moon, in which the face is completely in the shadow—the "invisible phase"; (2) the first quarter, with the eastern half illuminated; (3) the full moon, with the entire face illuminated; and (4) the last quarter, with the western half illuminated.

28. **(B)** A *high* indicates an area of high air pressure, while a *low* indicates an area of low air pressure. Weather can be predicted by measuring differences between pressures. A high usually indicates fair weather, whereas low pressure areas indicate storms and bad weather.

29. **(D)** The retina of the eye contains rods and cones; these are the photoreceptors of the eye, so named because of their shape. Rods are concerned with perception of gray to black in dim light, while cones respond to light of high intensity and are concerned with color perception. Nerve fibers from these receptors eventually converge to form the optic nerves leading to the brain.

30. **(C)** Malaria is a parasitic disease caused by protistans in the genus *Plasmodium*. Some of the life cycle stages of *Plasmodium* are passed in mosquitoes of the genus *Anopheles,* which transmit the disease.

31. **(B)** Archimedes' Principle indicates that an object will displace its weight in water. Thus, a 1000-ton ship would displace 1000 tons of water.

32. **(D)** A photoelectric cell works on the principle that light can be used to produce electric currents in some metals. When light energy strikes the metal (usually cesium) in the photoelectric cell, it is converted into electric energy. The cesium emits electrons. The greater the amount of light striking the metal, the more electric energy produced.

33. **(B)** A camera lens is convex; light passing through such a lens is bent toward the center of the lens. Light reflected near the object and passing through the thinner outer edges of a convex lens bends more than light passing through the thicker areas, and light passing through the exact center of the lens does not bend at all. Because light reflected from an object is focused through such a lens and bent, rather than passing in a straight line, as it would if passing through plain glass, the image formed is reversed and is smaller than the original object.

34. **(A)** The dandelion and maple fruits, containing seed(s), have modifications that enable them to be dispersed easily by air currents and stronger winds. These modifications are the "wings" of the maple fruit and the "hairs" of the dandelion fruit. Milkweed seeds also have such appendages for wind dispersal. The cocklebur fruit is spiny, which causes it to attach to animals for dispersal.

35. **(B)** The flour beetle belongs to the Order Coleoptera which, with approximately 340,000 described species, is the largest order of insects. The housefly belongs to the Order Diptera, containing approximately 100,000 described species. The grasshopper belongs to the Order Orthoptera, containing approximately 20,000 species. The cockroach belongs to the Order Blattaria, containing only 3,700 species.

36. **(D)** The layer of tissue known as *spongy mesophyll* found in each leaf of a tomato and other flowering plants absorbs CO_2 from the air for use in photosynthesis and releases O_2 produced as a byproduct of photosynthesis back into the air. The spongy mesophyll is therefore equivalent in function to an animal's lung whose function is to absorb O_2 from the air for use in cellular respiration and release CO_2 produced as a byproduct of cellular respiration back into the air.

37. **(B)** Photosynthesis is an endergonic reaction which uses $CO_2 + H_2O$ to produce simple sugar and O_2. It is driven by radiant energy from sunlight.

38. **(A)** Unicellular eukaryotes, including colonial forms, belong to the Kingdom *Protista*. The other organisms in this question belong to phyla in the Kingdom *Animalia,* all members of which are multicellular. Phylum *Annelida* includes segmented worms, such as the earthworm. Phylum *Porifera* includes sponges. Phylum *Arthropoda* includes animals such as insects, spiders, crabs, crayfish, and millipedes that have a chitinous exoskeleton and jointed appendages.

39. **(C)** Spiders are characterized by a two-part body and four pairs of legs, while insects have a three-part body and three pairs of legs.

40. **(D)** *Pitchblende* is a natural mineral that contains uranium and radium, as well as many other substances. Uranium also occurs in other minerals, such as carnotite.

41. **(A)** Hydrogen is the lightest element known, having an atomic weight of 1.008. The atom contains one proton, no neutrons, and one electron.

42. **(B)** Nitrogen composes nearly four-fifths of the air; oxygen nearly one-fifth. The remainder of air consists of other gases.

43. **(C)** Light travels at a speed of about 186,000 miles per second; the sun is approximately 93,000,000 miles from the earth. Thus, calculations (93,000,000 miles divided by 186,000 miles per second) show that it takes about 500 seconds, or a bit more than eight minutes, for light from the sun to reach the earth.

44. **(A)** Cirrus clouds are feathery, finely textured clouds occurring in feathery bands across the sky; these occur at the greatest heights and usually are the fastest moving. Nimbus, cumulus and stratus clouds are lower and slower.

45. **(B)** The earth makes one complete rotation on its axis (360 degrees) in 24 hours; 45 degrees is one-eighth of 360 degrees. Therefore, it would take one-eighth of 24 hours, or three hours, for the earth to rotate 45 degrees.

46. **(C)** The thyroid regulates metabolic rate under normal conditions. A deficiency of thyroid hormone will cause a low basal metabolism, while an excess of the hormone will increase the metabolic rate.

47. **(B)** A *peptide bond* is the covalent bond that links the nitrogen atom on the end of one amino acid molecule with the carbon atom on the opposite end of another amino acid molecule. A peptide bond is formed by removing a molecule of water from the two amino acid molecules (see the explanatory answer for question 23 in Science Test 2 for an explanation of dehydration synthesis). Therefore, inserting a water molecule between two amino acids linked by a peptide bond will break the bond by putting a hydrogen atom back onto the nitrogen atom of one amino acid and a hydroxyl ion (OH–) back onto the terminal carbon atom of the other amino acid. Breaking a bond between two molecules by inserting a water molecule between them is called *hydrolysis* and is a common way of digesting large organic molecules such as starches and proteins.

48. **(C)** Rickettsial diseases, such as Rocky Mountain spotted fever and typhus, are transmitted by arthropod vectors, such as ticks and fleas. The rickettsial pathogen, an obligate intracellular parasite, can be acquired by the vector when it bites an animal or human harboring or infected with the pathogen; the pathogen is then transmitted to a healthy person when bitten by the vector. With some of rickettsial diseases, a warm blooded animal, such as a rodent, can act as a reservoir from which the vector may acquire the pathogen and then transmit it to humans.

49. **(D)** Passive immunity involves administering an antibody (an antitoxin, in the case of diphtheria) to the patient. This immunity is temporary, since the patient's body is not stimulated to form antibodies, as it would be if an antigen were administered. The temporary immunity is considered *passive* because the body is not active in forming antibodies. If an antigen stimulates the body to form its own antibodies against it, the immunity produced is *active*. Passive immunity provides temporary protection to one who has been exposed to a disease, or a method of treatment until the patient's body has started producing its own antibodies if the disease has been contracted. Active immunity imparts more lasting protection.

50. **(C)** Group O blood lacks antigen A and antigen B. Although it can form antibodies against both A and B, it cannot stimulate the formation of antibodies against A and B. Persons of group O are known as *universal donors*. Group AB blood has both antigens A and B but cannot form antibodies against either. Persons of group AB are known as *universal recipients*. Since group O has neither antigen, and AB cannot form either antibody, the only safe transfusion of those listed is choice (C). Persons of group A contain antigen A and can form antibodies against antigen B; blood group B contains antigen B and can form antibodies against A.

51. **(A)** Synergism is a phenomenon in which the whole is greater than the sum of the individual parameters.

52. **(B)** Xylem, characterized in angiosperms by vessels, conducts material upward in the plant. Most of the material conducted upward is water that has been absorbed from the soil by the root system. The water contains dissolved minerals and may contain, especially in deciduous perennials in the spring, sugar that has been formed by the digestion of starch stored in the lower plant parts.

53. **(B)** The earth rotates 360 degrees on its axis every 24 hours. 60 degrees is one-sixth of 360 degrees; therefore, it would take one-sixth of 24 hours, or four hours, for the earth to rotate 60 degrees.

54. **(C)** The rocks of the *lithosphere,* the earth's crust, are made up mostly of eleven elements, plus trace amounts of others. These eleven elements occur almost entirely in the form of compounds rather than in the free state. Aluminum is the third most abundant element; only oxygen and silicon occur in greater quantities.

55. **(B)** Oxygen is the gas that supports combustion, or burning. Materials will not burn in an oxygen-free environment.

56. **(C)** Distillation involves *evaporation,* or changing the water from a liquid to a gaseous state (usually by heating), and collecting and *condensing* the gaseous water back to a liquid. The water, because it is in a gaseous state, is separated from any impurities since they cannot evaporate with the water.

57. **(B)** On the Fahrenheit scale, the boiling point of water is 212 degrees; the freezing point is 32 degrees. Subtracting 32 degrees from 212 degrees results in a difference of 180 degrees, the number of degrees between the boiling and the freezing points of water.

58. **(B)** *Static electricity* is a non-moving electrical charge that accumulates on the surface of an object. A substance that contains an equal number of *protons* (positively charged particles) and *electrons* (negatively charged particles) is electrically neutral. If electrons are gained or lost, the substance becomes charged. When one object loses electrons and becomes positively charged, another must gain electrons and become negatively charged. If electrons are not in motion, the electricity is static. However, warm, moist air is a good conductor of electricity; moisture collects on the surfaces of objects and conducts electrons away from the surface, preventing the object from becoming charged. Cold air acts as a good insulator, preventing the movement of electrons away from the object. Therefore, static electricity can best be felt on a cold, dry day, when the electrons can accumulate on an object or surface.

59. **(A)** Jupiter is the largest planet known in our solar system, and is known to have twelve moons, or satellites, revolving around it. Neptune and Pluto are the greatest distance from the earth: two moons are identified for Neptune, and knowledge about Pluto, the most distant planet, is incomplete. Mercury is difficult to study because of its closeness to the sun. The glare of the sun makes observations difficult during the day and the planet is very low in the sky at night. However, with present explorations and studies of our solar system resulting in the accumulation of more knowledge, changes in previously held concepts are taking place.

60. **(A)** Deserts of the earth generally occur on the west side of continents, as influenced by prevailing westerly winds and nearby mountains. As the earth rotates from west to east, winds that approach continents from the west side loose moisture in ascending mountains and evaporate moisture from the opposite side—resulting in dry regions known as deserts.

61. **(B)** Atmospheric moisture combines with oxides of carbon, nitrogen, and sulfur to produce acid rain, as illustrated by the following reactions

$$H_2O + CO_2 \rightarrow H_2CO_3$$

$$H_2O + 2NO_2 \rightarrow 2HNO_3$$

$$H_2O + SO_2 \rightarrow H_2SO_3$$

62. **(B)** As water is warmed, its solubility of oxygen decreases, resulting in a lower O_2 content and producing unfavorable conditions for animals.

63. **(D)** The pesticide DDT was banned from the United States during the 1970s because research studies had shown it to be present in milk, fatty tissues, and the eggs of eagles and other birds. It was also proven to be a biological concentration—building up to higher concentration in succeeding levels of food chains.

64. **(C)** The human body is composed primarily of oxygen, carbon, hydrogen, and nitrogen which comprise approximately 96 percent of the body's mass; with about 15 other elements comprising the rest.

65. **(B)** Glucose and fructose are isomers because they are composed of identical numbers of carbon, hydrogen and oxygen atoms, with different structural arrangements and different functional groups. The carbon-oxygen bonding

in glucose and fructose, form aldehydes and ketones, respectively.

66. **(D)** The approximate percentages of oxygen, carbon, nitrogen, and potassium in the human body are: 65, 18.5, 3.5, and 0.5, respectively.

67. **(B)** Density is defined as mass per unit volume ($D = m/v$). The mathematical relationship shows that when equal masses of two substances of different densities are compared, the one with greater density occupies less space (volume).

68. **(D)** A bull's eye rash near the bite site has been present in more than half of the reported cases of Lyme disease.

FINAL SCIENCE EXAMINATION ANSWER SHEET

1. Ⓐ Ⓑ Ⓒ Ⓓ	19. Ⓐ Ⓑ Ⓒ Ⓓ	37. Ⓐ Ⓑ Ⓒ Ⓓ	55. Ⓐ Ⓑ Ⓒ Ⓓ
2. Ⓐ Ⓑ Ⓒ Ⓓ	20. Ⓐ Ⓑ Ⓒ Ⓓ	38. Ⓐ Ⓑ Ⓒ Ⓓ	56. Ⓐ Ⓑ Ⓒ Ⓓ
3. Ⓐ Ⓑ Ⓒ Ⓓ	21. Ⓐ Ⓑ Ⓒ Ⓓ	39. Ⓐ Ⓑ Ⓒ Ⓓ	57. Ⓐ Ⓑ Ⓒ Ⓓ
4. Ⓐ Ⓑ Ⓒ Ⓓ	22. Ⓐ Ⓑ Ⓒ Ⓓ	40. Ⓐ Ⓑ Ⓒ Ⓓ	58. Ⓐ Ⓑ Ⓒ Ⓓ
5. Ⓐ Ⓑ Ⓒ Ⓓ	23. Ⓐ Ⓑ Ⓒ Ⓓ	41. Ⓐ Ⓑ Ⓒ Ⓓ	59. Ⓐ Ⓑ Ⓒ Ⓓ
6. Ⓐ Ⓑ Ⓒ Ⓓ	24. Ⓐ Ⓑ Ⓒ Ⓓ	42. Ⓐ Ⓑ Ⓒ Ⓓ	60. Ⓐ Ⓑ Ⓒ Ⓓ
7. Ⓐ Ⓑ Ⓒ Ⓓ	25. Ⓐ Ⓑ Ⓒ Ⓓ	43. Ⓐ Ⓑ Ⓒ Ⓓ	61. Ⓐ Ⓑ Ⓒ Ⓓ
8. Ⓐ Ⓑ Ⓒ Ⓓ	26. Ⓐ Ⓑ Ⓒ Ⓓ	44. Ⓐ Ⓑ Ⓒ Ⓓ	62. Ⓐ Ⓑ Ⓒ Ⓓ
9. Ⓐ Ⓑ Ⓒ Ⓓ	27. Ⓐ Ⓑ Ⓒ Ⓓ	45. Ⓐ Ⓑ Ⓒ Ⓓ	63. Ⓐ Ⓑ Ⓒ Ⓓ
10. Ⓐ Ⓑ Ⓒ Ⓓ	28. Ⓐ Ⓑ Ⓒ Ⓓ	46. Ⓐ Ⓑ Ⓒ Ⓓ	64. Ⓐ Ⓑ Ⓒ Ⓓ
11. Ⓐ Ⓑ Ⓒ Ⓓ	29. Ⓐ Ⓑ Ⓒ Ⓓ	47. Ⓐ Ⓑ Ⓒ Ⓓ	65. Ⓐ Ⓑ Ⓒ Ⓓ
12. Ⓐ Ⓑ Ⓒ Ⓓ	30. Ⓐ Ⓑ Ⓒ Ⓓ	48. Ⓐ Ⓑ Ⓒ Ⓓ	66. Ⓐ Ⓑ Ⓒ Ⓓ
13. Ⓐ Ⓑ Ⓒ Ⓓ	31. Ⓐ Ⓑ Ⓒ Ⓓ	49. Ⓐ Ⓑ Ⓒ Ⓓ	67. Ⓐ Ⓑ Ⓒ Ⓓ
14. Ⓐ Ⓑ Ⓒ Ⓓ	32. Ⓐ Ⓑ Ⓒ Ⓓ	50. Ⓐ Ⓑ Ⓒ Ⓓ	68. Ⓐ Ⓑ Ⓒ Ⓓ
15. Ⓐ Ⓑ Ⓒ Ⓓ	33. Ⓐ Ⓑ Ⓒ Ⓓ	51. Ⓐ Ⓑ Ⓒ Ⓓ	69. Ⓐ Ⓑ Ⓒ Ⓓ
16. Ⓐ Ⓑ Ⓒ Ⓓ	34. Ⓐ Ⓑ Ⓒ Ⓓ	52. Ⓐ Ⓑ Ⓒ Ⓓ	70. Ⓐ Ⓑ Ⓒ Ⓓ
17. Ⓐ Ⓑ Ⓒ Ⓓ	35. Ⓐ Ⓑ Ⓒ Ⓓ	53. Ⓐ Ⓑ Ⓒ Ⓓ	
18. Ⓐ Ⓑ Ⓒ Ⓓ	36. Ⓐ Ⓑ Ⓒ Ⓓ	54. Ⓐ Ⓑ Ⓒ Ⓓ	

FINAL SCIENCE EXAMINATION

70 QUESTIONS • TIME—70 MINUTES

Directions: After carefully reading each test item, select the best answer. Blacken the corresponding space on your answer sheet.

1. Of the following human traits, the one under both genetic and hormonal control is

   (A) hemophilia
   (B) color blindness
   (C) baldness
   (D) blood type

2. If a sexually reproducing animal has a diploid number of 12, how many chromosomes would a mature sperm have?

   (A) 3
   (B) 24
   (C) 4
   (D) 6

3. The tissue to which gland cells belong is

   (A) connective
   (B) epithelial
   (C) secretory
   (D) nerve

4. Of the following, which is closest to the speed of sound in air at sea level?

   (A) one-fifth mile per second
   (B) one-half mile per second
   (C) one mile per second
   (D) five miles per second

5. The general formula for the acetylene series of hydrocarbons is

   (A) $C_nH_{2n} + 2$
   (B) C_nH_{2n}
   (C) $C_nH_{2n} - 2$
   (D) none of the above

6. How many molecules of ATP are required to activate a molecule of glucose in glycolysis?

   (A) 2
   (B) 6
   (C) 3
   (D) none

7. The vitamin that helps clotting of the blood is

   (A) C
   (B) D
   (C) E
   (D) K

8. Each nucleotide in a DNA molecule contains

   (A) a sugar
   (B) a nitrogen base
   (C) a phosphate group
   (D) all of the above

9. The wavelength (nM) of the visible portion of the electromagnetic spectrum is in the range of

   (A) 350–700
   (B) 800–1000
   (C) 200–350
   (D) 550–900

10. A person is more buoyant when swimming in salt water than in fresh water because

    (A) the person keeps his or her head out of salt water
    (B) salt water has greater tensile strength
    (C) salt coats the person's body with a floating membrane
    (D) salt water is denser than an equal volume of fresh water

11. Two parameters (e.g. the volume and the temperature of a gas) are directly proportional if a constant value can be calculated from their

    (A) product
    (B) ratio
    (C) sum
    (D) difference

12. Cellular proteins are synthesized in
    (A) ribosomes
    (B) mitochondria
    (C) lysosomes
    (D) golgi

13. All of the following mechanisms affect the amount of glucose in the blood *except*
    (A) adrenalin secretion
    (B) insulin secretion
    (C) level of oxygen intake
    (D) level of physical activity

14. The most active mixing of many digestive juices occurs in the
    (A) stomach
    (B) duodenum
    (C) ileum
    (D) jejunum

15. A *cold-blooded* animal is one that
    (A) has a body temperature colder than that of other types of animals
    (B) uses heat from its blood to warm other tissues of the body, lowering the blood temperature
    (C) depends on external heat sources to regulate its body temperature
    (D) is incapable of regulating its body temperature

16. The basic mechanism of hereditary transmission is
    (A) sexual reproduction
    (B) polyploidy
    (C) separation of chromosomes
    (D) the mitotic mechanism

17. If the electrical voice waves produced by a whistle are formed in one second, what is the wave frequency demonstrated in the following figure?

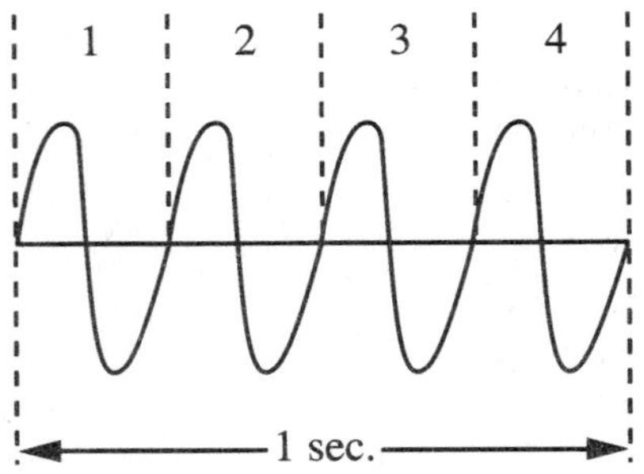

    (A) 4 hertz
    (B) 8 hertz
    (C) 12 hertz
    (D) 16 hertz

18. Of the following, the highest bactericidal activity of light occurs at a wavelength in angstrom units of
    (A) 2536
    (B) 3256
    (C) 5236
    (D) 6532

19. In the diagram below, the refraction of the light rays indicates that the lens is

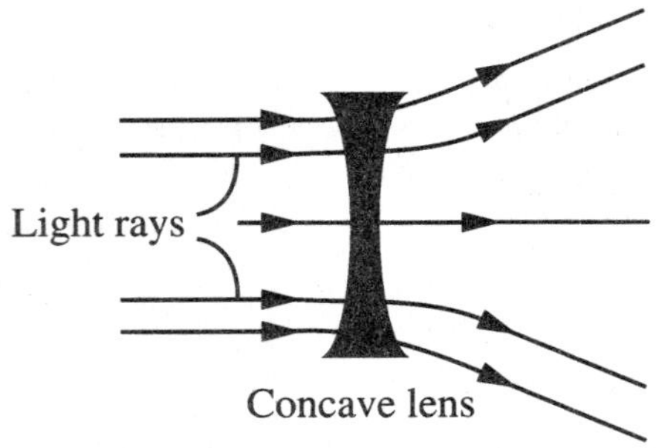

    (A) thicker in center than edges
    (B) thinner at center than edges
    (C) uniform in thickness
    (D) consistent in dimensions

20. A man hears the echo from a mountain wall five seconds after he has shouted. Of the following, the figure most nearly expressing the distance of the man from the mountain is
    (A) five miles
    (B) one mile
    (C) 900 yards
    (D) 1100 feet

21. Which of the following statements about wavelengths is true?
    (A) Visible wavelengths vary in lengths.
    (B) The wavelength of green is the longest.
    (C) Radio waves are electromagnetic waves shorter than infrared.
    (D) Infrared rays are shorter than red light rays.

22. An object appears white, or colorless, when it
    (A) absorbs the light reaching it
    (B) transmits only blue light
    (C) rejects all colors
    (D) reflects all colors at the same time

23. Another name for animal starch is

(A) cellulose
(B) lecithin
(C) glycogen
(D) chitin

24. Of the following, a human blood disease that has been definitely shown to be due to a hereditary factor or factors is

(A) pernicious anemia
(B) sickle cell anemia
(C) polycythemia
(D) leukemia

25. All of the following elements are major constituents of a cell *except*

(A) carbon
(B) potassium
(C) hydrogen
(D) phosphorus

26. If a machine listed for 1800 watts is plugged into a 110-volt system, approximately how many amps will it use?

(A) 6.6
(B) 13.0
(C) 16.0
(D) 19.8

27. The selection of algae as a possible source of additional food for man is based primarily on their ability to carry on

(A) fermentation
(B) digestion
(C) photosynthesis
(D) oxidation

28. Birds and bats are both flying, warm-blooded vertebrates. Yet they are *not* considered closely related because of the difference in their

(A) brain structure
(B) manner of feeding their young
(C) ability to see
(D) ability to hear

29. In eukaryotic cells, the phase of division which produces two daughter cells is

(A) G
(B) mitosis
(C) G_2
(D) cytokinesis

30. Of the following, one difference between frog and man is that the frog has no

(A) salivary glands
(B) thyroid gland
(C) pancreas
(D) adrenal gland

31. When a molecule of glucose in humans is degraded, the percent of its energy capable of generating ATP is nearest to

(A) 100
(B) 50
(C) 25
(D) 80

32. Velocity, defined as the rate of displacement of an object, is

(A) scalar
(B) inertia
(C) vector
(D) centripetal

33. The fundamental principle expressed by the Einstein Equation ($E = mc^2$) on mass-energy equivalency is that

(A) small mass = much energy
(B) small mass = little energy
(C) little energy = great mass
(D) all of the above

34. Exophthalmic goiter is caused by

(A) hypoactivity of the thyroid
(B) hyperactivity of the thyroid
(C) deficiency of vitamin A
(D) radioactive iodine

35. If other factors are compatible, a person who can most safely receive blood from any donor belongs to the basic blood group

(A) O
(B) A
(C) B
(D) AB

36. The Schick test indicates whether or not a person is probably immune to

(A) tuberculosis
(B) diptheria
(C) poliomyelitis
(D) scarlet fever

37. Evaporation of water is likely to be greatest on days of

(A) high humidity
(B) low humidity
(C) little or no wind
(D) low pressure

38. Of the following, the substance whose water solution will change the color of litmus from red to blue is

(A) $CuSO_4$
(B) K_2CO_3
(C) NaNO
(D) $Zn(NO_3)_2$

39. The percentage of oxygen by weight in $Al_2(SO_4)_3$ (atomic weights: Al = 27, S = 32, O = 16) is approximately

(A) 19
(B) 21
(C) 56
(D) 92

40. In backcrossing, a hybrid is always mated with

(A) its own parent
(B) another hybrid
(C) a pure dominant
(D) a pure recessive

41. Of the following processes, the one carried on exclusively by bacteria is

(A) maturing of cheese
(B) synthesis of antibiotics
(C) formation of humus
(D) synthesis of vitamin K in the intestines

42. Of the following, a structure found in mammals but *not* in reptiles is the

(A) lung
(B) brain
(C) diaphragm
(D) ventricle

43. The specific function of light energy in the process of photosynthesis is to

(A) activate chlorophyll
(B) split water
(C) reduce carbon dioxide
(D) form carbohydrates

44. The resistance of matter to changes in motion is

(A) elasticity
(B) inertia
(C) momentum
(D) inflexible

45. Some substances are transported across cell membranes by proteins known as

(A) ligases
(B) permeases
(C) hydrolases
(D) monomers

46. Which sequence correctly illustrates a food chain?

(A) algae-insect larvae-fish-man
(B) algae-fish-insect larvae-man
(C) insect larvae-algae-fish-man
(D) fish-insect larvae-algae-man

47. Grasses are usually pollinated by

(A) wind
(B) water
(C) birds
(D) insects

48. Among vertebrates the embryonic ectoderm gives rise to which of the following?

(A) nervous system
(B) digestive system
(C) skeletal system
(D) respiratory system

49. Generally, life depends directly or indirectly for food, energy, and oxygen upon

(A) parasitic organisms
(B) green plants
(C) fungi
(D) animals

50. The functions of plant roots may normally include all of the following *except*

(A) photosynthesis
(B) food storage
(C) absorption
(D) support

51. The weight in grams of 22.4 liters of nitrogen (atomic weight = 14) is

(A) 3
(B) 7
(C) 14
(D) 28

52. In the production of sounds, the greater the number of vibrations per second, the

(A) greater the volume
(B) higher the tone
(C) lower the volume
(D) lower the tone

53. A segment of a DNA molecule transcribes a base sequence, AGAUAU, on an mRNA codon. The compatible sequence on the tRNA anticodon is

(A) UUAGCG
(B) UCUAUA
(C) AAUAUA
(D) CGCAAA

54. Which of the following species will combine with a chloride ion to produce ammonium chloride?

(A) NH_3
(B) K^+
(C) NH_4^+
(D) Al^{+++}

55. Which one of the following characteristics represents a difference between plants and animals?

(A) organ systems
(B) specialization
(C) sexual reproduction
(D) cellular adaptation

56. Which one of the following graphs represents Boyle's Law?

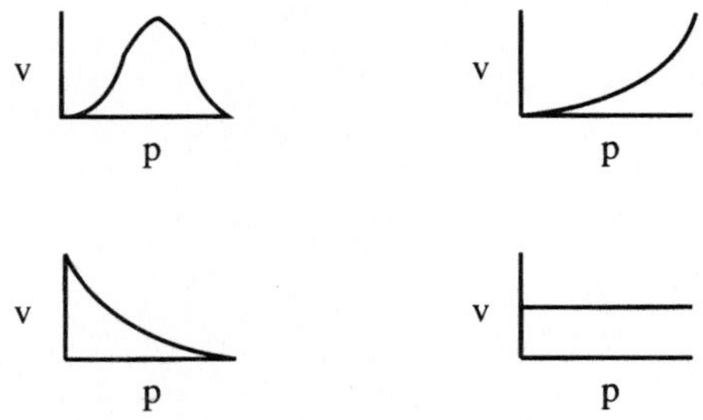

57. Which of the following minerals is restored to the soil by plants of the pea and bean family?

(A) sulfates
(B) nitrates
(C) carbonates
(D) phosphates

58. In humans, any hereditary defect caused by a gene on the Y chromosome would occur

(A) only in males
(B) only in females
(C) only if the gene were recessive
(D) about equally in males and females

59. There is no oxidation-reduction in a reaction involving

(A) single replacement
(B) double replacement
(C) simple decomposition
(D) direct combination of elements

60. A cross between two black guinea pigs yields 3 blacks and 1 white offspring. The white allele in the parents was

(A) dominant
(B) recessive
(C) sex-linked
(D) absent

61. The cellular organelle where respiratory reactions for the release of energy occurs is a

(A) centrosome
(B) chromosome
(C) chromoplast
(D) mitochondrion

62. Members of a population that are reproductively isolated from other populations form a

(A) race
(B) species
(C) community
(D) genus

63. The most efficient cellular respiratory process, in terms of energy-yield per molecule of glucose, is

(A) aerobic respiration
(B) anaerobic respiration
(C) fermentation
(D) phosphorylation

64. Which of the following is not a requirement for photosynthesis?
    (A) oxygen
    (B) carbon dioxide and water
    (C) sunlight
    (D) chlorophyll

65. A cellular organelle found in typical plant cells but not in typical animal cells is the
    (A) chloroplast
    (B) ribosome
    (C) mitochondrion
    (D) centrosome

66. In the absence of oxygen, plants and microbes convert pyruric acid into
    (A) alcohol and CO_2
    (B) lactic acid
    (C) CO_2 and H_2O
    (D) amino acids

67. Every cell contains
    (A) a cell membrane and cytoplasm
    (B) a cell wall and cytoplasm
    (C) a nucleus and cell wall
    (D) plastids and pigments

68. Digestion in humans is
    (A) extracellular
    (B) intracellular
    (C) vacuolar
    (D) intercellular

69. An example of an obligate intracellular parasitic microorganism is a
    (A) tapeworm
    (B) virus
    (C) bacterium
    (D) spirochaete

70. Which of the following substances is *not* transported by the blood?
    (A) oxygen
    (B) metabolic wastes
    (C) digestive enzymes
    (D) hormones

FINAL SCIENCE EXAMINATION ANSWER KEY

1. **C**
2. **D**
3. **B**
4. **A**
5. **C**
6. **A**
7. **D**
8. **D**
9. **A**
10. **D**
11. **B**
12. **A**
13. **C**
14. **B**
15. **C**
16. **C**
17. **A**
18. **A**
19. **B**
20. **C**
21. **A**
22. **D**
23. **C**
24. **B**
25. **B**
26. **C**
27. **C**
28. **B**
29. **D**
30. **A**
31. **B**
32. **C**
33. **A**
34. **B**
35. **D**
36. **B**
37. **B**
38. **B**
39. **C**
40. **D**
41. **D**
42. **C**
43. **A**
44. **B**
45. **B**
46. **A**
47. **A**
48. **A**
49. **B**
50. **A**
51. **D**
52. **B**
53. **A**
54. **C**
55. **A**
56. **B**
57. **B**
58. **A**
59. **B**
60. **B**
61. **D**
62. **B**
63. **A**
64. **C**
65. **A**
66. **A**
67. **A**
68. **A**
69. **B**
70. **C**

FINAL SCIENCE EXAMINATION EXPLANATORY ANSWERS

1. **(C)** All conditions are under genetic control; however, hereditary baldness is also under hormonal control. Baldness is expressed as a dominant characteristic in males but recessive in females because of the hormones present. Thus, a male and female may inherit the same genes for baldness, but the expression of the genes will depend on the sex hormones.

2. **(D)** Diploid cells in the testes undergo meiosis to reduce the chromosome number by $\frac{1}{2}$ to the haploid condition.

3. **(B)** There are only four basic kinds of tissues: epithelial, connective, muscle, and nerve. Gland cells are among the epithelial tissues that cover the internal and external surfaces of various parts of the body.

4. **(A)** The speed of sound in air varies slightly with temperature, increasing slightly as temperature increases. For convenience, the speed of sound in air is referred to as 1100 feet per second. This is an approximate value that can be used despite various conditions. 1100 feet is approximately one-fifth of a mile (one mile = 5280 feet).

5. **(C)** A member of the acetylene series is unsaturated, with a triple bond between two carbons. The formula for acetylene, for example, is H–C ≡ C–H; because of the triple bond between two carbons, the number of hydrogens is reduced by two. Thus, the general formula is $Cn_2H_2n - 2$.

6. **(A)** A molecule of glucose uses two molecules of ATP to supply activation energy to initiate the glycolytic pathway.

7. **(D)** Prothrombin is produced in insuffient quantities if there is a deficiency of vitamin K; prothrombin produces thrombin, which acts as an enzyme to convert fibrinogen to fibrin, the mesh that traps blood cells, forming the clot. Thus, if vitamin K is deficient, prothrombin is deficient, and clotting is delayed or does not occur.

8. **(D)** Each nucleotide of a DNA molecule contains a molecule of deoxyribose sugar, a nitrogen base, and a phosphate group, which is attached to the 3' carbon of one sugar molecule and the 5' carbon of a second sugar.

9. **(A)** The wavelength of energy in the electromagnetic spectrum ranges from 10^{-3} nM to 10^{14} nM, with visible light between 350 nM and 700 nM.

10. **(D)** The buoyancy of an object in water or air is determined by its *density* relative to the surrounding medium: thus objects less dense than the surrounding medium will float, and those more dense will sink. Salt water is denser than fresh water because of the much greater amount of dissolved substances. Therefore, a person will float more easily in salt water because there is a greater difference between the density of the person's body and that of the water.

11. **(B)** Two parameters are directly proportional if their ratio is a mathematical constant ($K = x/y$).

12. **(A)** Cellular proteins are synthesized at the ribosomes where codon triplets of m-RNA are paired with anticodon triplets of t-RNA to direct amino acid sequences.

13. **(C)** Insulin increases the permeability of the cell membrane to glucose, thus increasing the rate of glucose uptake by the cells from the bloodstream. Adrenalin promotes an increase in cardiac activity, respiratory rate, and the breakdown of glycogen (stored in the liver) to glucose, thus raising the glucose level of the blood. With physical activity, glucose is more rapidly utilized by cells, which must remove glucose from the blood, thus reducing the blood level of glucose.

14. **(B)** The digestion and absorption of most nutrients occurs in the *duodenum,* the first portion of the small intestine. Therefore, digestive juices are most active at this site.

15. **(C)** The term *cold-blooded* is commonly used in reference to animals such as reptiles that depend on external sources of heat to help regulate their body temperature. Cold-blooded animals, more properly called *ectotherms,* must bask in sunlight or lie on warm ground to raise their body temperature if it begins to fall. Conversely, they must lie in the shade or shelter beneath an object such as a rock to cool off their bodies if their internal temperature begins to rise too high. By contrast, warm-blooded animals, more properly called *endotherms,* are more or

less independent of external sources of heat, relying on a combination of heat generated by their metabolism and insulation on the surface of the body to keep their internal temperature constant.

16. **(C)** Chromosomes contain genetic material, or carry genes; the separation of the chromosomes of each pair is involved in *meiosis,* or reduction division, in the production of sexual reproductive cells. The *gametes* (egg and sperm) will each receive one-half the chromosomes carried by the parent, or one chromosome of each pair carried by the parent. Thus, the gametes will be *haploid.* When fertilization occurs, the zygote becomes *diploid,* having received one chromosome of each pair from each parent. Therefore, each individual inherits one-half of its chromosomes and genes from its father and one-half from its mother.

17. **(A)** A *hertz* can be defined as the number of wavelengths per second. A wave or wavelength is the distance between successive values, for example, from crest to crest. The diagram shows four waves in the one-second period, or four hertz.

18. **(A)** Light consists of colors of varying wavelengths. Visible light ranges from red, with a wavelength of about 7000 angstrom units, down to violet, with a wavelength of about 4000 angstroms. Ultraviolet has shorter wavelengths (150–3900 Å) and is bactericidal; the highest bactericidal activity occurs between 2000 Å and 3000 Å.

19. **(B)** The lens is concave; therefore, it is thicker at the edges. Light rays passing through a concave lens are refracted or bent outward, so they spread apart. A light ray passing through the center of the lens is not bent.

20. **(C)** Sound travels in air at a rate of approximately 1100 feet/second; in five seconds the sound will have traveled approximately 5500 feet. Half of that distance was to reach the mountain, and half was the return of the echo. Therefore, the man is about 2750 feet from the mountain (half of 5500 feet), or about 900 yards.

21. **(A)** Visible light consists of different colors of light, producing a spectrum of red (with the longest wavelength), orange, yellow, green, blue, indigo, and violet (with the shortest wavelength).

22. **(D)** White light consists of the colors or wavelengths of the visible spectrum—red, orange, yellow, green, blue, indigo, and violet. An object appears to be a certain color when it is reflecting light of this wavelength, and absorbing all others. A white object is reflecting all of the colors or wavelengths at the same time.

23. **(C)** Liver glycogen, which is a polymer of glucose molecules, is called animal starch.

24. **(B)** Persons with sickle cell anemia carry a variant hemoglobin molecule in the red blood cells, instead of the normal hemoglobin A. The production of hemoglobin is under genetic control.

25. **(B)** All elements listed are found in cells. Carbon, hydrogen, and phosphorus are three of the six major elements from which most organic molecules are built. Potassium is one of the five essential minor elements.

26. **(C)** An *ampere* (amp) is a unit for measuring the rate of flow of electricity. A *watt* is the metric unit of power; it is the power produced by 1 amp in a I volt circuit. Thus, the formula *watt* = *amp* × *volt*, can be used, or *amp* = *watt/volt*. If the problem is worked using this formula, the answer is (C), 16 amps.

27. **(C)** Photosynthesis is the process by which an organic, energy-containing compound (sugar or glucose) is produced from inorganic materials. This is a process basic to the production of organic compounds that can be used for food. Algae and other green plants exhibit photosynthesis.

28. **(B)** The presence of mammary glands for feeding young is the important characteristic of the class *Mammalia*. Birds are members of the class *Aves;* they do not nurse or suckle their young.

29. **(D)** Cytakineses is the stage in eukaryotic cell division in which the cytoplasm divides to produce daughter cells.

30. **(A)** The frog does not chew its food, and digestion of its food does not start in the mouth, as with man. Hence, salivary glands are not found in the frog. However, the endocrine system of the frog is basically like that of man, and the thyroid, pancreas, and adrenal glands are found in the frog as well as in man.

31. **(B)** Eukaryotic cells have high efficiency, relative to mechanical device. They are capable of extracting approximately 50 percent of the energy in glucose molecules for biological work.

32. **(C)** Vector quantities must have both magnitude and direction for complete description. An object cannot have a velocity without direction.

33. **(A)** The equation $E = mc^2$ demonstrates mass and energy are interchangeable and that small amounts of mass can yield large amounts of energy under specific conditions.

34. **(B)** The overproduction of the thyroid hormones causes a condition known as exophthalmic goiter, or Graves' disease. The thyroid may or may not be enlarged, but increased metabolic rate, protrusion of eyes (exophthalmus), increased blood pressure, increased heart rate, loss of weight, etc., are symptoms of Graves' disease. This disease may be treated by surgical removal of, or destruction of, a part of the thyroid gland.

35. **(D)** A person of blood group AB has antigen A and antigen B, but cannot produce antibodies against A or B. Therefore, such a person can receive blood from any of the four blood groups and is often called a "universal recipient."

36. **(B)** The Schick Test, developed by Bela Schick, is administered by injecting a weak solution of the diphtheria toxin cutaneously. A reddening of the site of injection indicates susceptibility to diphtheria; lack of reddening indicates immunity, indicating the presence of sufficient antitoxin to protect the person against diphtheria.

37. **(B)** *Evaporation* is the physical change of a substance from a liquid to a gas. The rate of movement of gas molecules into the air is more rapid in dry air or when the humidity is low, and decreases with increased humidity. The movement of air currents (wind) carries away the vapor above the surface of the liquid, thus increasing evaporation rate.

38. **(B)** K_2CO_3 in aqueous solution dissociates into potassium ions and carbonate ions. Water dissociates into hydrogen ions and hydroxyl ions. The carbonate ions can react with the hydrogen ions forming bicarbonate ions (HCO_3-). The removal of hydrogen ions will yield an excess of hydroxyl ions, making the solution basic, and raising the pH. Since litmus, an indicator in the range of pH 6–8, is red in acid solution and blue in basic solution, K_2CO_3 will cause a basic reaction.

39. **(C)** Of the 17 atoms making up a molecule of $Al_2(SO_4)_3$, there are two atoms of aluminum, three atoms of sulfur, and twelve atoms of oxygen (four oxygens in each of the three sulfate ions). The weight of the oxygen is 192; the total weight of the molecule is 342. Thus, the percentage of oxygen by weight is $\frac{192}{342}$, or 56 percent.

40. **(D)** To determine genotype of a hybrid, a pure recessive is always used in a test backcross. Any dominant trait carried by the hybrid parent will be expressed in some of the offspring; the recessive traits will also be expressed in some of the offspring, since the recessive parent cannot produce a dominant to mask it. Ratios and phenotypes will indicate the genotype of the hybrid parent.

41. **(D)** Maturing of cheese, formation of humus, and the synthesis of antibiotics can involve other kinds of organisms instead of, or in addition to, bacteria. The synthesis of vitamin K is a process performed by bacteria in the intestine and is not known to be performed by any other kind of organism.

42. **(C)** Reptiles do not possess a diaphragm, but have the other structures listed.

43. **(A)** Light activates the chlorophylls, causing the emission of electrons at high energy levels. The energy-rich electron can pass through a series of catalysts; the light energy is converted to chemical energy resulting in phosphorylation, etc.

44. **(B)** Inertia is the tendency of a body at resst or in motion to remain constant unless acted upon by an outside force.

45. **(B)** Permease are cellular proteins that transport substances across plasma membranes.

46. **(A)** In a food chain, algae are the primary "producers," occupying the bottom level of the food chain since they produce organic materials through photosynthetic processes. Insect larvae are some of the animals that can feed on algae; fish, which prey on animals such as insect larvae, are in turn consumed by man.

47. **(A)** Grasses are usually pollinated by wind; the grass flower typically does not attract insects or birds. Since grasses are mostly land plants, water would not play a significant role in their pollination.

48. **(A)** The *ectoderm* is the outer germ layer, which gives rise to the nervous and integumentary systems of the embryo.

49. **(B)** Only green plants can produce organic materials (food) from inorganic materials (carbon dioxide and water) through the process of photosynthesis. Oxygen and a by-product are returned to the air by means of this process. Animals may consume green plants (direct dependence) or may consume animals that consume green plants (indirect dependence) for food and energy.

50. **(A)** Photosynthesis occurs only in the presence of light and the chlorophylls. This means that photosynthesis occurs only in the green parts of plants that are exposed to light. Roots generally are not green and are subterranean organs; therefore, roots generally do not exhibit photosynthetic activity.

51. **(D)** One mole (gram molecular weight) of nitrogen is 28 grams, since two nitrogen atoms form a nitrogen molecule (N_2). One mole of gas occupies a volume of 22.4 liters at standard conditions.

52. **(B)** The frequency, or number of vibrations per second, determines pitch, or tone. The greater the frequency, the higher the pitch; the lower the frequency, the lower the pitch.

53. **(A)** In DNA and RNA molecules, adenine (A) must pair with thymine (T) or uracil (U). Guanine (G) always pairs with cytosine (C). This specificity is based on complementarity of molecular geometry, relative to the formation of double or triple bonds.

54. **(C)** The NH^+ species has a positive valence which has affinity for a negative chloride (Cl^-) ion.

55. **(A)** Although plants have tissues and organs that perform specific functions, these are not organized into organ systems such as one would find in animals, especially higher animals.

56. **(B)** Boyle's Law illustrates the relationship between the pressure and volume of a mass of gas at a fixed temperature. The law can be simply stated: at a given fixed temperature and mass of gas, pressure and volume are inversely proportional. For example, volume will increase as pressure decreases, or volume will decrease as pressure increases. Therefore, pressure × volume = a constant.

57. **(B)** Peas and beans are members of the legume family and have nitrogen-fixing bacteria in nodules on their roots. Nitrogen-fixing bacteria convert atmospheric gaseous nitrogen into nitrates, thus restoring nitrates to the soil. It is only in the form of nitrates that plants generally can obtain nitrogen from the soil.

58. **(A)** The male sex chromosome is referred to as the Y chromosome. It is inherited only by male offspring; thus, a male is XY and a female is XX, as far as inheritance of sex is concerned. Therefore, any gene located on the Y chromosome is inherited only by males since females will inherit an X from the male parent.

59. **(B)** Oxidation-reduction reactions are those in which one substance is oxidized by the loss of electrons, and another substance is reduced by the gain of electrons. In double replacement reactions, this does not occur. Ions are exchanged between reactants and do not lose or gain electrons.

60. **(B)** The cross indicates that the parents were heterozygous blacks (1 black and 1 white allele). The cross would yield 1 homozygous black, 2 heterozygous blacks, and 1 homozygous white offspring.

61. **(D)** The mitochondrion is called the powerhouse of the cell; most of the respiratory process involving the release of energy occurs in this organelle.

62. **(B)** Reproductive isolation is the major criterion for determination of speciation.

63. **(A)** Oxygen is a waste product of photosynthesis. Green plants use carbon dioxide and water as raw materials to produce sugar in the presence of chlorophyll and sunlight as follows:

$$CO_2 + H_2O \xrightarrow[\text{chlorophyll}]{\text{sunlight}} C_6H_{12}O_6 + O_2$$

64. **(C)** *Egestion* is the elimination of undigested wastes from the digestive tracts or cavity: enzymes are not involved in this process but are involved in the other processes named.

65. **(A)** Chloroplasts contain the chlorophylls, the green pigments, and are characteristic of green plants but not of animals.

66. **(A)** In the absence of oxygen, plants and microbes convert pyruvic acid into alcohol and carbon dioxide by a process called fermentation.

67. **(A)** The cell wall and plastids are characteristic of plant cells but not animal cells. A nucleus may not be present in some cells, such as mature human red blood cells. But all cells have cytoplasm surrounded by a plasma or cell membrane.

68. **(A)** Digestion in humans occurs primarily in the lumen of the stomach and small intestine where macromolecules are degraded to small molecules capable of being absorbed.

69. **(B)** A virus does not exhibit reproduction, synthesis, and other characteristics of life outside a living host cell; thus, it is an obligate intracellular parasite.

70. **(C)** Digestive enzymes pass directly from the gland or gland cells producing them to the site of digestion. Thus, they are not transported in the bloodstream as are the other substances named.

UNIT IV: READING COMPREHENSION

TECHNIQUES OF READING INTERPRETATION

Reading comprehension presents problems to many test-takers. To avoid this, make every effort to improve your ability to interpret reading passages.

First, understand that there are two aspects of success in reading interpretation:

1. reading speed
2. reading understanding

Too many individuals read with excellent comprehension but read too slowly. Remember, there is a time limit on your test. On the other hand, some people read rapidly, but, for reasons that we shall cite later, do not thoroughly understand what they are reading. Both speed of reading and comprehension of the material read are important during an exam. Let us, then, divide our discussion into two parts:

1. increasing reading speed
2. improving reading comprehension

GENERAL ADVICE

You were probably taught to read letter-by-letter; gradually, as you matured, you learned to read word-by-word. As an adult, however, you should be able to read a complete phrase as quickly as you once read just one letter. If you cannot do this, or if you have trouble understanding what you read, you should practice reading intensively.

There is no need to be discouraged if this is the case. Most students can increase the speed of their reading significantly with a little effort. The old idea that slow readers make up for their slowness by better comprehension of what they read has been proved untrue. Your ability to comprehend what you read should keep pace with your increase in speed. You can absorb as many ideas per page and get many more ideas per unit of reading time by applying specific techniques of reading.

It has been demonstrated that those who read best also read quickly. This is probably due to the fact that heavier concentration is required for rapid reading; and concentration is what enables a reader to grasp important ideas contained in the reading material.

A good paragraph generally has one central thought—that is, a *topic sentence*. Your main task is to locate and absorb that thought while reading the paragraph. The correct interpretation of the paragraph is based upon that thought, and not upon your personal opinions, prejudices, or preferences. If a selection consists of two or more paragraphs, its correct interpretation is based on the central idea of the entire passage. The ability to grasp the central idea of a passage can be acquired by practice—practice that will also increase the speed with which you read.

An important rule to follow in order to improve reading ability is to force yourself to increase your speed. Just as you once stopped reading letter-by-letter, now learn to stop reading word-by-word. Force yourself to read rapidly across the line of type, skimming it. Don't permit your eyes to stop for individual words; try instead to reconstruct the whole idea even if a word has been missed. Proceed quickly through the paragraph in this skimming fashion, without rereading or backtracking to a missed word.

If you find yourself failing to comprehend what you read, read the material over several times rapidly until you do understand. Do *not* slow down on rereading. At first, you may find yourself missing some of the ideas. With persistent practice, however, you will step up both your reading speed and your ability to comprehend what you read.

You may need to overcome certain handicaps or bad reading habits at once. Do not move your lips, pronounce words individually silently or aloud, or think of each word separately as you read. These habits can be overcome almost automatically if you learn to leap from phrase to phrase. You can synchronize your eye movements with your mind, both of which are a great deal nimbler than your lips.

Certain physical factors affect reading. You should always read sitting in a comfortable position, erect, with head slightly inclined. The light should be excellent, with both an indirect and a direct source available; direct light should come from behind you and slightly above your shoulder, in such a way that the type is evenly lit. Hold the reading matter at your own best reading distance and at a convenient height, so you don't stoop or squint. It goes without saying that if you need reading glasses, you should certainly use them.

INCREASING READING SPEED: CAUSES AND CURES OF SLOW READING

Cause #1: Word-by-word reading. Our earliest reading, since it is done aloud, is, of necessity, word-by-word reading. Unfortunately, this method of reading sometimes becomes so firmly implanted that it persists as a bad reading habit.

Cure: Use the *eye-span method.* Look at the first part of a sentence that consists of a thought-unit. Then, look for the next thought-unit, if there is another one in the same sentence—then, look for still another thought-unit. For example, consider this sentence:

Reading maketh a full man, conference a ready man, and writing an exact man. How many ideas are there in the sentence? Three. Now, employ the eyespan method in reading this sentence.

<u>Reading maketh a full man,</u>
EYE SPAN 1

<u>conference a ready man,</u>

EYE SPAN 2

<u>and writing an exact man.</u>
EYE SPAN 3

Cause #2: Vocalizing. Some readers move their lips or whisper while they read "silently." This practice slows down silent reading time considerably.

Cure: You must consciously refrain from moving your lips or whispering during silent reading. Have someone watch you while you read. Are you vocalizing?

Cause #3: One-speed reading. You should vary your reading speed according to what you are reading.

Cure: The pace of your reading should change not only from book to book, but even within a reading selection. Be flexible so that you can change speed from paragraph to paragraph, even from sentence to sentence. Adjust your reading rate according to the purpose for which you are reading. Scanning a passage for main ideas may be accomplished with rapid reading. Reading a novel for enjoyment would allow you to read at a medium rate. Reading to obtain detailed information would require you to read at a rather slow pace.

INCREASING READING COMPREHENSION

The following are good techniques to use on *any* reading interpretation question.

1. Read the selection through quickly to get the general sense.
2. Reread the selection, concentrating on the central idea.
3. Can you now pick out the *topic sentence* in each paragraph?

4. If the selection consists of more than one paragraph, determine the *central idea* of the entire selection.
5. Examine the four choices for each test item carefully yet rapidly. Eliminate immediately those choices that are far-fetched, ridiculous, irrelevant, false, or impossible.
6. Eliminate those choices that may be true but have nothing to do with the sense of the selection.
7. Check those few choices that now remain as possibilities.
8. Refer back to the original selection and determine which one of these remaining possibilities is best in view of
    a) information *stated* in the selection
    b) information *implied* in the selection
9. Be sure to consider only the facts *given or definitely implied* in the selection.
10. Be especially careful of trick expressions or catch-words, which sometimes destroy the validity of a seemingly acceptable answer. These include the expressions "under all circumstances," "at all times," "always," "under no conditions," "absolutely," "completely," and "entirely."

Avoid Traps

Trap #1. Sometimes the questions cannot be answered on the basis of the stated facts. You may be required to make a *deduction* from the facts given. Making a deduction requires you to draw conclusions from something already known.

Trap #2. Some reading passages are designed to arouse the reader's emotion, or describe situations with which the reader can identify. Be certain to base an answer selection on the information presented in the passage. Eliminate your personal opinions.

Trap #3. Many questions and the appropriate responses to these questions are based on important details that are nestled in the paragraph. Reread the paragraph as many times as necessary (keeping an eye on your watch) to find significant facts that will provide answers to the questions.

Get Plenty of Practice

Read:

(a) editorial pages of various newspapers

(b) book reviews (also drama and movie reviews)

(c) magazine articles

For each selection that you read, do the following:

(a) Jot down the main idea of the article.

(b) Look up the meanings of words you don't know or aren't sure of.

A Sample Question

Here is a sample question followed by analysis. Try to understand the process of arriving at the correct answer.

Too often, indeed, have scurrilous and offensive allegations by underworld figures been sufficient to blast the careers of irreproachable and incorruptible executives who, because of their efforts to serve the people honestly and faithfully, incurred the enmity of powerful political forces and lost their positions.

Judging from the contents of the preceding sentence, which conclusion might be most valid?

(A) The large majority of executives are irreproachable and incorruptible.
(B) Criminals often swear in court that honest officials are corrupt in order to save themselves.
(C) Political forces are always clashing with government executives.
(D) False statements by criminals sometimes cause honest officials the loss of their positions or the ruin of their careers.

Interpretation

Statement (A) can generally be said to be a true statement, but it cannot be derived from the paragraph. Nothing is said in the paragraph about "the large majority" of executives.

Statement (B) may also be a true statement and can, to a certain extent, be derived from the paragraph. However, the phrase "in order to save themselves" is not relevant to the sense of the paragraph, and even if it were, this choice does not sum up its central thought.

Statement (C) cannot be derived from the paragraph. The catch-word "always" makes this choice entirely invalid.

Statement (D) is the best conclusion that can be drawn from the contents of the paragraph, in light of the four choices given. It is open to no exceptions and adequately sums up the central thought of the paragraph.

Analysis of the Reading Comprehension Test Item

There are standardized tests designed to assess reading comprehension skills and provide an evaluation of the test-taker's independent reading level, instructional reading level, frustration reading level, and reading rate. Reading comprehension test items usually elicit a response that would indicate the test-taker's ability to identify directly stated details; indirectly stated details; main idea; inferences; and generalizations. Other target skills may include making judgments, drawing conclusions, and determining the author's purpose.

There are two types of reading comprehension test items. The first type is a long reading passage, usually a few paragraphs in length, followed by a series of questions. The second type is a short passage, usually a single paragraph in length, alongside one question. Several paragraphs in succession may treat the same topic, but the questions will always deal with the adjacent paragraph.

In order to determine your reading rate, the proctor will tell test-takers to stop after exactly one minute of exam time. Test-takers will then be asked to mark the point at which they were reading when they were told to stop, and this marking will be used for the determination.

Sample Questions # 1

The sample long reading passage below, followed by a set of six questions, will help you to analyze comprehension test items and to understand why a particular response is the correct or appropriate one.

Studying the questions before reading a passage will cause you to be more alert when reading the passage, that is, you will be aware of what information in the passage will best help you answer the questions. Now read the six questions at the end of the passage and then proceed to answer them. Note that the questions are followed by explanatory notes that indicate the skill addressed and strategies to use in your approach to a particular type of question.

"The Land of Frost and Fire" is no misnomer for the elliptic island republic in the North Atlantic known as Iceland. The island is so called because erupting volcanoes and steaming hot springs lie adjacent to its glaciers and ice fields. The official name of the country in Icelandic is Lydveldid Island, or the Republic of Iceland.

The "frost" is frigidly evident in the island's numerous ice fields that traverse the hoary landscape. Approximately one-eighth of the island is covered by glaciers. In the southeast, a glacier known as Vatnajokull makes an area of about 8550 square kilometers (about 3300 square miles). Iceland, just south of the Arctic Circle, has more than 120 glaciers.

Lydveldid Island's "fire" reaps from the many hot springs and spouting geysers that cloud the panorama of the seventeen-province republic. To add heat to the "fire" are some one hundred volcanoes including at least twenty-five that have erupted and been recorded in the annals of the island's autocratic history. Lava and rocks erupting from volcanoes have contoured much of the land. The central highlands reflect the barren wilderness of lava fields. Hekla in the southwest is the best-known Icelandic volcano because of its many eruptions. The years 1766, 1940, 1947, and 1980 mark its explosive appearances.

Thermal springs are also common in Iceland. The springs occur as geysers, sizzling mud lakes, and in various other forms. The most famous geyser here is Great Geysir, which is situated in southwest Iceland. The natives of this island of swift-flowing rivers boast of Geysir's spectacular and frequent eruptions occurring at irregular intervals of five to thirty-six hours. The torrid spring reportedly thrusts a column of boiling water upward to about sixty meters or two hundred feet.

Volcanic in origin, Iceland is indeed a land of contrast. Dazzling ice and jet black lava covering most of Iceland's surface attest to the appropriateness of its nickname—"Land of Frost and Fire."

1. Where are Iceland's hot springs and glaciers located?

   (A) in the central highlands
   (B) in the southwest
   (C) next to the glaciers
   (D) in the southeast

Explanatory Note: This is a directly stated detail question. When answering this type of question, always consider the *wh* word with which the question begins. *Who* can be answered by the name of a person. *When* is answered by a word or phrase that tells at what time or in what sequence something happens. *Why* is answered by a word or phrase that tells the reason something happens. *What* is usually answered by the name of a thing or event. *Which* is answered by choosing the correct person, place, or thing from two or more persons, places, or things. *Where* is answered by the name of a place or a phrase that describes the location of one person or thing in relation to another (spatial relationships). Finally, *how* should be considered with these question words. *How* is answered by the way in which something is done. Question 1 is a *where* question denoting a spatial relationship. The correct answer is C. Since adjacent means "next to" and encompasses the location of both the glaciers and geysers, this is the appropriate response. A, B, and D could be ruled out immediately because they do not describe the location of both the glaciers and the geysers.

2. An appropriate title for this passage would be

   (A) Volcanoes and Geysers
   (B) Iceland: The Island Republic
   (C) Iceland: A Land of Contrast
   (D) Thermal Springs

Explanatory Note: This is a main idea question. This type of question requires the test-taker to consider what the passage is mostly about. Read the question first. Then scan the entire passage to find out what it is mostly about. A word of caution: Some answer choices are merely details from the passage. It is not difficult to choose (C) as the best title.

3. It is apparent that this passage is intended to

   (A) inform
   (B) entertain
   (C) persuade
   (D) share an experience

Explanatory Note: The skill addressed in this question is identifying author's purpose. The test-taker must determine what the author is trying to accomplish by writing this selection. What kind of response does he or she want from the reader. If the reader can say that he or she enjoyed this passage or thought it was hilarious, obviously the passage was meant to entertain. If the reader's reaction is, "Well, I think I'll try that" or "I have to agree with that," the passage was written to persuade. If the passage is a narration or a storytelling written in the first person (I, me, my, myself—all references to the writer) the passage is probably aimed at sharing an experience. If the reader's reaction is, "I didn't know that," or "I never heard of this before," there is a good chance that the author intended to inform. The correct answer for this question is A, "inform."

4. The people of Iceland's sentiments toward the presence of geysers in their native land is one of

   (A) mixed emotions
   (B) pride
   (C) dread and fear
   (D) indifference

Explanatory Note: This question requires the test-taker to infer a meaning or idea. In other words, "read between the lines." In the fourth paragraph of this passage, it is mentioned that the natives "boast of Geysir's spectacular and frequent eruptions." Usually, people boast about something when they are proud of it. The correct response would therefore be, B, "pride."

5. According to this passage, Iceland's form of government at one time reflected

   (A) total rule by the state
   (B) rule by and for the people
   (C) rule by royalty
   (D) rule by dictator

Explanatory Note: This test question is an example of indirectly stated detail. In paragraph three of this passage the phrase "the annals of the island's autocratic history" appears. The adjective "autocratic," though irrelevant to the main idea of the passage, and even to the sentence in which it appears, does provide an informational detail. The term autocratic suggests government by one person having unlimited power. The correct answer therefore would be, D, "rule by dictator." In completing this type question, the test-taker should scan the passage to eliminate answer choices. Eliminate answer choices that are obviously related to the main idea, and in some cases, be careful of negative words in the question (no, not, not any).

6. Iceland is a difficult place to

   (A) grow crops
   (B) raise a family
   (C) get an education
   (D) start a business

Explanatory Note: Question 6 requires that you make a judgment or draw a conclusion. Since the passage does not mention family life, education, or industry, it would be safe to eliminate choices B, C, and D. The passage also does not mention agriculture; however it does describe the land as being "barren wilderness" and "covered by glaciers." These conditions are unsuitable for farming. Therefore, A, "grow crops," is an appropriate answer.

Sample Questions #2

Below are two sample short reading passages and questions, followed by analyses of the test items. Try to determine the answers on your own before reading the "Explanatory Note."

A

At birth, you more than likely weighed less than 10 pounds. As an adult you may weigh anywhere from 90 to 200 pounds or more. Obviously, there is much more of you as an adult. Despite your growth, the cells that comprise your adult body are no larger than those that made up your body in infancy. This means that your adult body is made up of billions more cells. You might question the source of these new cells. To satisfy your curiosity, they came from old cells via a process known as cell division.

(Answer Question 31)

31. The main idea of Paragraph A:

   (A) Most infants weigh less than 10 pounds.
   (B) Growth in human beings is accomplished by cell division.
   (C) Living cells increase in number by a process called cell division.
   (D) The cells that make up an adult body are larger than those of an infant body.

B

At a certain time during its existence, a cell divides into two cells. At the start of cell division, the nucleus becomes more dense and grainier than it was earlier. The grainy material, known as chromatin, eventually divides into short cordlike structures called chromosomes. The chromosomes travel through the cell, forming a double line near the center of the cell.

(Answer Question 32)

32. As a result of the movement of chromosomes through the cell,

    (A) A grainy material is formed
    (B) A cell divides into two cells
    (C) The chromatin divides into short, cordlike structures
    (D) A double line of them is formed near the center of the cell

Explanatory Note: In question number 31, you are clearly asked to find the main idea of Paragraph A. This means that you are to consider what the paragraph is mostly about. If you chose B, "Growth in human beings is accomplished by cell division," you have cited the correct response. A review or second reading of the paragraph will show that choice A could be supported by the paragraph; however, you should question the word "most." This statement merely provides a detail that leads to the principal concept. Choice C is factual, but it only supplies a major detail to the overall concept. Choice D, according to the paragraph, is incorrect information since the passage states that "despite your growth, the cells that comprise your adult body are no larger than those that made up your body in infancy." Answer B most clearly ties together the two remaining details (choices A and C) and states what the paragraph is mostly about.

Explanatory Note: In question number 32, the word "result" indicates a cause/effect response ("result" and "effect" are synonymous in this case). The paragraph clearly states that "the chromosomes travel through the cell, forming a double line near the center of the cell." (Paraphrase: *causing* a double line to form.) A review of the paragraph would prove that adding any of the activities described in responses A, B, or C to the question stem would not yield the proper sequence of the cell division process. Therefore, the correct answer is D.

READING IN THE CONTENT AREA

Efficient reading requires that the reader be flexible. As you read on page 264, "Increasing Reading Speed," it is necessary to adjust your reading rate according to the purpose for which you are reading. It is equally important to adapt your reading style to the material being read. Before investigating effective strategies to use in making such reading adjustments, it is necessary to examine and recognize the structure and patterns of writing unique to each subject area. This study of various reading materials will help you to get a feel for their differences and to determine which reading style to apply to any given reading task.

Reading comprehension test items are frequently designed to reflect the course content of the field of study targeted by the entrance examination. For instance, entrance exams for educational programs leading to health careers may feature reading passages that treat scientific topics and information.

Unlike the humanities—which deal with emotions, attitudes, and sympathies of human beings via the study of philosophy, religion, music, art, and literature—science is the accumulation of knowledge by means of the study, observation, and classification of data justifiable by general laws or concrete truths. Scientists look for and acquire information regarding forms and processes of nature. They search for an undistorted view of reality and, therefore, cannot allow their values, feelings, attitudes, beliefs, and prejudices—or those of society—to interfere with their work.

Due to the nature of the subject matter, a scientist's writings follow a certain style. Descriptions are very exacting, factual, and detailed. They are void of background mood or setting, and are unemotional. As you read scientific material, you must concentrate on the following reading skills:

1. Developing vocabulary
2. Finding the main concepts
3. Determining and remembering supporting details

4. Understanding the organization or major pattern of writing in science (examination, classification, generalization, problem solution, comparison or contrast, sequence)

5. Drawing conclusions

A review of the Verbal Ability section of this book will provide strategies for understanding and developing specialized scientific vocabulary. One method encourages vocabulary expansion through the use of a glossary, dictionary, thesaurus, etc., as well as through context clues. Another encourages the recognition of words that stand for concepts instead of facts. Other approaches include the study of word roots and affixes and the recognition of symbols.

The design or style of the text in science reading materials makes finding the main concepts simple. There are usually titles, opening comments in boldface type, headings, a summary, and questions at the end of the chapter or chapter section. In your initial reading, read only the text features just listed. This will allow you to explore and get a sense of the main ideas presented in the chapter, article, or selection. It will also prepare you for a second and closer reading.

Once you have identified the main ideas in a scientific passage, the next step in understanding what you are reading is to determine the supporting details. Supporting details answer the who, what, why, where, and when surrounding the main idea. Ask yourself these questions once you have completed a paragraph. In science, you should also question how much or to what extent.

Understanding the organization or major pattern of writing in science is vital to your reading comprehension. First of all, you should concentrate on examining the material you are about to read *before* you actually read it. Know the topic(s) that will be addressed and sum up the vocabulary in the particular reading selection. Next, check to see the type of writing pattern that stands out in the material. There are four:

> *Classification* places into groups and subgroups a variety of objects or areas. For instance, in the explanation of plant life, a writer may outline the classification of plants. The breakdown could begin with vascular and nonvascular and seedless nonvascular plants. From here the author could branch out to descriptions of mosses and liverworts, etc. In this pattern, watching for structural parts in order of importance is a must. Be aware of subheadings and all boldface type.
>
> *Process-description* requires you to be aware of what the process is and exactly how it works. Studying illustrations and diagrams are a big help here in this pattern.
>
> *Factual-statement* involves the presentation of facts to define things, to compare or contrast things, and to illustrate things. When reading for facts, remember that "fact" in the world of science means a statement that can be supported by scientific observation and experimentation and that has not yet been disproved. A fact defines something or explains its actions.
>
> *Problem-solving* usually appears in science passages that give an account of past scientific problems and discoveries achieved through experimentation. There are three helpful questions that you should ask yourself in analyzing a problem-solving passage: (1) What is the problem or question? (2) How does the author answer or respond to the question? (3) How do I know the question was answered?

Drawing conclusions is basic to the study of the sciences. A sound conclusion is a judgment based on facts. Consider what you need to know in order to make a sound judgment about something you read. Check the facts given. Think about what these facts are based on (experimentation, observation, etc.) to make certain of their reliability. Then consider the facts that are not given. Reread the passage to gather information that may be implied rather then stated. This method should help you in your test-taking venture. Speaking of tests, by now you have probably drawn some conclusions about the entrance exam you are about to take, and about the specialized vocabulary that may appear on it. However, do not conclude that scientific reading material is extremely difficult; instead, think of it as a kind of reading material that requires a very different approach. That should make it less forboding.

READING COMPREHENSION TESTS ANSWER SHEET

TEST 1: READING COMPREHENSION

1. Ⓐ Ⓑ Ⓒ Ⓓ	7. Ⓐ Ⓑ Ⓒ Ⓓ	13. Ⓐ Ⓑ Ⓒ Ⓓ
2. Ⓐ Ⓑ Ⓒ Ⓓ	8. Ⓐ Ⓑ Ⓒ Ⓓ	14. Ⓐ Ⓑ Ⓒ Ⓓ
3. Ⓐ Ⓑ Ⓒ Ⓓ	9. Ⓐ Ⓑ Ⓒ Ⓓ	15. Ⓐ Ⓑ Ⓒ Ⓓ
4. Ⓐ Ⓑ Ⓒ Ⓓ	10. Ⓐ Ⓑ Ⓒ Ⓓ	
5. Ⓐ Ⓑ Ⓒ Ⓓ	11. Ⓐ Ⓑ Ⓒ Ⓓ	
6. Ⓐ Ⓑ Ⓒ Ⓓ	12. Ⓐ Ⓑ Ⓒ Ⓓ	

TEST 2: READING COMPREHENSION

1. Ⓐ Ⓑ Ⓒ Ⓓ	5. Ⓐ Ⓑ Ⓒ Ⓓ
2. Ⓐ Ⓑ Ⓒ Ⓓ	6. Ⓐ Ⓑ Ⓒ Ⓓ
3. Ⓐ Ⓑ Ⓒ Ⓓ	7. Ⓐ Ⓑ Ⓒ Ⓓ
4. Ⓐ Ⓑ Ⓒ Ⓓ	8. Ⓐ Ⓑ Ⓒ Ⓓ

TEST 3: READING COMPREHENSION

1. Ⓐ Ⓑ Ⓒ Ⓓ	6. Ⓐ Ⓑ Ⓒ Ⓓ
2. Ⓐ Ⓑ Ⓒ Ⓓ	7. Ⓐ Ⓑ Ⓒ Ⓓ
3. Ⓐ Ⓑ Ⓒ Ⓓ	8. Ⓐ Ⓑ Ⓒ Ⓓ
4. Ⓐ Ⓑ Ⓒ Ⓓ	9. Ⓐ Ⓑ Ⓒ Ⓓ
5. Ⓐ Ⓑ Ⓒ Ⓓ	

TEST 4: READING COMPREHENSION

1. Ⓐ Ⓑ Ⓒ Ⓓ	6. Ⓐ Ⓑ Ⓒ Ⓓ
2. Ⓐ Ⓑ Ⓒ Ⓓ	7. Ⓐ Ⓑ Ⓒ Ⓓ
3. Ⓐ Ⓑ Ⓒ Ⓓ	8. Ⓐ Ⓑ Ⓒ Ⓓ
4. Ⓐ Ⓑ Ⓒ Ⓓ	9. Ⓐ Ⓑ Ⓒ Ⓓ
5. Ⓐ Ⓑ Ⓒ Ⓓ	10. Ⓐ Ⓑ Ⓒ Ⓓ

TEST 5: READING COMPREHENSION

1. Ⓐ Ⓑ Ⓒ Ⓓ
2. Ⓐ Ⓑ Ⓒ Ⓓ
3. Ⓐ Ⓑ Ⓒ Ⓓ
4. Ⓐ Ⓑ Ⓒ Ⓓ
5. Ⓐ Ⓑ Ⓒ Ⓓ
6. Ⓐ Ⓑ Ⓒ Ⓓ
7. Ⓐ Ⓑ Ⓒ Ⓓ
8. Ⓐ Ⓑ Ⓒ Ⓓ

TEST 6: READING COMPREHENSION

1. Ⓐ Ⓑ Ⓒ Ⓓ
2. Ⓐ Ⓑ Ⓒ Ⓓ
3. Ⓐ Ⓑ Ⓒ Ⓓ
4. Ⓐ Ⓑ Ⓒ Ⓓ
5. Ⓐ Ⓑ Ⓒ Ⓓ
6. Ⓐ Ⓑ Ⓒ Ⓓ

READING COMPREHENSION TESTS

TEST 1: READING COMPREHENSION

15 QUESTIONS • TIME—35 MINUTES

Directions: Carefully read the following paragraphs and then answer the accompanying questions, basing your answer on what is stated or implied in the paragraphs. When you have decided which choice is best, blacken the corresponding space on your answer sheet. There is only one best answer for each question.

TAKING IT TO HEART

A

Prior to 1628 when William Harvey published his book on the circulation of the blood and the operation of the heart, no one really knew or understood the function of the heart or how it worked. There was some speculation about it having something to do with the blood; however, people generally thought of it as the place in the body from which love and courage were generated.

(Answer Question 1)

1. Based upon Paragraph A, which of these statements is true?

   (A) One function of the heart is to generate love and courage in a human being.
   (B) The purpose and function of the heart was not understood until 1628.
   (C) Harvey published a book that dealt with performing operations on the heart.
   (D) The fact that the heart is instrumental in the circulation of the blood is merely speculation.

B

Until Harvey's discovery, no one was aware that the heart is one of the toughest muscles in the human body and one of the most awesome pumps in the world. It is the heart that pumps the blood throughout the body night and day. This mighty muscle, though only the size of a clenched fist, does enough work in one 24-hour period to lift a man weighing 150 pounds to an altitude of almost 1000 feet into the air.

(Answer Question 2)

2. According to Paragraph B, it is understood that:

   (A) The heart is a muscle that pumps blood throughout the body.
   (B) Harvey discovered the heart.
   (C) The heart can lift a man weighing 150 pounds to a height of 1000 feet.
   (D) All muscles in the human body perform as pumps.

C

Actually, the heart is two pumps, side by side—one on the right and one on the left. The right pump sends blood from the veins to the lungs. Then it pumps blood through the lungs to the pump on the left, which sends it through the body.

(Answer Question 3)

3. The main idea of Paragraph C:

   (A) The right pump of the heart sends blood from the veins to the lungs.
   (B) The pumps that make up the heart are situated side by side.
   (C) The left pump sends the blood through the body.
   (D) The heart is two pumps that work to send blood throughout the body.

D

Although the right- and left-hand sides of the heart are two different pumps with no direct connection between them, they squeeze and relax in just about the same rhythm. Together they pump approximately 13,000 quarts of blood through the body daily.

(Answer Question 4)

E

The most amazing thing about the heart is that it continues beating throughout life, resting only a fraction of a second after each beat. Considering that this entails 100,000 beats per day, the durability of this organ is undoubtedly phenomenal.

(Answer Question 5)

4. A point made in Paragraph D:

   (A) The human body contains 13,000 quarts of blood.
   (B) Despite the fact that they squeeze and relax in just about the same rhythm, the two pumps do not have a connection.
   (C) The rhythm of the two pumps is synchronized.
   (D) The two pumps operate as one.

5. Which statement is supported by Paragraph E?

   (A) The third part of the heartbeat is a period of rest.
   (B) A steady heartbeat is characteristic of a strong and healthy heart.
   (C) The heart beats about 70 times per minute.
   (D) You can easily detect your own heartbeat.

THE SKIN YOU'RE IN

F

The first thing you see when you look at the human body is the skin. The average adult human body is covered with about 18 square feet of skin. Skin varies in thickness. It is very thin over the eyelids and considerably thicker on the palms of the hands and the soles of the feet.

(Answer Question 6)

6. A conclusion that can be drawn from Paragraph F:

   (A) The skin is the one organ readily visible on the human body.
   (B) Adults have thicker skin than children.
   (C) Skin on the human body is thicker on parts of the body most likely to come in contact with foreign objects and surfaces.
   (D) 18 square feet of skin would be adequate to cover and protect all adult human beings.

G

The skin is composed of two layers. The outer layer of skin is called the epidermis. This name comes from ancient Greek meaning "outer layer." This layer is made up of dead, flattened cells which are continually sloughing off as we move around. The bottom of the epidermis is made of live cells that die and replace those that wear off on the surface. Throughout the body's lifetime, the under layer of skin continually creates new cells. This is the reason why cuts and scrapes heal in a short period of time.

(Answer Question 7)

7. From Paragraph G it may be inferred:

   (A) That the production of new cells constitutes healing in the human being.
   (B) The ancient Greeks were probably the first to study skin.
   (C) The bottom of the epidermis is comprised of flattened cells that gradually wear away.
   (D) Skin is the organ responsible for growth in the human body.

H

Beneath the outer layer is another layer called the dermis. This is a much deeper layer made entirely of living cells. There are several small blood vessels and nerve endings in the dermis. There are coiled tubes in this layer which open into the epidermis layer through openings called pores. The pores are the openings to the coiled tubes or sweat glands. Hairs, which grow out of the skin, are rooted in the dermis. They grow out of openings called hair follicles. Oil glands in the skin connected with the hair roots constantly oil the outer skin keeping it supple and strong.

(Answer Question 8)

8. Which statement is supported by Paragraph H?

   (A) The skin needs oil to remain pliant and durable.
   (B) The coiled tubes in the epidermis are actually pores.
   (C) Dry skin may be an indication of a problem in the hair follicle.
   (D) The epidermis provides the body with adequate temperature control.

I

The functions of the skin are numerous. The skin is a protective covering for the body that is airtight and waterproof. When it is unbroken it is a barrier to harmful bacteria. The coloring matter of the skin, known as pigment, serves to screen out certain harmful rays of the sun. The skin helps to regulate the temperature of the body and also functions as a sense organ. There are many nerve endings in the skin that caution us to stay away from things that are too hot or too cold and cause us to have a sense of touch. They enable us to detect sensation in our immediate surroundings and transmit impulses to the brain where the sensations are identified.

(Answer Question 9)

9. According to Paragraph I, it is understood that:

   (A) Skin coloring is the result of harmful rays of the sun.
   (B) Sensations are directly perceived by the skin.
   (C) The function of the skin is merely that of a protective covering.
   (D) The skin is a deterrent to harmful bacteria only if it is unbroken.

NURSING INTERVENTIONS

J

The term "nursing interventions" encompasses and describes activities that reflect nursing responsibility in the execution of health treatment. More specifically, it refers to nursing treatments, nursing observations, health teaching, and medical treatment performed by nurses. A nursing intervention is a single course of action intended to fulfill the unmet human needs that are ascertained from the patient's problem. A nursing diagnosis is, therefore, a prerequisite to implementing the appropriate care to meet the needs of the patient. It is apparent that in order to determine and initiate nursing intervention, one must have a scientific background and extensive education in nursing.

(Answer Question 10)

10. The main idea of Paragraph J:

    (A) The role of an individual who has a scientific and nursing education background and who performs a single course of action to satisfy the unmet human needs of a patient is known as nursing intervention.
    (B) A nursing diagnosis is synonomous with nursing intervention.
    (C) Nursing responsibility includes health teaching.
    (D) Nursing assessment is necessary for effective nursing intervention.

Blood Donors Available—No Thanks! I'll Do It Myself!

K

With the advent of AIDS and other communicable diseases, people are reluctant to submit to blood transfusions as a measure of medical treatment, even in emergency situations. Many individuals are opting to store their own blood in case it is ever needed.

(Continue to Paragraph L)

11. The accelerated interest in autologous transfusion is due to:

    (A) a lack of blood donors
    (B) an attempt to stimulate rapid production of new blood cells
    (C) the time-saving element in the event of emergency surgery
    (D) a rise in fear of communicable diseases

L

New blood cells are constantly being produced in the body. This is the reason that lost blood in a healthy person is replaced quickly. This rapid production of blood cells also enables a person to donate to others who might need blood. When blood is taken from one person and given to another, the procedure is called a homologous blood transfer. When a person' s own blood is used for transfusion, having been stored in anticipation of surgery, the procedure is known as autologous blood transfer. This blood is collected prior to surgery.

(Continue to Paragraph M)

12. This passage supports the concept:

    (A) Autologous transfer is a practical and easily accessible alternative to blood transfusion.
    (B) Any type of blood transfusion places a patient in a high-risk health situation.
    (C) Hemoglobin carries oxygen and carbon dioxide throughout the body.
    (D) Lost blood, even in a healthy person, is replaced only after a long period of time.

M

Though the concept of being transfused with one's own blood is very comforting, there are many factors that discourage the use of this technology. First is the expense of storing the blood. It has been estimated that the cost of safely storing the blood comes to approximately $200 per year. Another drawback is that a patient may be thousands of miles away from his or her blood supply or blood bank when the need for blood arises.

(Continue to Paragraph N)

13. From this passage it may be inferred:

    (A) Saline is a cleansing or sterilizing agent.
    (B) The storing of one's own blood supply is affordable for all.
    (C) Homologous transfusion requires blood typing and matching.
    (D) The option of autologous transfusion is not feasible in instances of elective surgery.

N

In an attempt to satisfy patients' requests to be transfused with their own blood, regardless of the medical emergency, doctors have developed two forms of autologous blood transfusion. One form utilizes suction devices to collect blood lost during surgery. After this blood has been cleansed, it may be put back into the body. Blood lost during surgery can also be collected with sponges. The sponges are then squeezed out into a container of saline solution, a kind of salt solution. This blood is processed within 15 minutes and is again introduced into the patient's circulation. Doctors believe that by using both methods they can retrieve up to 90 percent of blood that would otherwise be lost.

(Continue to Paragraph O)

O

Despite these efforts to make autologous blood transfer feasible for most patients, there still remain those situations that make it virtually impossible to collect blood. For instance, in the case of an auto accident victim, much blood is often lost before medical treatment is obtainable. To help in an incident such as this, doctors are researching ways to develop artificial hemoglobin that would temporarily transport oxygen and carbon dioxide throughout the body. Another solution to the problem that is being explored is the reproduction of a hormone that causes the body to produce blood cells much more rapidly than it would normally. This would mean that the body could replace most of its own blood and therefore reduce the need for transfusion. Even though researchers are doing extensive work to develop new techniques to protect people from blood tainted by disease, reserving one's own blood for future use seems to be the safest method of transfusion for now.

(Answer Questions 11–15)

14. A fact expressed in this passage is:
    (A) Artificial hemoglobin could permanently supply the body with oxygen and carbon dioxide.
    (B) Suction devices and sponges are two surgical implements used in the collection of blood lost during surgery.
    (C) Laser surgery is being used more frequently in an effort to minimize blood loss during surgery.
    (D) Autologous transfusion, in the event of surgery, requires that the blood always be collected prior to surgery.

15. This article suggests:
    (A) Homologous transfusions are on the decline.
    (B) The effort by researchers to protect patients from blood contaminated by disease cannot guarantee safe blood transfusion.
    (C) Autologous transfusion is impractical.
    (D) Surgical patients who are transfused autologously are assured a more rapid recovery.

TEST 2: READING COMPREHENSION

8 QUESTIONS • TIME—12 MINUTES

Directions: Carefully read the following passage and then answer the accompanying questions, basing your answers on what is stated or implied in the passage. When you have decided which choice is best, blacken the corresponding space on your answer sheet. There is only one best answer for each question.

Living organisms are unique, among the known forms of matter, because they are capable of creating their own specific highly organized structure out of substances taken from far more disorganized surroundings, and can transmit this capability to their offspring. Perhaps the oldest and most profound theoretical problem in biology is the effort to explain the curious paradox that, despite its unique capability for self-duplication and inheritance, a living organism is nevertheless a mixture of substances which are separately no more possessed of these properties than are the more prosaic molecules that never occur in living cells. This question has been at the root of a long train of experiments, debates, and speculations that began in classical times and continues unbroken through the development of present-day "molecular biology."

The basic issues are simply stated. If the component parts of a cell are not themselves alive, whence come the life-properties exhibited by the whole? Apart from the untenable notion of a mystic nonmaterial "vital force" which supposedly animates the otherwise dead substance of the cell, the debate has elicited two main positions: (a) There is, in fact, some special cellular component which possesses the fundamental attribute of self-duplication, and which is therefore a "living molecule" and the basic source of the life-properties of the cell. (b) The unique properties of life are inherently connected with the very considerable complexity of living substance and arise from interactions among its separable constituents which are not exhibited unless these components occur together in the complex whole. In this view, only the entire living cell is capable of self-duplication.

There is at this time a widespread impression that this issue has been resolved and that the cell does indeed contain a component—DNA—which, according to the theory of the "DNA code," possesses the basic attribute of life, self-duplication, and which guides the activities of all the inheritable processes of the cell.

The importance of this conclusion is self-evident, for it would answer, at last, the basic question of the origin of the unique properties of life, and, if correct, should lead to unprecedented technological control over these properties. It is appropriate, therefore, to ask what criteria are required to establish that a molecule, such as DNA, is capable of self-duplication, to examine the degree to which the available evidence meets such criteria, and to determine whether the undoubted importance of DNA in the biology of inheritance may be due to some properties other than those attributed to it by current theory.*

**Reprinted with permission of American Scientist. From "DNA and the Chemistry of Inheritances," by Barry Commoner, American Scientist 52, 1964.*

1. The chief conclusion to be derived from the foregoing considerations is that
   (A) self-duplication of living organisms is the result of the biochemical aspects of genetics
   (B) the origin of unique properties of life is a "vital force"
   (C) the relationships between reproduction and inheritance are mutually exclusive
   (D) self-duplication is a process of converting nonliving matter to living matter

2. In this passage, the author identifies the uniqueness of living organisms by which one of the following characteristics?
   (A) Similar life forms are created from separate substances possessing the properties of life.
   (B) Similar life forms are created from separate substances that do not possess the properties of life.
   (C) New organisms are reproduced from a single substance.
   (D) New organisms are produced from noncellular components.

3. The author's approach to the study of inheritance is

    (A) biological and chemical
    (B) ecological and biological
    (C) chemical and ecological
    (D) physical and biological

4. Which one of the following statements best describes the "DNA code" theory?

    (A) DNA acts as a catalyst in the creation of life.
    (B) DNA controls heredity but not cell reproduction.
    (C) The cell has the ability to synthesize DNA, which animates nonliving matter.
    (D) The cell contains DNA, a living molecule capable of self-duplication.

5. The basic issues regarding self-duplication presented in this passage include all of the following *except* the

    (A) role of living and nonliving matter in the creation of life
    (B) relationships between cellular parts and the complex whole
    (C) differences between genetic processes and reproduction in living organisms
    (D) paradox between the phenomenon of self-duplication and the biochemical processes involved in the creation of life

6. The ultimate purpose of research related to heredity is to

    (A) balance the relationships between living and nonliving matter
    (B) create life through artificial techniques
    (C) control inheritable processes of the cell
    (D) create unknown forms of life

7. The author's approach to the study of the DNA theory is to

    (A) apply the principles of molecular biology to the notion of "vital force"
    (B) establish criteria for judging the capabilities of DNA to self-duplicate
    (C) assume that DNA is the isolated factor of self-duplication and study genetic processes
    (D) confirm that the creation of organisms is a self-duplication process

8. The best title for this passage might be

    (A) *DNA, the Miracle of Life*
    (B) *Self-Duplication: The Mystery of Life*
    (C) *Differences Between Self-Duplication and Heredity*
    (D) *The Status of Genetic Research*

TEST 3: READING COMPREHENSION

9 QUESTIONS • TIME—12 MINUTES

Directions: Carefully read the following passage and then answer the accompanying questions basing your answers on what is stated or implied in the passage. When you have decided which choice is best, blacken the corresponding space on your answer sheet. There is only one best answer for each question.

Although there are many branches of chemistry, there is virtually nothing more important than the chemistry of plants and animals. Life and health rely on a branch of chemistry called biochemistry. The prefix "bio" derives from the Greek word for life. There are chemists who specialize solely in the science of nutrition. These chemists have found that certain kinds of food substances are necessary to nourish the body.

One important food group includes sugar and starch. Sugar and starch are compounds comprised of carbon, hydrogen, and oxygen. These compounds are called carbohydrates.

There are various kinds of sugar; glucose and sucrose are two. Glucose is found in the juice of some fruits and is represented by the formula $C_6H_{12}O_6$. Sucrose, as found in the sugar bowl on the breakfast table, is chemically more complex. Its formula is $C_{12}H_{22}O_{11}$.

Starch is known by the formula $C_6H_{10}O_5$. It is a polymer, a giant molecule made up of many units. Starch exists mostly in foods such as bread, rice, potatoes, corn, and cereals. By joining molecules of water to the starch units, the sugars can be formed. What happens is the atoms of hydrogen and oxygen in water add on to those in the starch units. The process is similar to addition in arithmetic.

Example:	$C_6H_{12}O_5$	(StarchUnit)
	H_2O	(Water Added)
	$C_6H_{12}O_6$	(Glucose)

Starch and sugar must be introduced into the bloodstream in order to be used by the body. This can be accomplished easily with sugars since they dissolve in water and pass readily through the wall of the intestines to the blood vessels that are all around it. Starch, however, must be changed into sugar before it can dissolve. This change is made possible by the digestive juices which simply add a water molecule onto each starch unit, yielding glucose. The glucose can then be carried into the blood stream like any sugar.

It is understood that food is burned in the body just as diesel oil or gasoline is burned in an engine. However, the fundamental or basic concepts of biochemistry explained in this passage attest to the fact that the chemical action in human beings is much more intricate and complex.

1. According to this passage:

   (A) Biochemists are concerned solely with the life of plants.
   (B) Sugar and starch are not considered carbohydrates.
   (C) There are only two kinds of sugar.
   (D) Sugar and starch belong to the same food group.

2. It could be concluded that

   (A) starches are soluble in water
   (B) compounds are made up of two or more elements
   (C) glucose is a complex sugar
   (D) formulas represent elements

3. In comparing the formulas for glucose and starch, it should be noted that

   (A) sucrose does not contain hydrogen
   (B) they contain equal molecules of water
   (C) glucose contains two atoms more of hydrogen and one atom more of oxygen than starch
   (D) neither contain oxygen

4. Table sugar is made up of

   (A) 11 atoms of carbon, 22 atoms of hydrogen, and 11 atoms of oxygen
   (B) 6 atoms of carbon, 12 of hydrogen, and 6 of oxygen
   (C) 12 atoms of carbon, 22 of hydrogen, and 11 of oxygen
   (D) 12 atoms of carbon, 24 atoms of hydrogen, and 12 atoms of oxygen

5. Carbohydrates contain the elements

   (A) carbon, hydrogen, and oxygen
   (B) oxygen, carbon, and nitrogen
   (C) carbon, hydrogen, and phosphorus
   (D) oxygen, sulfur, and phosphorus

6. Fruits, rice, and cereal all contain

   (A) starch
   (B) carbohydrates
   (C) sugar
   (D) sucrose

7. Based on this passage, it may be inferred that bread is converted to

   (A) starch by the body
   (B) sugar by the body
   (C) complex sugar by the body
   (D) sucrose by the body

8. Nutrients are carried throughout the body by means of

   (A) the stomach
   (B) the small intestine
   (C) the circulatory system
   (D) oxygen

9. It could be concluded that scientists who specialize in the science of nutrition are in fact

   (A) pharmacists
   (B) geochemists
   (C) biochemists
   (D) nuclear chemists

TEST 4: READING COMPREHENSION

10 QUESTIONS • TIME—13 MINUTES

Directions: Carefully read the following passage and then answer the accompanying questions, basing your answers on what is stated or implied in the passage. When you have decided which choice is best, blacken the corresponding space on your answer sheet. There is only one best answer for each question.

With the recent use of DNA (deoxyribonucleic acid) as a means of providing evidence in a number of world-renowned criminal cases, the general public views this carrier of genetic information as a modern day scientific discovery. However, a glimpse at the history of DNA will prove the notion of a "modern day miracle" quite to the contrary.

To investigate the discovery of DNA, one would have to research the laboratory and work of the Swiss biochemist, Johan Friedrich Miescher, back in 1868. Miescher had been involved in the study of the cell nucleus, the round control center which contains the chromosomes as well as other elements. He believed that cells were made of protein and attempted to break down this protein with a digestive enzyme. As Miescher continued this investigation, he was perplexed by the fact that the enzyme would break down the cell but not the nucleus. He then launched an investigation of the substance that comprised the cell. As he analyzed it, he saw that it contained large amounts of a strange material that was very unlike protein. Miescher chose to call this substance nuclein. He had no idea of its significance, nor did he recognize that he had discovered what came to be known in later years as nucleic acid. Nucleic acid is the chemical family to which DNA belongs.

In 1944 a team of scientists from the Rockefeller Institute proved for the first time that DNA was the carrier of hereditary information. Oswald T. Avery, Colin M. MacLeod, and Maclyn McCarty accomplished this by extracting some of the DNA in pure form from a bacterium and substituting it for a defective gene in another related bacterium.

Some ten years later, the intricate molecular structure of DNA was described by Harvard biochemist James D. Watson and physicist Francis Crick of Great Britain. However, prior to this, scientist Rosalind Franklin discovered that the DNA molecule was a strand of molecules in a spiral form. Dr. Franklin demonstrated that the spiral was so large that it was most likely formed by two spirals. Ultimately, Franklin determined that the structure of DNA is similar to the handrails and steps of a spiral staircase.

Equipped with the work and findings of Rosalind Franklin and others, Watson and Crick were able to construct a model of a DNA molecule. This model depicted the sides or "handrails" of the DNA molecules as being made up of two twisted strands of sugar and phosphate molecules. The "stairs" that hold the two sugar phosphate strands apart are made up of molecules called nitrogen bases.

All of this data supports the fact that DNA is by no means a "new discovery"; however, what is the significance of it at all? Why is DNA important to you? The answer is that all of the characteristics you possess are affected by the DNA in your cells. It controls the color of your eyes, the color of your hair, and whether or not you have a tolerance for dairy products. These characteristics are known as traits. The way your traits appear depends on tire kinds of proteins your cells make. DNA stores the blueprints for making the proteins. Your DNA is uniquely different from that of anyone else on earth, and you are identifiable by these proteins.

1. It could be concluded that

   (A) Watson and Crick discovered DNA
   (B) the strands of DNA take the form of a double hexagon
   (C) DNA is as unique to individuals as a fingerprint
   (D) Miescher's analysis of nuclein resulted directly in the discovery of DNA

2. From this passage it may be deduced that enzymes are

   (A) unstable
   (B) ineffective
   (C) catalysts
   (D) solutions

3. It may be inferred that an individual's DNA determines

   (A) whether or not he/she can digest milk
   (B) whether or not he/she is immune to the common cold
   (C) an individual's choice of residential location
   (D) a person's inclination toward dishonesty

4. The types of protein produced by a cell are controlled by the DNA contained in its

   (A) nitrogen bases
   (B) nucleus
   (C) cell wall
   (D) sugar phosphate bands

5. It is implied that proteins are

   (A) the control center of the cell
   (B) blueprint of the cell
   (C) the storage center of the cell
   (D) the building blocks of a cell

6. A reference to the "spiral staircase" constitutes a description of

   (A) the molecular structure of proteins
   (B) the molecular structure of digestive enzymes
   (C) the molecular structure of RNA
   (D) the molecular structure of DNA

7. Digestive enzymes are effective in breaking up

   (A) nuclein
   (B) DNA
   (C) all chemical compounds
   (D) protein

8. The word "nucleus" refers to

   (A) the round control center of the cell
   (B) the walls of the cell
   (C) a strand of molecules
   (D) a helix

9. The scientific disciplines used in determining the structure of the DNA molecule include biology, chemistry, and

   (A) geneology
   (B) serologly
   (C) physics
   (D) embryology

10. As described in this passage, "model" means

   (A) an exhibitor of fashion
   (B) a physical form representing a concept
   (C) a miniature version of an existing object
   (D) a person on whom an artist bases his/her rendition

TEST 5: READING COMPREHENSION

8 QUESTIONS • TIME—13 MINUTES

Directions: Carefully read the following passage and then answer the accompanying questions, basing your answers on what is stated or implied in the passage. When you have decided which choice is best, blacken the corresponding space on your answer sheet. There is only one best answer for each question.

The pituitary gland is a small gland, about the size of an acorn or cherry, that lies at the base of the brain. It was once thought to be the "master gland" of the body, since its secretions appeared to influence the activity of all other endocrine glands. However, it is now known that other glands, especially the thyroid and adrenal glands, influence the pituitary gland.

The pituitary gland consists of two lobes: anterior and posterior. The anterior lobe secretes several different hormones. One of these, the *somatotropic* or growth hormone, regulates the growth of the skeleton. If an oversecretion of this hormone occurs during the growing years, tremendous height may be attained. This condition is called *giantism*. Circus giants, over 8 feet tall, weighing over 300 pounds and wearing size 30 shoes, are examples of this disorder. If the oversecretion occurs during adult life, the bones of the face and hands thicken, since they cannot grow in length. However, the organs and the soft tissues enlarge tremendously. This condition is known as *acromegaly*. Victims of this disorder have greatly enlarged jawbones, noses, hands and fingers.

Somatotropic hormone deficiency results in a *pituitary dwarf*, or midget. These individuals are perfectly proportioned "men in miniature." They are quite different from the thyroid dwarf in that they have normal intelligence.

Another hormone secretion of the anterior lobe of the pituitary gland, the *gonadotropic* hormone, influences the development of the reproductive organs. It also influences hormone secretion of the ovaries and testes. The gonadotropic hormone, together with the sex hormones, causes the sweeping changes that occur during adolescence, when a child becomes an adult.

Other secretions of the anterior lobe of the pituitary gland include hormones that stimulate the secretion of milk in the mammary glands (*lactogenic* hormone), the activity of the thyroid gland (*thyrotropic* hormone), and the parathyrotropic glands (*parathyrotropic* hormone).

ACTH is a secretion of the anterior lobe of the pituitary gland and stimulates the outer part, or *cortex*, of the adrenal glands. The adrenals, in turn, secrete hormones responsible for the control of certain phases of carbohydrate, fat, and protein metabolism, and the salt and water balance in the body.

The adrenal cortex also yields hormones that control the production of some kinds of white corpuscles and the structure of connective tissue. When ACTH is given to patients with leukemia, a dramatic but, unfortunately, temporary improvement occurs. Its effects in arthritis treatment are somewhat more encouraging. Good results in the treatment of asthma and other allergies with ACTH have been reported. Even though ACTH may not give permanent cures to these diseases, its use may lead the way to the discovery of their actual causes.

The posterior lobe of the pituitary gland produces two hormones: (1) *pitressin,* which helps regulate the amount of water in the blood and the blood pressure; and (2) *pitocin,* which stimulates smooth muscles. It is administered following childbirth to cause contraction of the muscles of the uterus, thus preventing blood loss.

1. A hormone is

   (A) an important gland
   (B) a kind of medicine
   (C) a chemical secretion
   (D) a kind of germ

2. Which of the following is not a secretion of the pituitary gland?

   (A) somatotropin
   (B) gonadotrophin
   (C) pitocin
   (D) adrenalin

3. Which of the following will affect the age at which a person reaches puberty?

   (A) sex hormones
   (B) somatotrophin
   (C) lactogenic hormone
   (D) none of these

4. Cretinism results in a stunted body and a dull, stupid mentality. It is caused by a defect in which gland?

   (A) pituitary
   (B) adrenal
   (C) thyroid
   (D) parathyroid

5. The circus giant of over 8 feet in height probably got too much somatotrophic hormone when he was

   (A) an infant
   (B) a teenager
   (C) a young adult
   (D) an older adult

6. A cure for leukemia is

   (A) a pituitary hormone
   (B) an adrenal hormone
   (C) a cortexial hormone
   (D) none of these

7. A cow which failed to have enough lactogenic hormone would probably

   (A) fail to become pregnant
   (B) become overly fat
   (C) lose a lot of weight
   (D) not give any milk

8. A person admitted to a hospital with swollen limbs due to too much water in the joints may be suffering from

   (A) improper functioning of the adrenal gland
   (B) overactivity of the pituitary gland
   (C) underactivity of the pituitary gland
   (D) too much pitressin

TEST 6: READING COMPREHENSION

6 QUESTIONS • TIME—8 MINUTES

Directions: Carefully read the following passage and then answer the accompanying questions, basing your answers on what is stated or implied in the passage. When you have decided which choice is best, blacken the corresponding space on your answer sheet. There is only one best answer for each question.

PET (positron emission tomography) is a sort of a Geiger counter for the brain. It displays in living color which regions are active during remembering, thinking, and other mental tasks. PET scans, in other words, show the brain recalling and cogitating.

PET was developed in 1972. Currently, six American laboratories use it in research. The procedure for administering a PET scan requires the scientist to inject radioactive water into the volunteer's bloodstream. The water, though radioactive, is safe. The "hot blood" makes its way to the brain. Active regions of the brain use more blood than inactive areas, so they illuminate with radioactivity that is captured on special detectors surrounding the person's head.

Researchers use this new "window on the mind" to observe and monitor all regions of the brain. They can tune into motor functions controlled by the cerebrum, monitor the reception and processing of sensory information in the cerebral cortex (where higher thinking takes place), and observe the formation of long-term memory in the hippocampus. The scan provides information on the activity in the amygdala, a center of emotions where scent perceptions are gathered, and in the cerebellum, where balance is controlled.

Numerous studies of the brain have been conducted using PET. One study proved the brain to be "pretty nimble when it comes to switching circuits." Common nouns were shown to 11 adult volunteers. The volunteers were asked to respond with an appropriate verb. For instance, "car" might elicit "drive." This exercise resulted in four areas of the brain lighting up, including the cerebellum and part of the cortex. After 15 minutes of practice, the same nouns were used again to test the same volunteers. None of the original areas lit up. Only the brain's motor system, which controls muscles, showed activity. It appears that if the brain knows the answer cold, it does not have to think much. However, when the subjects encountered a new list of nouns, the original thinking areas lit up again. The sudden change would indicate that when a task is novel and requires conscious thought, the brain calls on resources extremely different from those required for the simple repetition of a word.

1. PET permits neuroscientists to
   - (A) study an individual's vocabulary skills
   - (B) perform various surgical procedures on the brain
   - (C) monitor the activity in the different regions of the brain
   - (D) alter the function of the hippocampus

2. The term "hot blood" refers to
   - (A) blood circulation in the amygdala, a center of emotions
   - (B) blood injected with radioactive water
   - (C) blood transfused at elevated temperatures
   - (D) blood located at the base of the brain

3. The hippocampus
   - (A) receives and processes sensory information
   - (B) controls balance
   - (C) forms long-term memories
   - (D) controls motor function

4. One experiment conducted suggests that
   - (A) cognition is not exactly subtle
   - (B) one can essentially rearrange the brain, and in only 15 minutes
   - (C) the hippocampus is not the site of visual memory
   - (D) The subject's level of intelligence is directly related to the extent of brain activity observable

5. In this reading passage, positron emission tomography is compared to

   (A) a Geiger counter
   (B) previous methods used to scan the brain
   (C) a recalling/cogitating catalyst
   (D) a new type of x-ray

6. The study described in this passage would

   (A) support an argument for the brain's ability to handle learned tasks without conscious thought
   (B) dispel the idea that someone speaks without thinking
   (C) suggest that a visual image etches a channel in the cortex
   (D) prove that there is little activity in the cerebellum

READING COMPREHENSION TESTS ANSWER KEY

TEST 1: READING COMPREHENSION

1. **B**	4. **B**	7. **A**	10. **A**	13. **A**
2. **A**	5. **C**	8. **A**	11. **D**	14. **B**
3. **D**	6. **C**	9. **D**	12. **C**	15. **B**

TEST 2: READING COMPREHENSION

1. **A**	3. **A**	5. **C**	7. **B**
2. **B**	4. **D**	6. **C**	8. **B**

TEST 3: READING COMPREHENSION

1. **D**	3. **C**	5. **A**	7. **B**	9. **C**
2. **B**	4. **A**	6. **B**	8. **C**	

TEST 4: READING COMPREHENSION

1. **C**	3. **A**	5. **D**	7. **D**	9. **C**
2. **C**	4. **B**	6. **D**	8. **A**	10. **B**

TEST 5: READING COMPREHENSION

1. **C**	3. **A**	5. **B**	7. **D**
2. **D**	4. **C**	6. **D**	8. **A**

TEST 6: READING COMPREHENSION

1. **C**	3. **C**	5. **A**
2. **B**	4. **B**	6. **A**

Part III

PRACTICE FOR ALLIED HEALTH SCHOOL ENTRANCE EXAMINATIONS

UNIT V: VERBAL ABILITY

VERBAL ABILITY TESTS ANSWER SHEET

TEST 1: SYNONYMS

1. Ⓐ Ⓑ Ⓒ Ⓓ	10. Ⓐ Ⓑ Ⓒ Ⓓ	19. Ⓐ Ⓑ Ⓒ Ⓓ	28. Ⓐ Ⓑ Ⓒ Ⓓ
2. Ⓐ Ⓑ Ⓒ Ⓓ	11. Ⓐ Ⓑ Ⓒ Ⓓ	20. Ⓐ Ⓑ Ⓒ Ⓓ	29. Ⓐ Ⓑ Ⓒ Ⓓ
3. Ⓐ Ⓑ Ⓒ Ⓓ	12. Ⓐ Ⓑ Ⓒ Ⓓ	21. Ⓐ Ⓑ Ⓒ Ⓓ	30. Ⓐ Ⓑ Ⓒ Ⓓ
4. Ⓐ Ⓑ Ⓒ Ⓓ	13. Ⓐ Ⓑ Ⓒ Ⓓ	22. Ⓐ Ⓑ Ⓒ Ⓓ	31. Ⓐ Ⓑ Ⓒ Ⓓ
5. Ⓐ Ⓑ Ⓒ Ⓓ	14. Ⓐ Ⓑ Ⓒ Ⓓ	23. Ⓐ Ⓑ Ⓒ Ⓓ	32. Ⓐ Ⓑ Ⓒ Ⓓ
6. Ⓐ Ⓑ Ⓒ Ⓓ	15. Ⓐ Ⓑ Ⓒ Ⓓ	24. Ⓐ Ⓑ Ⓒ Ⓓ	33. Ⓐ Ⓑ Ⓒ Ⓓ
7. Ⓐ Ⓑ Ⓒ Ⓓ	16. Ⓐ Ⓑ Ⓒ Ⓓ	25. Ⓐ Ⓑ Ⓒ Ⓓ	34. Ⓐ Ⓑ Ⓒ Ⓓ
8. Ⓐ Ⓑ Ⓒ Ⓓ	17. Ⓐ Ⓑ Ⓒ Ⓓ	26. Ⓐ Ⓑ Ⓒ Ⓓ	35. Ⓐ Ⓑ Ⓒ Ⓓ
9. Ⓐ Ⓑ Ⓒ Ⓓ	18. Ⓐ Ⓑ Ⓒ Ⓓ	27. Ⓐ Ⓑ Ⓒ Ⓓ	

TEST 2: ANTONYMS

1. Ⓐ Ⓑ Ⓒ Ⓓ Ⓔ	8. Ⓐ Ⓑ Ⓒ Ⓓ Ⓔ	15. Ⓐ Ⓑ Ⓒ Ⓓ Ⓔ	22. Ⓐ Ⓑ Ⓒ Ⓓ Ⓔ	29. Ⓐ Ⓑ Ⓒ Ⓓ Ⓔ
2. Ⓐ Ⓑ Ⓒ Ⓓ Ⓔ	9. Ⓐ Ⓑ Ⓒ Ⓓ Ⓔ	16. Ⓐ Ⓑ Ⓒ Ⓓ Ⓔ	23. Ⓐ Ⓑ Ⓒ Ⓓ Ⓔ	30. Ⓐ Ⓑ Ⓒ Ⓓ Ⓔ
3. Ⓐ Ⓑ Ⓒ Ⓓ Ⓔ	10. Ⓐ Ⓑ Ⓒ Ⓓ Ⓔ	17. Ⓐ Ⓑ Ⓒ Ⓓ Ⓔ	24. Ⓐ Ⓑ Ⓒ Ⓓ Ⓔ	
4. Ⓐ Ⓑ Ⓒ Ⓓ Ⓔ	11. Ⓐ Ⓑ Ⓒ Ⓓ Ⓔ	18. Ⓐ Ⓑ Ⓒ Ⓓ Ⓔ	25. Ⓐ Ⓑ Ⓒ Ⓓ Ⓔ	
5. Ⓐ Ⓑ Ⓒ Ⓓ Ⓔ	12. Ⓐ Ⓑ Ⓒ Ⓓ Ⓔ	19. Ⓐ Ⓑ Ⓒ Ⓓ Ⓔ	26. Ⓐ Ⓑ Ⓒ Ⓓ Ⓔ	
6. Ⓐ Ⓑ Ⓒ Ⓓ Ⓔ	13. Ⓐ Ⓑ Ⓒ Ⓓ Ⓔ	20. Ⓐ Ⓑ Ⓒ Ⓓ Ⓔ	27. Ⓐ Ⓑ Ⓒ Ⓓ Ⓔ	
7. Ⓐ Ⓑ Ⓒ Ⓓ Ⓔ	14. Ⓐ Ⓑ Ⓒ Ⓓ Ⓔ	21. Ⓐ Ⓑ Ⓒ Ⓓ Ⓔ	28. Ⓐ Ⓑ Ⓒ Ⓓ Ⓔ	

VERBAL ABILITY TESTS

TEST 1: SYNONYMS

35 QUESTIONS • TIME—20 MINUTES

Directions: In each sentence below, one word is italicized. For each sentence, select the option which best (or most nearly) corresponds in meaning with the italicized word.

1. It has been recommended that this system be used in place of *traditional* types.

   (A) unfamiliar
   (B) usual
   (C) flexible
   (D) general

2. In our society, irresponsible behavior often leads to a monetary *penalty.*

   (A) arrangement
   (B) gratification
   (C) punishment
   (D) precaution

3. He spent the *allotted* study time to complete his assignments.

   (A) authorized
   (B) designated
   (C) agreed
   (D) alerted

4. The Senate passed the farmland *preservation* bill.

   (A) maintenance
   (B) stratagem
   (C) exordium
   (D) incumbency

5. It was apparent that he had attempted to *concoct* an alibi.

   (A) inculcate
   (B) conceal
   (C) reveal
   (D) fabricate

6. The City Council could have avoided this *scenario* by passing the ordinance.

   (A) preliminary plan
   (B) obliteration
   (C) veneration
   (D) deficiency

7. The Superior Court judge *imposed* the sentence.

   (A) indicated
   (B) granted
   (C) perpetuated
   (D) inflicted

8. The researchers will run a *comparative* series of tests.

   (A) objective
   (B) relative
   (C) subjective
   (D) scientific

9. Geologists *assure* us that our earth is a few billion years old.

   (A) guarantee
   (B) instruct
   (C) inform
   (D) advise

10. He was determined to *foil* the scheme of his opponent.

    (A) heighten
    (B) secure
    (C) disencumber
    (D) thwart

11. The examiner *purported* to be an official representative.

    (A) addressed
    (B) claimed
    (C) propitiated
    (D) conciliated

12. The ship carried refugees of every *persuasion.*

    (A) mediocrity
    (B) sort
    (C) prospectus
    (D) compendium

13. The child could not *recollect* the incident.
    (A) remember
    (B) dubitate
    (C) interrogate
    (D) illumine

14. The Supreme Court *rescinded* the law.
    (A) complicated
    (B) inveigled
    (C) revoked
    (D) accepted

15. The implementation of the plan was given *scant* consideration.
    (A) audacious
    (B) fervid
    (C) little
    (D) clothed

16. The key speaker in his lengthy presentation *scoffed* at religion.
    (A) exonerated
    (B) amplified
    (C) confuted
    (D) mocked

17. She completed the *sprint* with a sudden surge of energy.
    (A) relaxation
    (B) adventure
    (C) run
    (D) convergence

18. The content of the message was *urgent.*
    (A) privileged
    (B) amendable
    (C) pressing
    (D) absolved

19. A *simulated* rescue mission was conducted by the forest rangers.
    (A) pretended
    (B) superficial
    (C) stimulated
    (D) simultaneous

20. A *histamine* is released from the tissues when the cells are injured.
    (A) A histone
    (B) An amine
    (C) A stimulant
    (D) An isoenzyme

21. Her quickening gait seemed regulated by the *pulse* of the big city.
    (A) utility
    (B) pace
    (C) reverence
    (D) solace

22. The language of the publication is *unsophisticated* but informative.
    (A) ponderous
    (B) elaborate
    (C) simple
    (D) superficial

23. All the evidence presented pointed to *willful* execution of a crime.
    (A) deliberate
    (B) eminent
    (C) amicable
    (D) remorseful

24. There is no *provision* for deadlines in the contract.
    (A) improvement
    (B) convenience
    (C) aggregation
    (D) stipulation

25. The furnishings *impart* an air of elegance to the room.
    (A) communicate
    (B) indemnify
    (C) reinforce
    (D) disguise

26. She exhibited great *valor* in handling the emergency.
    (A) ingeniousness
    (B) courage
    (C) discretion
    (D) optimism

27. Various courses were *fused* in the revision of the curriculum.
    (A) required
    (B) implicated
    (C) combined
    (D) involved

28. Production of complex molecules is accomplished by *replication.*

    (A) duplication
    (B) synthesis
    (C) fixation
    (D) reproduction

29. The task of choosing one from so many qualified applicants *bewildered* the employer.

    (A) perplexed
    (B) aggravated
    (C) subdued
    (D) infuriated

30. The revision of the city plan incorporated adjustments in the projected *modes* of transportation.

    (A) increments
    (B) expenditures
    (C) means
    (D) modifications

31. The politician sought to *aggrandize* himself at the expense of the people.

    (A) exhaust
    (B) subjugate
    (C) sacrifice
    (D) exalt

32. The newcomer made an effort to *mingle* with the crowd.

    (A) argue
    (B) mix
    (C) disrupt
    (D) flout

33. If an organization's programs were described as *philanthropic*, the programs would be

    (A) primitive
    (B) deleterious
    (C) extraneous
    (D) benevolent

34. If the traits of a nation's leader were *covetous*, they were

    (A) greedy
    (B) exemplary
    (C) disparate
    (D) adventitious

35. Rabbits *breed* offspring rapidly.

    (A) raise
    (B) gather
    (C) propagate
    (D) destroy

TEST 1: SYNONYMS ANSWER KEY

1. **B**
2. **C**
3. **D**
4. **A**
5. **D**
6. **A**
7. **D**
8. **B**
9. **A**
10. **D**
11. **B**
12. **B**
13. **A**
14. **C**
15. **C**
16. **D**
17. **C**
18. **C**
19. **A**
20. **B**
21. **B**
22. **C**
23. **A**
24. **D**
25. **A**
26. **B**
27. **C**
28. **A**
29. **A**
30. **C**
31. **D**
32. **B**
33. **D**
34. **A**
35. **C**

TEST 2: ANTONYMS

30 QUESTIONS • TIME—15 MINUTES

Directions: Read each question carefully and consider all possible answers. When you have decided which choice is best, blacken the corresponding space on your answer sheet. There is only one best answer for each question.

1. IMMUTABLE:
   (A) erudite
   (B) abject
   (C) changeable
   (D) fantastic
   (E) aura

2. DUCTILE:
   (A) feted
   (B) alluvial
   (C) stubborn
   (D) abnormal
   (E) belabor

3. FASTIDIOUS:
   (A) factitious
   (B) absurd
   (C) indifferent
   (D) sloppy
   (E) chary

4. TEMERITY:
   (A) affinity
   (B) cherubim
   (C) humility
   (D) degenerate

5. ITINERANT:
   (A) animosity
   (B) metaphor
   (C) perpetrator
   (D) resident
   (E) cerebrum

6. TACITURN:
   (A) malevolent
   (B) loquacious
   (C) paltry
   (D) opaque
   (E) morbid

7. NEFARIOUS:
   (A) grotesque
   (B) virtuous
   (C) jovial
   (D) pious
   (E) cerement

8. OBSEQUIOUS:
   (A) harbinger
   (B) bold
   (C) heredity
   (D) quaff
   (E) falchion

9. OSTENTATION:
   (A) emulsion
   (B) languid
   (C) modesty
   (D) kilogram
   (E) bey

10. CONTENTION:
    (A) equation
    (B) guild
    (C) oblivion
    (D) pacification
    (E) bream

11. IMPUTATION:
    (A) assiduous
    (B) radiant
    (C) challis
    (D) raiment
    (E) vindication

12. BENIGN:
    (A) cayenne
    (B) relevant
    (C) robot
    (D) malevolent
    (E) precarious

13. COHERENT:

(A) perspicacious
(B) zephyr
(C) weal
(D) chaotic
(E) changeling

14. DEPREDATION:

(A) plethoric
(B) gloss
(C) restoration
(D) usher
(E) trochal

15. PROVOCATIVE:

(A) sedentary
(B) capricious
(C) vindictive
(D) tawny
(E) pacifying

16. SUBMISSION:

(A) authorized
(B) defiance
(C) assignment
(D) defeat
(E) belabor

17. AFFLUENT:

(A) immigrant
(B) junction
(C) insufficient
(D) kin
(E) clandestine

18. CHURLISH:

(A) exiguous
(B) laudable
(C) cheerful
(D) maternal
(E) civet

19. SYMMETRY:

(A) invocation
(B) madrigal
(C) distortion
(D) satyr
(E) cilia

20. DULCET:

(A) extrinsic
(B) optimistic
(C) unanimous
(D) acerbate
(E) chiffonette

21. PIQUANT:

(A) factitious
(B) vain
(C) insipid
(D) vulture
(E) chromatic

22. OPPORTUNE:

(A) dialectical
(B) mutable
(C) clinch
(D) weird
(E) inexpedient

23. PETULANT:

(A) irascible
(B) cheerful
(C) uncouth
(D) abnormal
(E) closure

24. SAVORY:

(A) apathy
(B) clandestine
(C) pliant
(D) unpalatable
(E) capillary

25. SATIATED:

(A) satirical
(B) centaur
(C) gorgeous
(D) delectable
(E) hungry

26. RECLUSIVE:

(A) empyreal
(B) obscure
(C) gregarious
(D) rustication
(E) chilblain

27. COURTEOUS:
    (A) flaccid
    (B) emollient
    (C) insolent
    (D) scrupulous
    (E) chaffinch

28. USURP:
    (A) succinct
    (B) predict
    (C) pacify
    (D) clematis
    (E) donate

29. ACRIMONIOUS:
    (A) alluvial
    (B) apocalyptic
    (C) concourse
    (D) harmonious
    (E) carcanet

30. SKEPTIC:
    (A) cryptic
    (B) bigot
    (C) discursive
    (D) eminent
    (E) caricature

TEST 2: ANTONYMS ANSWER KEY

1. **C**	11. **E**	21. **C**
2. **C**	12. **D**	22. **E**
3. **D**	13. **D**	23. **B**
4. **C**	14. **C**	24. **D**
5. **D**	15. **E**	25. **E**
6. **B**	16. **B**	26. **C**
7. **B**	17. **C**	27. **C**
8. **B**	18. **C**	28. **E**
9. **C**	19. **C**	29. **D**
10. **D**	20. **D**	30. **B**

UNIT VI: QUANTITATIVE ABILITY

QUANTITATIVE ABILITY TESTS ANSWER SHEET

TEST 1: NONVERBAL ARITHMETIC

1. Ⓐ Ⓑ Ⓒ Ⓓ	7. Ⓐ Ⓑ Ⓒ Ⓓ	13. Ⓐ Ⓑ Ⓒ Ⓓ
2. Ⓐ Ⓑ Ⓒ Ⓓ	8. Ⓐ Ⓑ Ⓒ Ⓓ	14. Ⓐ Ⓑ Ⓒ Ⓓ
3. Ⓐ Ⓑ Ⓒ Ⓓ	9. Ⓐ Ⓑ Ⓒ Ⓓ	
4. Ⓐ Ⓑ Ⓒ Ⓓ	10. Ⓐ Ⓑ Ⓒ Ⓓ	
5. Ⓐ Ⓑ Ⓒ Ⓓ	11. Ⓐ Ⓑ Ⓒ Ⓓ	
6. Ⓐ Ⓑ Ⓒ Ⓓ	12. Ⓐ Ⓑ Ⓒ Ⓓ	

TEST 2: PROBLEM SOLVING

1. Ⓐ Ⓑ Ⓒ Ⓓ	7. Ⓐ Ⓑ Ⓒ Ⓓ	13. Ⓐ Ⓑ Ⓒ Ⓓ
2. Ⓐ Ⓑ Ⓒ Ⓓ	8. Ⓐ Ⓑ Ⓒ Ⓓ	14. Ⓐ Ⓑ Ⓒ Ⓓ
3. Ⓐ Ⓑ Ⓒ Ⓓ	9. Ⓐ Ⓑ Ⓒ Ⓓ	15. Ⓐ Ⓑ Ⓒ Ⓓ
4. Ⓐ Ⓑ Ⓒ Ⓓ	10. Ⓐ Ⓑ Ⓒ Ⓓ	
5. Ⓐ Ⓑ Ⓒ Ⓓ	11. Ⓐ Ⓑ Ⓒ Ⓓ	
6. Ⓐ Ⓑ Ⓒ Ⓓ	12. Ⓐ Ⓑ Ⓒ Ⓓ	

TEST 3: ALGEBRA

1. Ⓐ Ⓑ Ⓒ Ⓓ	5. Ⓐ Ⓑ Ⓒ Ⓓ
2. Ⓐ Ⓑ Ⓒ Ⓓ	6. Ⓐ Ⓑ Ⓒ Ⓓ
3. Ⓐ Ⓑ Ⓒ Ⓓ	7. Ⓐ Ⓑ Ⓒ Ⓓ
4. Ⓐ Ⓑ Ⓒ Ⓓ	8. Ⓐ Ⓑ Ⓒ Ⓓ

TEST 4: QUANTITATIVE COMPARISONS

1. Ⓐ Ⓑ Ⓒ Ⓓ	6. Ⓐ Ⓑ Ⓒ Ⓓ	11. Ⓐ Ⓑ Ⓒ Ⓓ	16. Ⓐ Ⓑ Ⓒ Ⓓ
2. Ⓐ Ⓑ Ⓒ Ⓓ	7. Ⓐ Ⓑ Ⓒ Ⓓ	12. Ⓐ Ⓑ Ⓒ Ⓓ	17. Ⓐ Ⓑ Ⓒ Ⓓ
3. Ⓐ Ⓑ Ⓒ Ⓓ	8. Ⓐ Ⓑ Ⓒ Ⓓ	13. Ⓐ Ⓑ Ⓒ Ⓓ	18. Ⓐ Ⓑ Ⓒ Ⓓ
4. Ⓐ Ⓑ Ⓒ Ⓓ	9. Ⓐ Ⓑ Ⓒ Ⓓ	14. Ⓐ Ⓑ Ⓒ Ⓓ	19. Ⓐ Ⓑ Ⓒ Ⓓ
5. Ⓐ Ⓑ Ⓒ Ⓓ	10. Ⓐ Ⓑ Ⓒ Ⓓ	15. Ⓐ Ⓑ Ⓒ Ⓓ	20. Ⓐ Ⓑ Ⓒ Ⓓ

QUANTITATIVE ABILITY TESTS

TEST 1: NONVERBAL ARITHMETIC

14 QUESTIONS • TIME—20 MINUTES

Directions: Read each question carefully and consider all possible answers. When you have decided which choice is best, blacken the corresponding space on your answer sheet. There is only one best answer for each question.

1. What fraction of a whole is the shaded area in Figure 1?

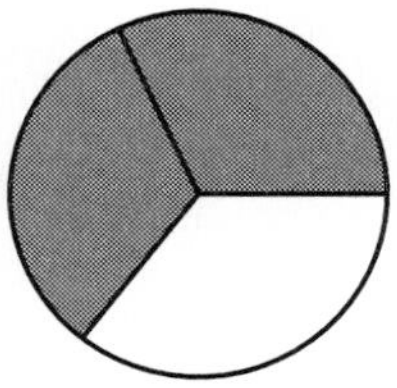

(A) $\frac{1}{2}$

(B) $\frac{3}{4}$

(C) $\frac{2}{3}$

(D) $\frac{2}{5}$

2. Which of the following equations demonstrates that Figure 2 and Figure 3 are equivalent?

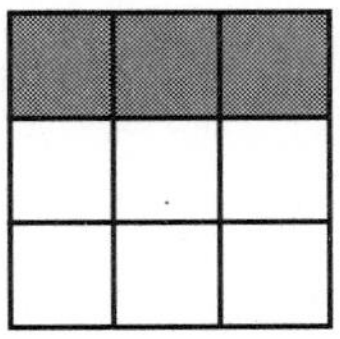

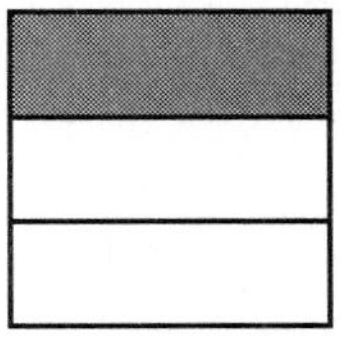

(A) $\frac{3}{9} = \frac{1}{3}$

(B) $\frac{9}{3} = \frac{3}{1}$

(C) $\frac{3}{9} = \frac{3}{3}$

(D) $\frac{9}{3} = \frac{1}{3}$

3. Select the answer that represents reduction of the fraction $\frac{630}{140}$ to the lowest term.

(A) $\frac{70}{2}$

(B) $\frac{70}{4}$

(C) $\frac{2}{9}$

(D) $\frac{9}{2}$

4. Which one of the following equations is correct for building up the fraction $\frac{3}{8}$ to have a denominator of 24?

(A) $\frac{3}{8} = 3 \times \frac{3}{8} \times 3 = \frac{9}{24}$

(B) $\frac{3}{8} = 3 \times \frac{24}{8} \times 24 = \frac{9}{24}$

(C) $\frac{8}{24} = 8 \times \frac{3}{1} \times 24 = \frac{24}{24}$

(D) $\frac{3}{24} = 3 \times \frac{1}{3} \times 8 = \frac{1}{24}$

5. Which of the following equations expresses the whole number 6 as an equivalent fraction with a denominator of 5?

(A) $\frac{6}{5} = 6 \times \frac{5}{5} \times 5 = \frac{30}{25}$

(B) $\frac{6}{5} = 6 \times \frac{1}{5} \times 1 = \frac{6}{5}$

(C) $\frac{6}{1} = 6 \times \frac{5}{1} \times 5 = \frac{30}{5}$

(D) $\frac{6}{1} = 5 \times \frac{1}{6} \times 1 = \frac{5}{6}$

6. The product of $\frac{5}{3} \times \frac{2}{7}$ equals

(A) $\frac{6}{35}$

(B) $\frac{35}{6}$

(C) $\frac{21}{10}$

(D) $\frac{10}{21}$

7. The product of $\frac{25}{36} \times \frac{16}{20}$ equals

(A) $\frac{10}{8}$

(B) $\frac{8}{10}$

(C) $\frac{9}{5}$

(D) $\frac{5}{9}$

8. $\frac{3}{4}$ divided by $\frac{5}{2}$ equals

(A) $\frac{10}{3}$

(B) $\frac{3}{10}$

(C) $\frac{20}{6}$

(D) $\frac{6}{20}$

9. Select the correct answer for $\frac{72}{50} \times \frac{200}{35}$

(A) $\frac{63}{250}$

(B) $\frac{250}{63}$

(C) $\frac{288}{35}$

(D) $\frac{35}{288}$

10. A 12 ounce bottle has 7 ounces of liquid in it. What fraction of the bottle is filled?

(A) $\frac{3}{4}$

(B) $\frac{1}{2}$

(C) $\frac{7}{12}$

(D) $\frac{12}{7}$

11. What is the solution to the problem, $\frac{2}{9} + \frac{5}{4} - \frac{3}{8}$?

(A) $\frac{72}{60}$

(B) $\frac{60}{72}$

(C) $\frac{72}{49}$

(D) $\frac{49}{72}$

12. When you multiply $2\frac{1}{3} \times 1\frac{1}{2}$, the answer is

(A) $3\frac{1}{3}$

(B) $3\frac{1}{2}$

(C) $2\frac{1}{5}$

(D) $2\frac{2}{6}$

13. Change $2\frac{1}{2} \times 3\frac{1}{3}$ to a simple fraction. The answer is

(A) $\frac{3}{4}$

(B) $\frac{4}{3}$

(C) $\frac{1}{3}$

(D) $\frac{1}{4}$

14. Which one of the following options is a solution to the problem $5\frac{3}{4} + 6\frac{5}{9}$?

(A) $12\frac{5}{12}$

(B) $11\frac{15}{36}$

(C) $12\frac{11}{36}$

(D) $11\frac{8}{13}$

TEST 1: NONVERBAL ARITHMETIC ANSWER KEY

1. **B**
2. **A**
3. **D**
4. **A**
5. **C**
6. **D**
7. **D**
8. **B**
9. **A**
10. **C**
11. **D**
12. **B**
13. **A**
14. **C**

TEST 1: NONVERBAL ARITHMETIC EXPLANATORY ANSWERS

1. **(B)** Since the whole is divided into 3 units, the denominator is 3. There are 2 units shaded, so the numerator is 2. The shaded part is $\frac{2}{3}$ of the whole.

2. **(A)** Figure 1 is divided into 9 parts, and is a square. The shaded part can be represented by the fraction $\frac{3}{4}$. Figure 2 is divided in 3 parts, and is also a square. The fraction $\frac{1}{3}$ represents the shaded part, $\frac{3}{9}$ and $\frac{1}{3}$ represents the same part of the whole and are therefore equivalent, $\frac{3}{9} = \frac{1}{3}$.

3. **(D)** $\frac{630}{140} = (70 \times 9)/(70 \times 2) = \frac{9}{2}$

4. **(A)** Multiply both parts by the same number. 8 multiplied by what number will give 24. Answer: divide 24 by 8 = 3. The denominator and the numerator are multiplied by 3 = $\frac{9}{24}$.

5. **(C)** Use the same process as number 4.

   $\frac{6}{1} = 6 \times \frac{5}{1} \times 5 = \frac{30}{5}$

6. **(D)** Multiply numerators and denominators.

   $\frac{5}{3} \times \frac{2}{7} = 5 \times \frac{2}{3} \times 7 = \frac{10}{21}$

7. **(D)** Reduce and perform the multiplication.

   $\frac{25}{36} \times \frac{16}{20} = \frac{25}{36} \times \frac{4}{5}$ (divide by 4)

   $\frac{25}{36} \times \frac{4}{5}$ (divide by 5)

   $\frac{5}{36} \times \frac{4}{1}$ (divide by 4)

   $\frac{5}{9} \times \frac{1}{1} = 5 \times \frac{1}{9} \times 1 = \frac{5}{9}$

8. **(B)** Invert the divisor and change the operation to multiplication, reduce, and perform the multiplication.

   $\frac{3}{4} \div \frac{5}{2} = \frac{3}{4} \times \frac{2}{5}$

   $\frac{3}{4} \times \frac{2}{5}$ (divide by 2)

   $\frac{3}{2} \times \frac{1}{5} = \frac{3}{10}$

9. **(A)** Use the same procedure as number 8.

   $\frac{72}{50} \div \frac{200}{35} = \frac{72}{50} \times \frac{35}{200}$

   $\frac{72}{50} \times \frac{35}{200}$ (divide by 8)

   $\frac{9}{50} \times \frac{35}{25}$ (divide by 5)

   $\frac{9}{50} \times \frac{7}{5} = \frac{63}{250}$

10. **(C)** The bottle (whole) is divided into 12 ounces (the denominator) of which 7 ounces (the numerator) is filled. Thus $\frac{7}{12}$ of the bottle is filled.

11. **(D)** Find the lowest common denominator (LCD) build up each fraction to have 72 as denominator, perform addition and subtraction as indicated.

    The least common multiple (LCM) of 9 and 6 is 18.

    LCM of 18 and 8 is 72

    Therefore, LCD = 72

    $\frac{2}{9} = 2 \times \frac{8}{9} \times 8 = \frac{16}{72}$

    $\frac{5}{6} = 5 \times \frac{12}{6} \times 12 = \frac{60}{72}$

    $\frac{3}{8} = 3 \times \frac{9}{8} \times 9 = \frac{27}{72}$

    $16 + 60 - \frac{27}{72} = \frac{49}{72}$

12. **(B)** Change both mixed numbers into improper fractions and multiply:

$$2\frac{1}{3} \times 1\frac{1}{2} = \frac{7}{3} \times \frac{3}{2}$$

$$\frac{7}{3} \times \frac{3}{2} = \frac{7}{2} = 3\frac{1}{2}$$

13. **(A)** Use the same procedure as no. 12.

$$2\frac{1}{2} \div 3\frac{1}{3} = \frac{5}{2} \div \frac{10}{3}$$

$$\frac{5}{2} \times \frac{3}{10} = \frac{1}{2} \times \frac{3}{2} = \frac{3}{4}$$

14. **(C)** Add the whole numbers and fractional parts separately. Change improper fraction to a mixed number, then add

$$5\frac{3}{4} + 6\frac{5}{9} = 11 + \frac{3}{4} + \frac{5}{9}$$

$$= 11 + \frac{27}{36} + \frac{20}{36} \text{ (LCD = 36)}$$

$$= 11 + \frac{47}{36}$$

$$= 11 + 1\frac{11}{36} = 12\frac{11}{36}$$

TEST 2: PROBLEM SOLVING

15 QUESTIONS • TIME—20 MINUTES

Directions: Read each question carefully and consider all possible answers. When you have decided which choice is best, blacken the corresponding space on your answer sheet. There is only one best answer for each question.

1. If there are 245 sections in a city containing five boroughs, the average number of sections for each of the five boroughs is

   (A) 50 sections
   (B) 49 sections
   (C) 47 sections
   (D) 59 sections

2. If, in that same city, a section has 45 miles of street to plow after a snowstorm and nine plows are used, each plow will cover an average of how many miles?

   (A) 7 miles
   (B) 6 miles
   (C) 8 miles
   (D) 5 miles

3. If a crosswalk plow engine is run five minutes a day for ten days in a given month, how long will it run in the course of this month?

   (A) 50 minutes
   (B) $1\frac{1}{2}$ hours
   (C) 1 hour
   (D) 30 minutes

4. If the city uses 1500 men in manual street cleaning and half as many more to load and drive trucks, the total number of men used is

   (A) 2200
   (B) 2520
   (C) 2050
   (D) 2250

5. If, of 186 summonses issued, 100 were issued to first offenders, then there were how many summonses issued to other than first offenders?

   (A) 68
   (B) 90
   (C) 86
   (D) 108

6. A sanitation man is 40 feet behind a sanitation truck. There is a second sanitation truck 90 feet behind the first truck. How much closer is the man to the first truck than to the second?

   (A) 30 feet
   (B) 50 feet
   (C) 10 feet
   (D) 70 feet

7. If a flushing machine has a capacity of 1260 gallons, how many gallons will it contain when it is two-thirds full?

   (A) 809 gallons
   (B) 750 gallons
   (C) 630 gallons
   (D) 840 gallons

8. If an employee earns $160.00 a week and has deductions of $8.00 for the pension fund, $12.00 for medical insurance, and $29.60 withholding tax, his take-home pay will be

   (A) $110.40
   (B) $108.60
   (C) $102.00
   (D) $98.40

9. A city department uses 25 twenty-cent, 35 thirty-cent, and 350 forty-cent metered postage units each day. The total cost of stamps used by the department in a five-day period is

   (A) $29.50
   (B) $155.00
   (C) $290.50
   (D) $777.50

10. In 1975, a school bought 500 dozen pencils at 40 cents per dozen. In 1978, only 75 percent as many pencils were bought as were bought in 1975, but the price per dozen was 20 percent higher than the 1975 price. The total cost of the pencils bought in 1978 was

    (A) $180.00
    (B) $187.50
    (C) $240.00
    (D) $250.00

11. If the average cost of sweeping a square foot of a small town's street is $0.75, the cost of sweeping 100 square feet is

    (A) $7.50
    (B) $750
    (C) $75
    (D) $70

12. If a sanitation department scow is towed at the rate of three miles an hour, how many hours will it need to go 28 miles?

    (A) 10 hours 30 minutes
    (B) 12 hours
    (C) 9 hours 20 minutes
    (D) 9 hours 15 minutes

13. If a man is 60 feet away from a sanitation truck, how many feet nearer is he to the truck than a second truck that is 100 feet away?

    (A) 60 feet
    (B) 40 feet
    (C) 50 feet
    (D) 20 feet

14. Six gross of special drawing pencils were purchased for use in a city department. If the pencils were used at the rate of 24 a week, the maximum number of weeks that the six gross of pencils would last is

    (A) 6 weeks
    (B) 12 weeks
    (C) 24 weeks
    (D) 36 weeks

15. A cogwheel having eight cogs plays into another cogwheel having 24 cogs. When the small wheel has made 42 revolutions, how many has the larger wheel made?

    (A) 14
    (B) 20
    (C) 16
    (D) 10

TEST 2: PROBLEM SOLVING ANSWER KEY

1. **B**
2. **D**
3. **A**
4. **D**
5. **C**
6. **C**
7. **D**
8. **A**
9. **D**
10. **A**
11. **C**
12. **C**
13. **B**
14. **D**
15. **A**

TEST 2: PROBLEM SOLVING EXPLANATORY ANSWERS

1. **(B)** To find the *average* number of sections per borough, divide:

   245 sections divided by 5 boroughs = 49

   49 sections/borough

2. **(D)** Total miles = 45

   Number of plows = 9

   To find the *average* number of miles, divide:

   45 miles divided by 9 plows = 5 miles/plow

   Average = 5 miles

3. **(A)** Total time per day = 5 minutes

   Total days per month = 10 days

   Total time per month=

   $$\frac{5 \text{ minutes}}{\text{day}} \times \frac{10 \text{ days}}{\text{month}} = \frac{50 \text{ minutes}}{\text{month}}$$

4. **(D)** Total number for street cleaning = 1500
   Half that number load and drive = + 750
   2250

   2250 men used

5. **(C)** Total issued = 186
   Subtract:
   First Offenders = –100
   Other-than-first offenders 86

6. **(C)** The second truck is 90 feet – 40 feet = 50 feet from the man. The first truck is 40 feet from the man. The first truck is 50 feet – 40 feet = 10 feet closer than the second truck.

7. **(D)** Total capacity = 1260 gallons

   $\frac{2}{3}$ of 1260 is $\frac{2}{3} \times 1260$

   $= \frac{2520}{3}$

   = 840 gallons

8. **(A)** Total earnings = $160.00

   Deductions = $ 8.00 pension

   = $ 12.00 medical insurance
   = $ 29.60 withholding tax
   = $ 49.60 total deductions

   The take-home pay can be found by subtracting the total deduction from the salary.

   $160.00 – $49.60 = $110.40

   Take-home pay = $110.40

9. **(D)** *Stamps per day* *Cost per day*

Stamps per day		*Cost per day*
25/day × $0.20	=	5.00
35/day × $0.30	=	10.50
350 × $0.40	=	140.00
Total cost/day	=	$155.50

   For five days, 5 × $155.50 = $777.50

   Total cost = $777.50

10. **(A)** Total number of pencils bought in 1975 was 500 dozen at 40 cents a dozen; in 1978, 75 percent of the 500 dozen were bought at a 20 percent increase in price.

    First, find how many pencils were bought in 1978. Do this by multiplying:

    500 × 0.75 = 375 dozen were bought in 1978

    Now find the price per dozen. You know that it was 20 percent more than 40 cents:

    $0.40 × 0.20 increase = $0.08 or 8¢ increase in price

    So the price per dozen is:

    40¢ + 8¢ = 48¢ or $0.48

    To find the cost, multiply the number of dozens of pencils by the cost per dozen.

    375 dozen × $0.48/dozen = $180

    Total cost for 1978 = $180

11. **(C)** If it cost $0.75 to sweep one square foot, to find the cost for 100 square feet, multiply:

    100 square feet × 0.75 per square foot = $75

    Total cost = $75

12. **(C)** It takes one hour to tow a scow three miles. Find the time to tow the scow 28 miles by dividing:

    28 miles ÷ 3 miles/hour = $9\frac{1}{3}$ hours

    $\frac{1}{3}$ hour × 60 minutes/hour

    = 20 minutes

    Note: 1 hour = 60 minutes. To change hours to minutes multiply the fraction of an hour by 60 minutes/hour.

    It takes nine hours, 20 minutes to tow the scow 28 miles.

13. **(B)**

Truck to the other truck	100 feet
Truck to the man	– 60 feet
	40 feet

    The difference is 40 feet.

14. **(D)** One gross = 144 pencils

    6 gross = 144/gross × 6 gross = 864 pencils (on hand)

    If 24 pencils are used each week, divide to find the number of weeks they will last:

    864 divided by 24/week = 36 weeks

    Supplies would last 36 weeks.

15. **(A)** If the cogs on two wheels are sized and spaced the same, the smaller of the two wheels will turn faster than the larger one—the fewer cogs a wheel has, the more revolutions it makes. The number of cogs is, therefore, inversely proportional to the number of revolutions.

    The smaller wheel will make 3 revolutions for every 1 revolution the larger wheel makes. So when the smaller wheel makes 42 revolutions, the larger wheel will make 42 divided by 3 = 14 revolutions.

TEST 3: ALGEBRA

8 QUESTIONS • TIME—20 MINUTES

Directions: Read each question carefully and consider all possible answers. When you have decided which choice is best, blacken the corresponding space on your answer sheet. There is only one best answer for each question.

1. In the equation $4a + 5 = 13$, a equals

   (A) 4
   (B) 2
   (C) 7
   (D) 6

2. In the equation $\frac{10}{m} - 8 = \frac{5}{3}$, m equals

   (A) $\frac{10}{3}$
   (B) $\frac{3}{10}$
   (C) $\frac{30}{29}$
   (D) $\frac{29}{30}$

3. In the equation $3c^2 = 75d^4$, c equals

   (A) $\pm 5d^2$
   (B) $\pm 5d^4$
   (C) $\pm 25d^2$
   (D) $\pm 25d^4$

4. If two moles of compound A react with 5 moles of compound B to form 3 moles of compound C, then how many moles of A are required to react completely with 7 moles of B?

   (A) 5.7
   (B) 2.8
   (C) 7.5
   (D) 8.2

5. A car traveling at x mph takes 5 hours to go from city A to city B. Traveling at $x - 15$ mph, the car makes the return trip in six and two-thirds hours. What was the speed of the car on the return trip?

   (A) 60 mph
   (B) 55 mph
   (C) 50 mph
   (D) 45 mph

6. In 1997, a particular item A cost $2,500. In 1998, the price of A went up 20% because of inflation while in early 1999 there was a 10% increase in the price of A over its 1998 price. In June of 1999, A was put on sale with a 30% decrease in price. What was the sale price of A?

   (A) 2500
   (B) 2400
   (C) 2310
   (D) 2110

7. In the expression $\log_4 \frac{1}{16} = x$, what is the value of x?

   (A) −2
   (B) −4
   (C) +2
   (D) +4

8. What is the volume of a sphere of a radius 3 centimeters?

   (A) 119.05 cc
   (B) 113.04 cc
   (C) 106.00 cc
   (D) 101.08 cc

TEST 3: ALGEBRA ANSWER KEY

1. **B**
2. **C**
3. **A**
4. **B**
5. **D**
6. **C**
7. **A**
8. **B**

TEST 3:ALGEBRA EXPLANATORY ANSWERS

1. **(B)** $4a + 5 - 5 = 13 - 5$

   $4a = 8$

   $\frac{4a}{4} = \frac{8}{4}$

   $a = 2$

2. **(C)** $\frac{10}{m(3m)} - 8(3m) = (5/3)(3m)$

   $30 - 24m = 5m$

   $30 = 29m$

   $m = \frac{30}{29}$

3. **(A)** $c^2 = 25d^4$

   $\sqrt{c^2} = \sqrt{25d^4}$

   $c = \pm 5d^2$

4. **(B)** In a chemical reaction, the quantities of reactants/products are directly proportional.

   Let $x_1 = 2$ moles of A and $y_1 = 5$ moles of B.

   Then x_2 = number of moles of A and $y_2 = 7$ moles of B such that:

   $\frac{5}{2} = \frac{7}{x_2}$; $x_2 = 2.8$ moles of A

5. **(D)** Since displacement = (speed)(time), $d = vt$, speed and time are inversely proportional for a constant displacement. Let $v1 = x$ mph and $t1 =$ 5 hours; $v2 = x - 15$mph and $t2 = 6\frac{2}{3}$ hours = $\frac{20}{3}$ hours. Since both displacements are the same

   $5x = 6\frac{2}{3}(x - 15)$

   $5x = \frac{20}{3}(x - 15)$

   $15x = 20x - 300$

   $3(5x) = 3(\frac{20}{3})(x - 15)$

   $300 = 5x$

   $15x = 20(x - 15)$

   $x = 60$mph, speed from A to B

   $x - 15 = 45$mph is the speed on the return trip

6. **(C)** Sale price (1999) = \$2,310

   1997: Cost of A = \$2,500

   1998: Cost of A = \$2,500 + $\frac{20}{100} \times$ \$2,500 = \$3,000

   1999: Cost of A = \$3,000 + $\frac{10}{100} \times$ \$3,000 = \$3,300

   Sale Price (1999) = \$3,300 − $\frac{30}{100} \times$ \$3,300 = \$2,310

7. **(A)** $\log_4 \frac{1}{16} = x$

   $4x = \frac{1}{16}$

   $x = -2$

8. **(B)** $v = \frac{4}{3} r^3$

   Because $r = 3$ and $= 3.14$, $v = 4/3\ r^3 =$ $\frac{4}{3}(3.14)(3^3) = 113.04$

TEST 4: QUANTITATIVE COMPARISONS

20 QUESTIONS • TIME—30 MINUTES

Common Information: In each question, information concerning one or both of the quantities to be compared is given in the ITEM column. A symbol that appears in any column represents the same thing in Column A as it does in Column B.

Figures: Assume that the position of points, angles, regions, and so forth, are in the order shown; that the lines shown as straight are indeed straight; that figures lie in a plane unless otherwise indicated. Figures accompanying questions are intended to provide information you can use in answering the questions. However, unless a note states that a figure is drawn to scale, you should solve the problems by using your knowledge of mathematics, NOT by estimating sizes by sight or by measurement.

Directions: For each of the following questions, two quantities are given: one in Column A and one in Column B. Compare the two quantities and mark your answer sheet with the correct, lettered conclusion. These are your options:

A: the quantity in Column A is the greater;

B: the quantity in Column B is the greater;

C: the two quantities are equal;

D: the relationship cannot be determined from the information given.

Item	Column A	Column B
1.	5% of 34	The number that 34 is 5% of
2. 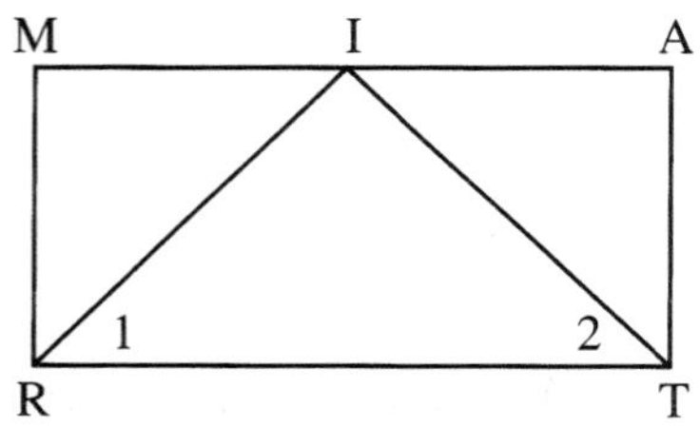 $\angle 1 < \angle 2$	IR	IT
3. $4 > x > -3$	$\frac{x}{3}$	$\frac{3}{x}$
4.	$\frac{2}{3} + \frac{3}{7}$	$\frac{16}{21} - \frac{3}{7}$

Item	Column A	Column B
5. 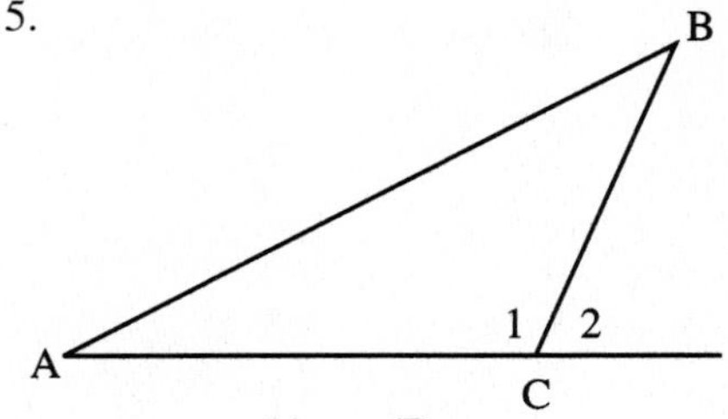 $\angle A > \angle B$; $\angle 1 < \angle A + \angle B$	$\angle A + \angle B$	$\angle 2$
6. y = an odd integer	The numerical value of y^2	The numerical value of y^3
7.	$8 + (6 \div 3) - 7(2)$	$6 + (8 \div 2) - 7(3)$
8.	$\frac{3}{4}$ of $\frac{9}{9}$	$\frac{9}{9} \times \frac{3}{4}$
9. 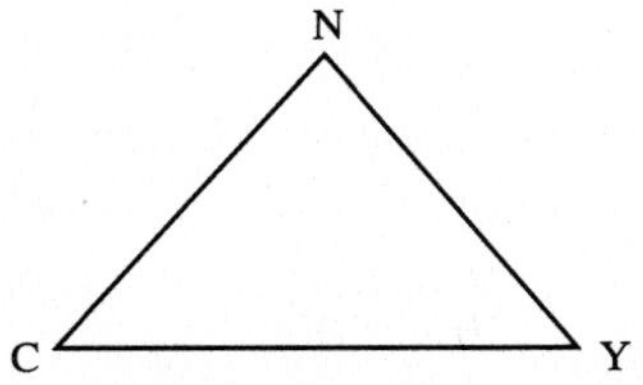 NC = NY; $\angle N > \angle C$	NC	CY
10. 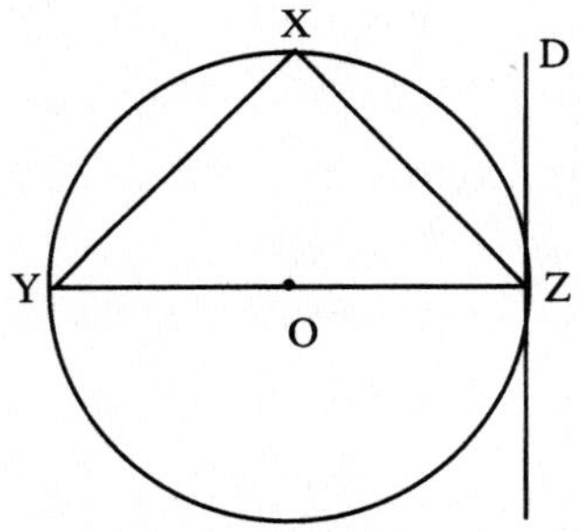 ΔXYZ is inscribed in circle O and DZ is tangent to circle O.	$\angle YXZ$	$\angle DZY$
11.	A given chord in a given circle.	The radius of the same circle.
12. 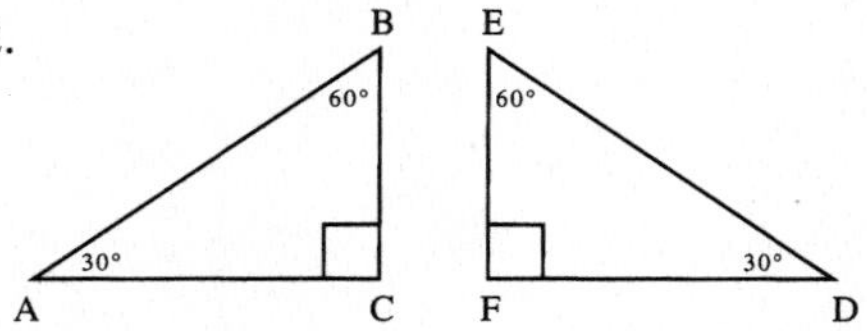	BC	FD
13.	$4 + (3 \times 2) - 7$	$(8 \div 2) + 3 - 1$
14.	50% of $\frac{4}{5}$	$\frac{4}{5}$ of $\frac{1}{2}$

Item		Column A	Column B
15.	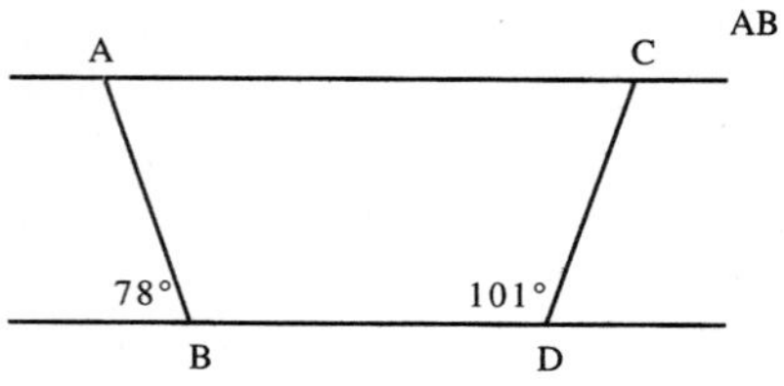 AC $\parallel$ BD	AB	CD
16.		$0.01 \div .1$	$0.01 \times .1$
17.	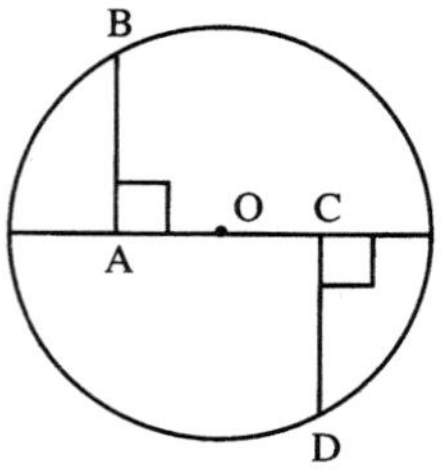 OA > OC	AB	CD
18.		The number that 6 is 20% of	10% of 300
19.	$3x + 2y = -1;\ 2x + 3y = 1$	The numerical value of x	The numerical value of y
20.	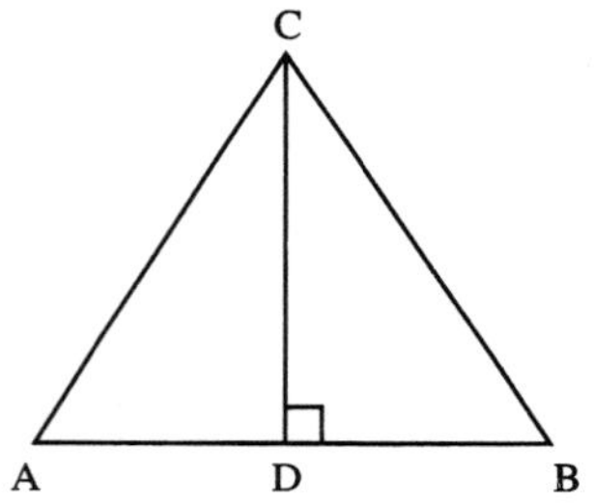 $CD \perp AB;\ \angle A > \angle B$	AC	CB

TEST 4: QUANTITATIVE COMPARISONS ANSWER KEY

1. **B**
2. **A**
3. **D**
4. **A**
5. **C**
6. **D**
7. **A**
8. **C**
9. **B**
10. **C**
11. **D**
12. **D**
13. **B**
14. **C**
15. **A**
16. **A**
17. **B**
18. **C**
19. **B**
20. **B**

TEST 4: QUANTITATIVE COMPARISONS EXPLANATORY ANSWERS

1. **(B)** 5% of 34 = 34 × 0.05 = 1.7

   The number that 34 is 5% of = 5% of n = 34

   $0.05n = 34$

   $n = \frac{34}{0.05}$

   $n = 0.05.$

   $n = 680$

   $$\begin{array}{r} 680. \\ 34.00. \\ \underline{30} \\ 40 \\ \underline{40} \\ 00 \\ \underline{00} \end{array}$$

   680 < 1.7

2. **(A)** In a triangle the greater side lies opposite the greater angle. ∠2 > ∠1 (given)

   IR > IT

3. **(D)** Since x could be any number from –3 to 4, the values of the fractions are impossible to determine.

4. **(A)** $\frac{2}{3} + \frac{3}{7} = \frac{14}{21} + \frac{9}{21}$

   $= \frac{23}{21}$

   $\frac{16}{21} - \frac{3}{7} = \frac{16}{21} - \frac{9}{21}$

   $= \frac{7}{21}$

5. **(C)**

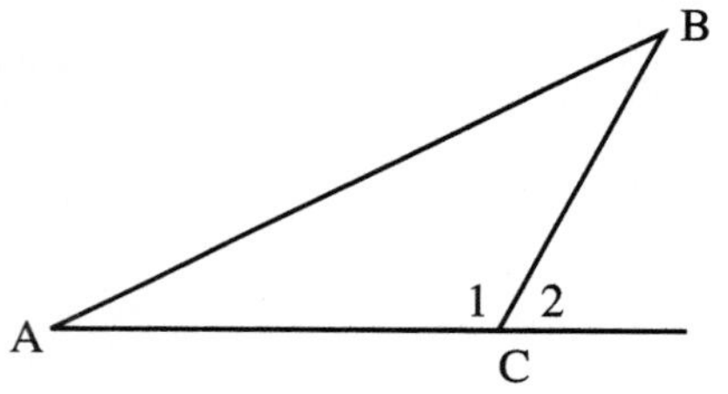

∠2 = ∠A + ∠B (an exterior angle of a triangle is equal to the sum of the two interior remote angles)

6. **(D)** There is not enough information given; y could equal 1, which would make both quantities equal; or y could be greater than 1, which would make y^3 greater than y^2. If y were a negative integer, then y^2 would be greater than y^3.

7. **(A)** $8 + (6 \div 3) - 7(2) = 8 + 2 - 14$

   $= 10 - 14$

   $= -4$

   $6 + (8 \div 2) - 7(3) = 6 + 4 - 21$

   $= 10 - 21$

   $= -11$

8. **(C)** $\frac{3}{4} \cdot \frac{9}{9} = \frac{3}{4}$

   $\frac{9}{9} \cdot \frac{3}{4} = \frac{3}{4}$

9. **(B)**

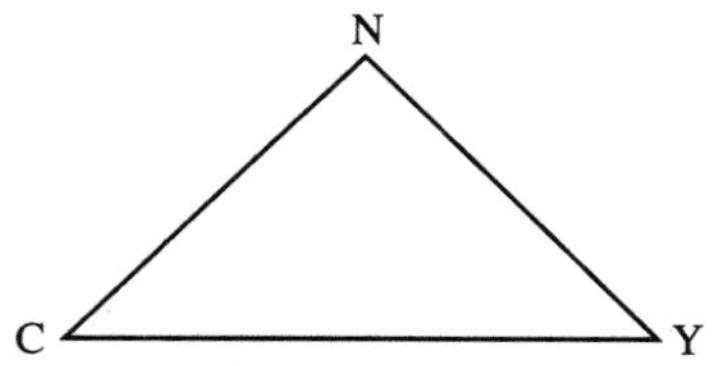

NC = NY given

∠C = ∠Y angles opposite equal sides are equal

∠N < ∠C given

∠N < ∠Y substitution

CY < NC the greater side lies opposite the greater angle

10. **(C)**

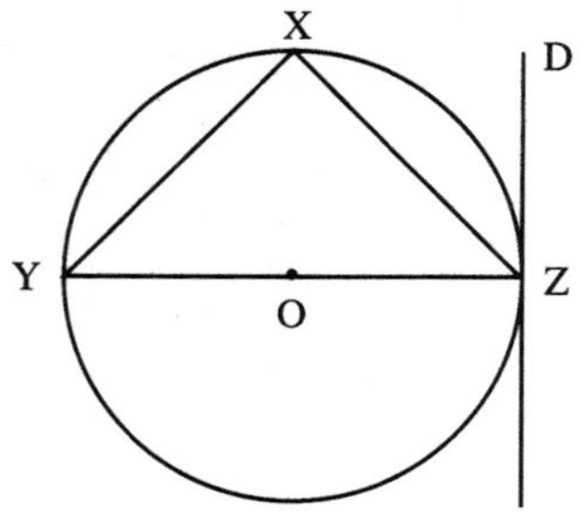

∠YXZ = 90° an angle inscribed in a semicircle equals 90°

∠DZY = 90° a radius is perpendicular to a tangent at their point of contact

11. **(D)** Impossible to determine from the information given. The radius could be less than, equal to, or greater than the chord.

12. **(D)** Since there are three unknown sides on both triangles, the length of BC or FD is impossible to determine.

13. **(B)** $4 + 3 \times 2 - 7 = 4 + 6 - 7$

    $= 10 - 7$

    $= 3$

    $8 \div 2 + 3 - 1 = 4 + 3 - 1$

    $= 7 - 1$

    $= 6$

14. **(C)** 50% of $\frac{4}{5} = \frac{1}{2} \times \frac{4}{5}$

    $= \frac{2}{5}$

    $\frac{4}{5}$ of $\frac{1}{2} = \frac{4}{5} \times \frac{1}{2}$

    $= \frac{2}{5}$

15. **(A)** The shortest line between two parallel lines is a line perpendicular to both lines. Therefore if there are two transversals between parallel lines, the one whose angle of intersection with the parallel lines is further from 90° is the longer transversal.

    $\angle B = 90° - 78° = 12°$

    $\angle D = 101° - 90° = 11°$

    $\therefore AB > CD$

16. **(A)** $0.01 \div 0.1 = 0.1$

    $0.01 \times 0.1 = 0.001$

17. **(B)** If two perpendiculars are drawn from the circumference of a circle to a diameter of the same circle the one that is closer to the center of the circle will be longer.

18. **(C)** The number that 6 is 20% of:

    20% of $n = 6$

    $0.20n = 6$

    $n = 6 \div 0.2$

    $n = 30$

    $10\% \times 300$

    0.10×300

    $= 30$

19. **(B)**

    $$\begin{aligned} 3(3x + 2y &= -1) \\ \underline{2(2x + 3y} &\underline{= \;\;1)} \\ 9x + 6y &= -3 \\ \underline{-(4x + 6y} &\underline{= \;\;2)} \\ 5x &= -5 \\ x &= -1 \end{aligned}$$

    $$\begin{aligned} 3x + 2y &= -1 \\ 3(-1) + 2y &= -1 \\ -3 + 2y &= -1 \\ 2y &= 2 \\ y &= 1 \end{aligned}$$

20. **(B)** $\angle A > \angle B$ given

    CB > AC In a triangle the greater side lies opposite the greater angle.

UNIT VII: BIOLOGY

BIOLOGY TESTS ANSWER SHEET

TEST 1: CELLS, STRUCTURE, AND FUNCTION

1. Ⓐ Ⓑ Ⓒ Ⓓ	11. Ⓐ Ⓑ Ⓒ Ⓓ	21. Ⓐ Ⓑ Ⓒ Ⓓ	31. Ⓐ Ⓑ Ⓒ Ⓓ
2. Ⓐ Ⓑ Ⓒ Ⓓ	12. Ⓐ Ⓑ Ⓒ Ⓓ	22. Ⓐ Ⓑ Ⓒ Ⓓ	32. Ⓐ Ⓑ Ⓒ Ⓓ
3. Ⓐ Ⓑ Ⓒ Ⓓ	13. Ⓐ Ⓑ Ⓒ Ⓓ	23. Ⓐ Ⓑ Ⓒ Ⓓ	33. Ⓐ Ⓑ Ⓒ Ⓓ
4. Ⓐ Ⓑ Ⓒ Ⓓ	14. Ⓐ Ⓑ Ⓒ Ⓓ	24. Ⓐ Ⓑ Ⓒ Ⓓ	34. Ⓐ Ⓑ Ⓒ Ⓓ
5. Ⓐ Ⓑ Ⓒ Ⓓ	15. Ⓐ Ⓑ Ⓒ Ⓓ	25. Ⓐ Ⓑ Ⓒ Ⓓ	35. Ⓐ Ⓑ Ⓒ Ⓓ
6. Ⓐ Ⓑ Ⓒ Ⓓ	16. Ⓐ Ⓑ Ⓒ Ⓓ	26. Ⓐ Ⓑ Ⓒ Ⓓ	36. Ⓐ Ⓑ Ⓒ Ⓓ
7. Ⓐ Ⓑ Ⓒ Ⓓ	17. Ⓐ Ⓑ Ⓒ Ⓓ	27. Ⓐ Ⓑ Ⓒ Ⓓ	37. Ⓐ Ⓑ Ⓒ Ⓓ
8. Ⓐ Ⓑ Ⓒ Ⓓ	18. Ⓐ Ⓑ Ⓒ Ⓓ	28. Ⓐ Ⓑ Ⓒ Ⓓ	38. Ⓐ Ⓑ Ⓒ Ⓓ
9. Ⓐ Ⓑ Ⓒ Ⓓ	19. Ⓐ Ⓑ Ⓒ Ⓓ	29. Ⓐ Ⓑ Ⓒ Ⓓ	39. Ⓐ Ⓑ Ⓒ Ⓓ
10. Ⓐ Ⓑ Ⓒ Ⓓ	20. Ⓐ Ⓑ Ⓒ Ⓓ	30. Ⓐ Ⓑ Ⓒ Ⓓ	40. Ⓐ Ⓑ Ⓒ Ⓓ

TEST 2: CELL METABOLISM

1. Ⓐ Ⓑ Ⓒ Ⓓ	6. Ⓐ Ⓑ Ⓒ Ⓓ	11. Ⓐ Ⓑ Ⓒ Ⓓ	16. Ⓐ Ⓑ Ⓒ Ⓓ
2. Ⓐ Ⓑ Ⓒ Ⓓ	7. Ⓐ Ⓑ Ⓒ Ⓓ	12. Ⓐ Ⓑ Ⓒ Ⓓ	17. Ⓐ Ⓑ Ⓒ Ⓓ
3. Ⓐ Ⓑ Ⓒ Ⓓ	8. Ⓐ Ⓑ Ⓒ Ⓓ	13. Ⓐ Ⓑ Ⓒ Ⓓ	18. Ⓐ Ⓑ Ⓒ Ⓓ
4. Ⓐ Ⓑ Ⓒ Ⓓ	9. Ⓐ Ⓑ Ⓒ Ⓓ	14. Ⓐ Ⓑ Ⓒ Ⓓ	19. Ⓐ Ⓑ Ⓒ Ⓓ
5. Ⓐ Ⓑ Ⓒ Ⓓ	10. Ⓐ Ⓑ Ⓒ Ⓓ	15. Ⓐ Ⓑ Ⓒ Ⓓ	20. Ⓐ Ⓑ Ⓒ Ⓓ

TEST 3: CELL REPRODUCTION AND GENETICS

1. Ⓐ Ⓑ Ⓒ Ⓓ	6. Ⓐ Ⓑ Ⓒ Ⓓ	11. Ⓐ Ⓑ Ⓒ Ⓓ	16. Ⓐ Ⓑ Ⓒ Ⓓ
2. Ⓐ Ⓑ Ⓒ Ⓓ	7. Ⓐ Ⓑ Ⓒ Ⓓ	12. Ⓐ Ⓑ Ⓒ Ⓓ	17. Ⓐ Ⓑ Ⓒ Ⓓ
3. Ⓐ Ⓑ Ⓒ Ⓓ	8. Ⓐ Ⓑ Ⓒ Ⓓ	13. Ⓐ Ⓑ Ⓒ Ⓓ	18. Ⓐ Ⓑ Ⓒ Ⓓ
4. Ⓐ Ⓑ Ⓒ Ⓓ	9. Ⓐ Ⓑ Ⓒ Ⓓ	14. Ⓐ Ⓑ Ⓒ Ⓓ	19. Ⓐ Ⓑ Ⓒ Ⓓ
5. Ⓐ Ⓑ Ⓒ Ⓓ	10. Ⓐ Ⓑ Ⓒ Ⓓ	15. Ⓐ Ⓑ Ⓒ Ⓓ	20. Ⓐ Ⓑ Ⓒ Ⓓ

TEST 4: HUMAN ANATOMY AND PHYSIOLOGY

1. Ⓐ Ⓑ Ⓒ Ⓓ	26. Ⓐ Ⓑ Ⓒ Ⓓ	51. Ⓐ Ⓑ Ⓒ Ⓓ	76. Ⓐ Ⓑ Ⓒ Ⓓ
2. Ⓐ Ⓑ Ⓒ Ⓓ	27. Ⓐ Ⓑ Ⓒ Ⓓ	52. Ⓐ Ⓑ Ⓒ Ⓓ	77. Ⓐ Ⓑ Ⓒ Ⓓ
3. Ⓐ Ⓑ Ⓒ Ⓓ	28. Ⓐ Ⓑ Ⓒ Ⓓ	53. Ⓐ Ⓑ Ⓒ Ⓓ	78. Ⓐ Ⓑ Ⓒ Ⓓ
4. Ⓐ Ⓑ Ⓒ Ⓓ	29. Ⓐ Ⓑ Ⓒ Ⓓ	54. Ⓐ Ⓑ Ⓒ Ⓓ	79. Ⓐ Ⓑ Ⓒ Ⓓ
5. Ⓐ Ⓑ Ⓒ Ⓓ	30. Ⓐ Ⓑ Ⓒ Ⓓ	55. Ⓐ Ⓑ Ⓒ Ⓓ	80. Ⓐ Ⓑ Ⓒ Ⓓ
6. Ⓐ Ⓑ Ⓒ Ⓓ	31. Ⓐ Ⓑ Ⓒ Ⓓ	56. Ⓐ Ⓑ Ⓒ Ⓓ	81. Ⓐ Ⓑ Ⓒ Ⓓ
7. Ⓐ Ⓑ Ⓒ Ⓓ	32. Ⓐ Ⓑ Ⓒ Ⓓ	57. Ⓐ Ⓑ Ⓒ Ⓓ	82. Ⓐ Ⓑ Ⓒ Ⓓ
8. Ⓐ Ⓑ Ⓒ Ⓓ	33. Ⓐ Ⓑ Ⓒ Ⓓ	58. Ⓐ Ⓑ Ⓒ Ⓓ	83. Ⓐ Ⓑ Ⓒ Ⓓ
9. Ⓐ Ⓑ Ⓒ Ⓓ	34. Ⓐ Ⓑ Ⓒ Ⓓ	59. Ⓐ Ⓑ Ⓒ Ⓓ	84. Ⓐ Ⓑ Ⓒ Ⓓ
10. Ⓐ Ⓑ Ⓒ Ⓓ	35. Ⓐ Ⓑ Ⓒ Ⓓ	60. Ⓐ Ⓑ Ⓒ Ⓓ	85. Ⓐ Ⓑ Ⓒ Ⓓ
11. Ⓐ Ⓑ Ⓒ Ⓓ	36. Ⓐ Ⓑ Ⓒ Ⓓ	61. Ⓐ Ⓑ Ⓒ Ⓓ	86. Ⓐ Ⓑ Ⓒ Ⓓ
12. Ⓐ Ⓑ Ⓒ Ⓓ	37. Ⓐ Ⓑ Ⓒ Ⓓ	62. Ⓐ Ⓑ Ⓒ Ⓓ	87. Ⓐ Ⓑ Ⓒ Ⓓ
13. Ⓐ Ⓑ Ⓒ Ⓓ	38. Ⓐ Ⓑ Ⓒ Ⓓ	63. Ⓐ Ⓑ Ⓒ Ⓓ	88. Ⓐ Ⓑ Ⓒ Ⓓ
14. Ⓐ Ⓑ Ⓒ Ⓓ	39. Ⓐ Ⓑ Ⓒ Ⓓ	64. Ⓐ Ⓑ Ⓒ Ⓓ	89. Ⓐ Ⓑ Ⓒ Ⓓ
15. Ⓐ Ⓑ Ⓒ Ⓓ	40. Ⓐ Ⓑ Ⓒ Ⓓ	65. Ⓐ Ⓑ Ⓒ Ⓓ	90. Ⓐ Ⓑ Ⓒ Ⓓ
16. Ⓐ Ⓑ Ⓒ Ⓓ	41. Ⓐ Ⓑ Ⓒ Ⓓ	66. Ⓐ Ⓑ Ⓒ Ⓓ	91. Ⓐ Ⓑ Ⓒ Ⓓ
17. Ⓐ Ⓑ Ⓒ Ⓓ	42. Ⓐ Ⓑ Ⓒ Ⓓ	67. Ⓐ Ⓑ Ⓒ Ⓓ	92. Ⓐ Ⓑ Ⓒ Ⓓ
18. Ⓐ Ⓑ Ⓒ Ⓓ	43. Ⓐ Ⓑ Ⓒ Ⓓ	68. Ⓐ Ⓑ Ⓒ Ⓓ	93. Ⓐ Ⓑ Ⓒ Ⓓ
19. Ⓐ Ⓑ Ⓒ Ⓓ	44. Ⓐ Ⓑ Ⓒ Ⓓ	69. Ⓐ Ⓑ Ⓒ Ⓓ	94. Ⓐ Ⓑ Ⓒ Ⓓ
20. Ⓐ Ⓑ Ⓒ Ⓓ	45. Ⓐ Ⓑ Ⓒ Ⓓ	70. Ⓐ Ⓑ Ⓒ Ⓓ	95. Ⓐ Ⓑ Ⓒ Ⓓ
21. Ⓐ Ⓑ Ⓒ Ⓓ	46. Ⓐ Ⓑ Ⓒ Ⓓ	71. Ⓐ Ⓑ Ⓒ Ⓓ	96. Ⓐ Ⓑ Ⓒ Ⓓ
22. Ⓐ Ⓑ Ⓒ Ⓓ	47. Ⓐ Ⓑ Ⓒ Ⓓ	72. Ⓐ Ⓑ Ⓒ Ⓓ	97. Ⓐ Ⓑ Ⓒ Ⓓ
23. Ⓐ Ⓑ Ⓒ Ⓓ	48. Ⓐ Ⓑ Ⓒ Ⓓ	73. Ⓐ Ⓑ Ⓒ Ⓓ	98. Ⓐ Ⓑ Ⓒ Ⓓ
24. Ⓐ Ⓑ Ⓒ Ⓓ	49. Ⓐ Ⓑ Ⓒ Ⓓ	74. Ⓐ Ⓑ Ⓒ Ⓓ	99. Ⓐ Ⓑ Ⓒ Ⓓ
25. Ⓐ Ⓑ Ⓒ Ⓓ	50. Ⓐ Ⓑ Ⓒ Ⓓ	75. Ⓐ Ⓑ Ⓒ Ⓓ	100. Ⓐ Ⓑ Ⓒ Ⓓ

BIOLOGY TESTS

TEST 1: CELLS, STRUCTURE, AND FUNCTION

40 QUESTIONS • TIME—30 MINUTES

Directions: Read each question carefully and consider all possible answers. When you have decided which choice is best, blacken the corresponding space on your answer sheet. There is only one best answer for each question.

1. Which movement requires carrier proteins but no direct cellular energy?

   (A) diffusion
   (B) osmosis
   (C) dialysis
   (D) facilitated transport

2. When coffee is dissolved in water, the coffee is the

   (A) tonicity
   (B) solute
   (C) colloid
   (D) solvent

3. Which term denotes the movement of glucose molecules from an area of lower concentration to an area of higher concentration?

   (A) osmosis
   (B) diffusion
   (C) dialysis
   (D) active transport

4. You place a cell in a solution of substance *x* and water. Substance *x* is always present in the cell, but you do not know the concentration ratio in either case. The cell increases in size. What is the tonicity of the solution in which you placed the cell?

   (A) hypotonic
   (B) isotonic
   (C) hypertonic
   (D) none of the above

5. Substance *x* passes through a plasma membrane easily. What phrase best describes the probable nature of the substance?

   (A) It is hydrophilic and non-polar.
   (B) It is hydrophobic and polar.
   (C) It is hydrophilic and polar.
   (D) It is hydrophobic and non-polar.

6. Cells which contain more dissolved salts and sugars than the surrounding solution are called

   (A) isotonic
   (B) hypertonic
   (C) hypotonic
   (D) osmosis

7. The glycoprotein covering the plasma membrane of an animal cell is involved in

   (A) osmosis
   (B) cell-to-cell recognition
   (C) cell movement
   (D) organic acid production

8. You are watching an amoeba engulf another organism. This process is an example of

   (A) receptor-mediated endocytosis
   (B) facilitated transport
   (C) pinocytosis
   (D) phagocytosis

9. The concentration of glucose in blood cells is lower than the concentration of glucose in liver cells. During active transport, glucose moves from blood cells into the liver. Which organelle would you expect to find in large numbers in the liver?

   (A) Golgi bodies
   (B) endoplasmic reticulum
   (C) ribosomes
   (D) mitochondria

10. If a red blood cell is placed in sea water, it will be in what kind of solution?

    (A) isotonic
    (B) hypotonic
    (C) hypertonic
    (D) facilitated diffusion

11. Plasmolysis is a term describing

(A) cytoplasmic movement
(B) cells which become turgid
(C) cellular shrinkage which occurs when cells are immersed in hypertonic solution
(D) amoeboid movement

12. The movement of substances from lesser concentration to higher concentration is called

(A) osmosis
(B) diffusion
(C) active transport
(D) pinocytosis

13. Which particular structure is present in both eucaryotic and procaryotic cells?

(A) membrane bound nucleus
(B) mitochondria
(C) plastids
(D) cell membrane

14. Chloroplasts are examples of plastids.

(A) True
(B) False

15. The endoplasmic reticulum and the Golgi body are found in prokaryotes but not eukaryotes.

(A) True
(B) False

16. There are two types of endoplasmic reticulum (ER): rough ER and smooth ER.

(A) True
(B) False

17. As you try to mix water and oil in your salad dressing they do not mix because

(A) water is hydrophillic and oil is hydrophobic
(B) water is polar and oil is nonpolar
(C) both are hydrophillic
(D) none of the above

18. Plant cells differ from animal cells in that plant cells

(A) have a glycoprotein covering their plasma membrane.
(B) have a cell wall and animal cells do not.
(C) have mitochondria and animal cells do not.
(D) do not have a nucleus.

19. Which cell type is characterized by the lack of a true nucleus and the absence of membrane-bound organelles?

(A) animal cell type
(B) plant cell type
(C) fungal cell type
(D) prokaryotic cell

20. The cytoskeleton within the cell is thought to function

(A) in a structural capacity
(B) in positioning certain enzymes in close proximity for increased efficiency
(C) as a means of enhancing secretion of metabolites within the cell
(D) both a and b

21. Which organelle is associated with hydrolytic enzymes and is sometimes referred to as a "suicide bag?"

(A) Golgi apparatus
(B) lysosome
(C) mitochondrion
(D) ribosome

22. Which kingdom contains **only** unicellular organisms?

(A) Monera
(B) Plantae
(C) Protista
(D) Fungi

23. The virus belongs to which one of the following kingdoms?

(A) Monera
(B) Plantae
(C) Protista
(D) none

24. Organisms which live on dead organic matter are called

(A) parasites
(B) carnivorous
(C) autotroph
(D) saprophytes

25. Which one of the following is a procaryotic cell?

(A) amoeba
(B) cheek cell
(C) elodea leaf cell
(D) gleocapsa

26. The presence of which of the following structures would definitely distinguish a cell as being an eucaryote?

    (A) cell membrane
    (B) cytoplasm
    (C) nucleus
    (D) cell wall

27. A friend of yours in his bedroom sneaks a cigarette, which is forbidden in his household. His mother comes to the door, knocks, and says "You have three minutes to get rid of that thing." She knew what was going on because of the process of

    (A) intuition
    (B) osmosis
    (C) facilitated transport
    (D) diffusion

28. Pinocytosis is the process of

    (A) enclosing a food source or other substance in a membrane and bringing it into a cell.
    (B) enclosing a liquid substance in a membrane and bringing it into the cell.
    (C) enclosing a manufactured substance in a membrane and secreting it from the cell.
    (D) binding a substance and a receptor and bringing it into the cell.

29. The AIDS virus is transported in bodily fluids. The Surgeon General of the United States sends out information about the disease and its transmission. In one section, there is a recommendation that one should use latex (a form of plastic) condoms rather than those made of natural membranes. This recommendation is probably based upon the principal of

    (A) diffusion
    (B) facilitated transport
    (C) active transport
    (D) varied selectively, permeability of membranes

30. The plasma membrane of the eukaryotic cell determines selectively which substances can enter and leave the cell. Such a membrane is said to be

    (A) impermeable
    (B) selectively permeable
    (C) isotonic
    (D) hypotonic

31. What primarily determines the shape of cells that lack cell walls?

    (A) microfubules and microfilaments
    (B) nucleus
    (C) endoplasmic reticulum (ER)
    (D) ribosomes

32. Which pair of organelles is responsible for energy supply to eukaryotic cells?

    (A) ribosomes and mitochondria
    (B) chloroplasts and mitochondria
    (C) nuclei and ribosomes
    (D) mitochondria and nuclei

33. Where in the single-celled organism *Euglena* would you expect to find the greatest concentration of mitochondria?

    (A) near the site of flagellum insertion
    (B) near the nucleus
    (C) near the site of lysosome production
    (D) within the chloroplasts

34. You collect some pond water and filter out the different organisms into separate jars. You add no food to the water, but one kind of organism is still alive long after the others have died. That species is best described as being

    (A) autotrophic
    (B) hydrophilic
    (C) autonomous
    (D) heterotrophic

35. Which kingdom consists of eukaryotic, heterotrophic, multicellular organisms?

    (A) Monera
    (B) Protista
    (C) Animalia
    (D) Plantae

36. When you mix salt with water, what is the water called?

    (A) solute
    (B) solvent
    (C) solution
    (D) ionizer

37. Which storage area comprises up to 90 percent of a plant's cell volume?

    (A) vacuole
    (B) leucoplast
    (C) chloroplast
    (D) Golgi body

38. With which organelle is the synthesis of ATP associated?

(A) ribosome
(B) plastid
(C) mitochondrion
(D) lysosome

39. Which organism is a procaryote?

(A) plant
(B) blue-green algae
(C) fungi
(D) amoeba

40. The plasma membrane is soluble to

(A) lipids
(B) proteins
(C) acids
(D) nucleic acids

TEST 1: CELLS, STRUCTURE, AND FUNCTION ANSWER KEY

1. **D**	11. **C**	21. **B**	31. **A**
2. **B**	12. **C**	22. **A**	32. **B**
3. **D**	13. **D**	23. **D**	33. **A**
4. **A**	14. **A**	24. **D**	34. **A**
5. **D**	15. **B**	25. **D**	35. **C**
6. **B**	16. **A**	26. **C**	36. **B**
7. **B**	17. **B**	27. **D**	37. **A**
8. **D**	18. **B**	28. **B**	38. **C**
9. **D**	19. **D**	29. **D**	39. **B**
10. **C**	20. **D**	30. **B**	40. **A**

TEST 1: CELLS, STRUCTURE, AND FUNCTION EXPLANATORY ANSWERS

1. **(D)** In facilitated diffusion, large molecules and ions diffuse through channels within membrane proteins. The process requires no input of energy on the part of the cell, since materials move down a concentration gradient. Facilitated diffusion occurs more rapidly when the temperature is higher, and when the concentration gradient is steeper.

2. **(B)** In a solution the solid particles dissolved are called solutes. For example, in a sugar solution, the water is the solvent, and sugar is a solute.

3. **(D)** In active transport, the transport proteins move a solute against its concentration gradient. Active transport does not proceed spontaneously. It requires an energy (ATP) input.

4. **(A)** A cell immersed in a solution with a lower concentration of dissolved materials (solutes) is in a hypotonic environment. The concentration of water is higher outside of the cell than inside. Under these conditions, water diffuses into the cell.

5. **(D)** Substance x is hydrophobic and nonpolar, so it can easily pass through the membrane due to the phospholipid structure of the membrane.

6. **(B)** A cell is hypertonic when it has higher solute concentration and less water concentration compared to the outside solution which has more water and less solute (hypotonic), so the water will diffuse inside the cell.

7. **(B)** On the outside of the membrane, short carbohydrate chains are covalently linked to the protruding proteins. The carbohydrates are thought to play a role in the adhesion of cells to one another and in the "recognition" of molecules that interact with the cell (such as hormones, antibodies and viruses).

8. **(D)** Macromolecules and fluid cross cellular membranes by bulk transport, in which the transported materials are contained within vesicles and do not mix with other materials of the cytoplasm. There are two forms of bulk transport: endocytosis and exocytosis. Endocytosis of a solid is known as phagocytosis.

9. **(D)** In active transport, energy (ATP) is needed. Mitochondria is the main organelle for ATP synthesis.

10. **(C)** Red blood cells have 0.9% salt solution whereas sea water has more solute than red blood cells, so it is a hypertonic solution compared to red blood cells.

11. **(C)** If any cell is placed in a hypertonic solution, the cell loses its water, dehydrates and dies, because the cell is hypotonic (more water) compared to outside solutions.

12. **(C)** The movement of materials against a concentration gradient need energy. (See number 3.)

13. **(D)** Every living organism is covered by a cell membrane.

14. **(A)** There are three different kinds of plastids present in the plant cells. Chloroplast is one of them.

15. **(B)** Procaryote cells do not have membrane bound organelles.

16. **(A)** Endoplasmic reticulum are of two kinds, one of which has ribosomes on their surface and is called rough ER; and the other without ribosomes is called smooth ER.

17. **(B)** Water is a polar molecule whereas oil is a non polar molecule. Water molecules have a slightly negative charge in one side and slightly positive charge in other side but lipid molecules do not have any charges.

18. **(B)** All plant cells have an outer rigid covering called cell wall made up of polysaccharide cellulose; but animals do not have cell walls only cell membranes.

19. **(D)** Procaryote cell, (example bacteria and blue-green algae) do not have a membrane bound nucleus but have naked DNA in the cytoplasm.

20. **(D)** The cytoskeleton is a web of fibrous protein that extends throughout the cell. It alters the shape of a cell, moves the whole cell from one place to another and pushes or pulls organelles.

21. **(B)** Lysosomes are essentially membrane bags that enclose hydrolytic enzymes which are involved in breaking down proteins, polysaccharides and lipids. If the lysosomes break open, the cell itself will be destroyed, because the enzymes they carry are capable of hydrolyzing all the major types of molecules found in a living cell.

22. **(A)** In five kingdom classification, all procaryote organisms belong to kingdom Monera. All procaryotes are unicellular.

23. **(D)** Virus is not a living cell; a submicroscopic, non-cellular particle composed of a nucleic acid core and a protein coat, reproducing only within a host, so it does not belong to any living kingdom.

24. **(D)** Some bacteria and fungi feed on dead organic matter to get their energy (saphros means rotten, putrid; and bios, life)

25. **(D)** Amoeba, check cells, elodea leaf all are eucaryotic and have membrane bound organelles, etc. Gleocapsa is a blue-green algae.

26. **(C)** Membrane bound nucleus is the major organelle of eucaryote cell. All living organisms have cell membrane, and cytoplasm, and some have cell wall.

27. **(D)** Diffusion is the tendency of materials to move down a concentration gradient. For example, perfume molecules escaping from an open bottle, for example, move away from one another. The molecules continue to diffuse until they are evenly dispersed throughout the room. Same thing happen with cigarette smoke.

28. **(B)** There are two forms of endocytosis, depending on the kind of material brought into the cell. Endocytosis of fluid is known as pinocytosis.

29. **(D)** All cells can exist as distinct entities because of the cell membrane, which regulates the passage of materials into and out of the cell. Latex membrane is used so it does not allow the HIV virus to pass through the membrane, so people will not get infected with the HIV virus.

30. **(B)** Membranes control the types of molecules that can pass into and out of the cell and organelles. This is because cell membranes are permeable to certain molecules and impermeable to others, a phenomenon known as selectively permeable.

31. **(A)** Three different types of filaments have been identified as major participants in the cytoskeletons: microtubules, microfilaments and intermediate filaments. It maintains the shape of the cell, enables it to move, anchors its organelles and directs its traffic.

32. **(B)** Both mitochondria and chloroplast are energy producing organelles. Mitochondria release the energy from food as a form of ATP and chloroplasts pick up the solar energy and convert it to chemical energy (ATP).

33. **(A)** Flagellum is constantly in motion; it needs a large quantity of energy, and mitochondria is the organelle which is the energy source of the cell.

34. **(A)** Autotrophic organisms such as plants, all algae, and some bacteria are able to synthesize their own organic food by using CO_2, H_2O, and sunlight.

35. **(C)** All animals are multicellular, have membrane bound organelles, and they cannot make their food from CO_2, H_2O, and sunlight.

36. **(B)** The liquid part of the solution is called solvent.

37. **(A)** A plant cell is characterized by a central vacuole, which stores materials and gives support. A typical central vacuole contains sugars, organic acids, proteins, inorganic ions, pigments, and toxic waste products, which might otherwise interfere with cellular activities.

38. **(C)** Mitochondrion is the powerhouse of the cell. It produces maximum amounts of chemical energy (ATP) for sustaining life.

39. **(B)** Blue-green algae are always small and single-celled and do not have membrane bound organelles.

40. **(A)** Membranes are composed of a phospholipid bilayer of molecules interspersed with protein molecules. Any kind of non-polar molecule such as lipids or some other organic solvents (ether, acetone, etc.) can easily pass through the lipid layer of membrane.

TEST 2: CELL METABOLISM

19 QUESTIONS • TIME—15 MINUTES

Directions: Read each question carefully and consider all possible answers. When you have decided which choice is best, blacken the corresponding space on your answer sheet. There is only one best answer for each question.

1. The process whereby muscle cells produce lactic acid is called

   (A) aerobic respiration
   (B) glycolysis
   (C) fermentation
   (D) electron transport chain

2. During aerobic respiration, which one of the following substances is released?

   (A) 22 ATP
   (B) 32 ATP
   (C) 2 ATP
   (D) 36 ATP

3. The final electron and hydrogen acceptor in aerobic respiration is

   (A) NAD
   (B) FAD
   (C) Co-enzyme
   (D) Oxygen

4. In exergonic reactions, the energy is

   (A) used
   (B) stored
   (C) released
   (D) lost

5. Most human enzymes function best in the temperature range of

   (A) 5–15 degrees C
   (B) 20–30 degrees C
   (C) 35–40 degrees C
   (D) 45–50 degrees C

6. Vitamins are important to the human diet because they are incorporated into

   (A) enzyme substitutes
   (B) ATP
   (C) co-enzymes
   (D) inhibitors

7. Energy can exist in many forms. Which is a true form of energy?

   (A) sound
   (B) light
   (C) diffusion
   (D) both a and b

8. Stored energy is referred to as

   (A) activation energy
   (B) kinetic energy
   (C) potential energy
   (D) electrical energy

9. Noncyclic-photophosphorylation takes place inside the

   (A) stroma
   (B) cytoplasm
   (C) thylakoids
   (D) golgi bodies

10. The products of the light reaction of photosynthesis are

    (A) Carbohydrate, CO_2
    (B) $NADPH_2$ + ATP + O_2
    (C) PGAL + CO_2 + H_2O
    (D) starch + CO_2

11. The dark reaction of photosynthesis takes place in

    (A) thylakoids
    (B) cytoplasm
    (C) stroma
    (D) grana

12. Respiration is inhibited by

    (A) glucose
    (B) sodium fluoride
    (C) sodium pyruvate
    (D) yeast

13. Aerobic cellular respiration is more important to sustain life than anaerobic because it produces

    (A) more pyruvic acid
    (B) more sugar
    (C) more energy
    (D) more lactic acid

14. Which organelle is responsible for oxygen production?

    (A) mitochondria
    (B) cilia
    (C) golgi body
    (D) chloroplasts

15. An organic catalyst which enhances the chemical reaction is called

    (A) a fat
    (B) a lactic acid
    (C) a polysaccharide
    (D) an enzyme

16. The first stage of aerobic cellular respiration is

    (A) electron transport chain
    (B) Kreb's cycle
    (C) glycolysis
    (D) light reaction

17. Which of the following is not produced during glycolysis?

    (A) NADH
    (B) FADH
    (C) pyruvate^2
    (D) ATP

18. Glycolysis occurs in the

    (A) nucleus
    (B) mitochondrion
    (C) plasma membrane
    (D) cytoplasm

19. For the aerobic pathway, electron transport systems are located in the

    (A) cytoplasm
    (B) golgi bodies
    (C) lysosomes
    (D) mitochondrion

TEST 2: CELL METABOLISM ANSWER KEY

1. **C**
2. **D**
3. **D**
4. **C**
5. **C**
6. **C**
7. **D**
8. **C**
9. **C**
10. **B**
11. **C**
12. **B**
13. **C**
14. **D**
15. **D**
16. **C**
17. **B**
18. **D**
19. **D**

TEST 2: CELL METABOLISM EXPLANATORY ANSWERS

1. **(C)** This is the process by which a glucose molecule is changed to two molecules of pyruvic acid with the liberation of a small amount of energy. In the absence of oxygen, pyruvic acid can be converted to ethanol or to one of several organic acids, of which lactic is the most common. This process is called fermentation.

2. **(D)** In the first stage, aerobic respiration (glycolysis) produces 2 ATP. In the second stage (Kreb's cycle) it produces 2 ATP. During the final stage (electron transport chain) it produces 32 ATP.

3. **(D)** During the final stage, electron transport, the loaded coenzymes (NADH and $FADH_2$) give up hydrogen and electrons. As the electrons pass through the transport systems, energy is released, indirectly giving ATP formation. Oxygen accepts the electrons and hydrogen at the end of the transport system and combined they form water.

4. **(C)** The reactants of some reactions have more energy than the products. Many such reactions release energy that cells can use, which is what happens during aerobic respiration.

5. **(C)** Each type of enzyme functions best within a certain temperature range. The chemical reaction rates decrease sharply when the temperature becomes too high. Humans usually die when their internal body temperature reaches 44°C (112°F) because it destroys the shape of the enzyme and thereby stops the metabolism.

6. **(C)** The enzyme helpers called coenzymes are complex organic molecules, many of which are derived from vitamins. These coenzymes can pick up hydrogen atoms that are liberated during glucose breakdown.

7. **(D)** Energy is a capacity to make things happen or to do work. There are different forms of energy.

8. **(C)** The stored form of energy is called potential energy. Example is glucose molecule; when it breaks down it releases a large quantity of chemical energy to do work.

9. **(C)** All the pigments are present inside the thylakoids. SO, the chlorophyll molecules and other pigments pick up the solar energy, convert it to chemical energy as a form of ATP and NADPH, and release oxygen during the non-cyclic light reaction.

10. **(B)** During non-cyclic light reactions, energy from the sun drives the formation of ATP (which carries energy) and NADPH (which carries hydrogen and electrons). Oxygen is a by-product of photosynthesis.

11. **(C)** The light independent reactions are the "synthesis" part of photosynthesis. ATP molecules deliver the required energy for the reaction. NADPH molecules deliver the required hydrogen and electrons and carbon dioxide diffuses inside the stronin. Then it forms the energy rich molecule glucose (the process is called dark reaction).

12. **(B)** Sodium fluoride is an enzyme inhibitor in glycolysis, so it inhibits the breakdown of glucose molecules during respiration and stops the formation of energy.

13. **(C)** Because aerobic respiration produces 36 ATP compared to anaerobic which only release 2 ATP.

14. **(D)** The organelle chloroplast is responsible for photosynthesis, which produces O_2 and the energy-rich molecule carbohydrate.

15. **(D)** All enzymes are protein molecules and protein is one of the organic molecules necessary for sustaining life.

16. **(C)** The first stage of cellular respiration where glucose is broken down step by step to form 2 pyruvic acid taking place inside the cytoplasm, is called glycolysis.

17. **(B)** In glycolysis only one coenzyme, NAD^+, is necessary. But in Kreb's cycle both NAD^+ and FAD^+ are necessary.

18. **(D)** The first stage of respiration, the breaking down of the glucose molecules, always takes place inside the cytoplasm because all the enzymes are there for the reaction.

19. **(D)** Electron transport systems and neighboring channel proteins serve as the machinery. These are embedded in the inner membrane that divides mitochondrion into two compartments.

TEST 3: CELL REPRODUCTION AND GENETICS

20 QUESTIONS • TIME—15 MINUTES

Directions: Read each question carefully and consider all possible answers. When you have decided which choice is best, blacken the corresponding space on your answer sheet. There is only one best answer for each question.

1. If body cells of cows contain a total of 40 chromosomes, sperm and egg cells of cows contain how many chromosomes total?

   (A) 10
   (B) 20
   (C) 25
   (D) 40

2. Codominance occurs when

   (A) both the alleles in a heterozygote are expressed phenotypically in an individual
   (B) expression of 2 different alleles alternates from one generation to the next
   (C) a heterozygote expresses an intermediate phenotype
   (D) offspring exhibit several different phenotypic expressions of a single trait

3. Mitosis in a single human cell usually results in the formation of

   (A) 2 diploid cells
   (B) 2 haploid cells
   (C) 4 diploid cells
   (D) 4 haploid cells

4. Meiosis in a single human cell usually results in the formation of

   (A) 2 diploid cells
   (B) 2 haploid cells
   (C) 4 diploid cells
   (D) 4 haploid cells

5. If you reproduce sexually, you produce gametes via

   (A) fertilization
   (B) mitosis
   (C) meiosis
   (D) recombination

6. If you reproduce asexually, you produce offspring via

   (A) fertilization
   (B) mitosis
   (C) meiosis
   (D) recombination

7. According to Mendel's Law of Segregation, an organism with the genotype Aa

   (A) produces only gametes containing the A allele
   (B) produces only gametes containing the a allele
   (C) half the time produces gametes containing A, and half the time a
   (D) three-quarters of the time produces gametes containing A, and one-quarter of the time a

8. What type of allele is expressed in the phenotype of only a homozygous individual?

   (A) incompletely dominant
   (B) haploid
   (C) recessive
   (D) dominant

9. The sex of a human child is determined by the sex chromosome from

   (A) the mother
   (B) the father
   (C) both parents
   (D) neither parents

10. Cell division occurs most rapidly in

    (A) heart tissue
    (B) muscle tissue
    (C) nervous tissue
    (D) cancerous tissue

11. If the sperm cells of a fish have 30 chromosomes, the body cell of the fish has

    (A) 80 chromosomes
    (B) 60 chromosomes
    (C) 120 chromosomes
    (D) none of the above

12. A condition resulting from the presence of an extra twenty-first chromosome is

    (A) hemophilia
    (B) the Rh-positive condition
    (C) phenylketonuria
    (D) Down syndrome

13. A woman who is a heterozygous carrier for a sex-linked recessive gene will pass it to

    (A) all of her sons
    (B) all of her daughters
    (C) all children
    (D) one-half of her sons and one-half of her daughters

14. Persons who have hemophilia cannot produce

    (A) new red blood cells
    (B) normally shaped red blood cells
    (C) functional blood clotting factors
    (D) white blood cells

15. Which of the following is an example of a sex-linked genetic disorder?

    (A) Tay-Sachs disease
    (B) cystic fibrosis
    (C) Turner's Syndrome
    (D) hemophilia

16. In the case of the sex-linked trait red-green color-blindness, which one of the following cannot occur?

    (A) a carrier mother passing the gene on to her son
    (B) a carrier mother passing the gene on to her daughter
    (C) a color-blind father passing the gene on to his son
    (D) a color-blind father passing the gene on to his daughter

17. The genotype for a man who has blue eyes and hemophilia is

    (A) $x^by\ x^hy$
    (B) bb hh
    (C) bb x^hy
    (D) Bbh

18. If both the parents have blood type AB, what will be the blood types of offspring?

    (A) A
    (B) AB
    (C) A, AB, and B
    (D) O

19. Which blood type would be a universal donor?

    (A) A
    (B) AB
    (C) B
    (D) O

20. Males that tend to be tall and have strong criminal records have which of the following sex chromosomes?

    (A) XXY
    (B) XY
    (C) XYY
    (D) XYXY

TEST 3: CELL REPRODUCTION AND GENETICS ANSWER KEY

1. **B**
2. **A**
3. **A**
4. **D**
5. **C**
6. **B**
7. **C**
8. **D**
9. **B**
10. **D**
11. **B**
12. **D**
13. **D**
14. **C**
15. **D**
16. **C**
17. **C**
18. **C**
19. **D**
20. **C**

TEST 3: CELL REPRODUCTION AND GENETICS EXPLANATORY ANSWER

1. **(B)** The adult bodies of most plants and animals consist of diploid (2n) rather than haploid (n) cells. A gamete (male sperm and female egg) is always a haploid cell, which means it has one set of chromosomes formed by meiosis of germ cells (2n). So if the germ cell is 40, the gamete will be 20.

2. **(A)** When two alternative alleles are fully apparent in a hybrid, with both phenotypes showing in the organism, we say that the hybrids exhibit codominance. Blood typing of humans provides an excellent example of codominance. The AB blood type inherits an A allele and a B allele. Neither allele is dominant over the other; therefore codominance causes a new blood type AB.

3. **(A)** The blood cells of humans divide by mitosis. In mitosis the diploid number of chromosomes is maintained and the resulting daughter cells are identical to the parent cell.

4. **(D)** Meiosis is the nuclear division which reduces the number of chromosomes in the resulting cells by half. Meiosis is necessary for the production of gametes or sex cells and results in 4 non-identical haploid cells (sperms and eggs).

5. **(C)** The first part of sexual reproduction is meiosis where the germ cells divide and produce four haploid gametes.

6. **(B)** Asexual reproduction occurs without sex and transfers the genes of just one parent to each offspring; it produces offspring that are genetically identical to one another and to their single parent by the process of mitosis.

7. **(C)** The first pattern of inheritance discovered by Mendel was the law of segregation. This law describes how the two copies of each gene segregate (separate) during meiosis so that just one copy ends up in each gamete (sperm and egg).

8. **(D)** The dominant will always show the dominant characteristic in their phenotype.

9. **(B)** The sex chromosome of a mother is always XX and the father XY. So, the sex of the child depends on whether he or she gets X or Y from the father. If the child gets X from the father and X from the mother, she will be a female. If the child gets Y from the father and X from the mother, the child will be a male.

10. **(D)** In normal cells, the cell division is controlled by two sets of genes: one set stimulates and the other set suppresses. In cancer, defective genes may overstimulate cell division or fail to halt cell division.

11. **(B)** Sperm cells are haploid (N), which are formed by meiosis of germ cells (2N). So if the haploid is 30, then germ cells should be 60.

12. **(D)** A person with Down Syndrome has three copies in chromosome #21 rather than two copies. The extra chromosome affects practically every part of the body.

13. **(D)** If we do the Punnet square for a woman who is a heterozygous carrier for sex-linked recessive gene and married to a normal man, half of her sons and half of her daughters will receive this gene.

    X^CX—Girl with recessive gene

    X^CY—Boy with recessive gene

    XY—normal boy

    XX—normal girl

14. **(C)** Hemophilia is one of the disorders caused by a Y-linked recessive allele. Many genes in many chromosomes contribute to normal blood clotting, but two gene loci in the Y chromosome are responsible for the two most common clotting disorders—hemophilia A and hemophilia B.

15. **(D)** Hemophilia is a sex-linked disorder because the defective gene is present in the Y sex chromosome.

16. **(C)** The sex-linked trait is present in the X chromosome. So, the father cannot pass the gene to his son because the son always receives the Y chromosome from his father, not the X chromosome.

17. **(C)** The blue gene is the autosomal recessive trait, whereas hemophilia is the sex-linked recessive trait. To get the blue eyes, the person should have two blue-eyes recessive genes. If the person is male, he needs only one recessive gene for hemophilia.

18. **(C)** If both parents are AB, they can only produce two different kinds of gametes (sperm and eggs), A and B. So the blood types of children will be A, AB, and B.

19. **(D)** Blood type O has neither A nor B polysaccharides (antigen) for antibodies to attack.

20. **(C)** Non-dysjunction of sex chromosomes (XY) in a man produces four types of abnormal sperms. When these abnormal sperm (YY) fertilizes normal X carrying chromosomes, they produce abnormal genotypes (XYY).

TEST 4: HUMAN ANATOMY AND PHYSIOLOGY

100 QUESTIONS • TIME—75 MINUTES

Directions: Read each question carefully and consider all possible answers. When you have decided which choice is best, blacken the corresponding space on your answer sheet. There is only one best answer for each question.

1. The ___ system picks up fluid leaked from blood vessels, houses white blood cells and is highly involved in mechanisms of immunity.

   (A) urinary
   (B) endocrine
   (C) integumentary
   (D) lymphatic

2. The major muscle component of inspiration is the

   (A) diaphragm
   (B) external intercostal muscles
   (C) internal intercostal muscles
   (D) abdominal muscles

3. Skin, nails and hair are components of the ___ system.

   (A) integumentary
   (B) lymphatic
   (C) skeletal
   (D) endocrine

4. Water reabsorption in the collecting duct of the kidneys is controlled by ___ from the posterior pituitary.

   (A) oxytocin
   (B) ADH
   (C) epinephrine
   (D) aldosterone

5. Most homeostatic control mechanisms are

   (A) positive feedback mechanisms
   (B) negative feedback mechanisms
   (C) neural mechanisms
   (D) endocrine mechanisms

6. The most important structure(s) in the routine control of respiration is/are the

   (A) trachea
   (B) irritant receptors
   (C) peripheral chemoreceptors
   (D) central chemoreceptors

7. A ___ plane is a vertical plane that divides the body into left and right parts.

   (A) frontal
   (B) transverse
   (C) sagittal
   (D) coronal

8. Cardiac output is equal to

   (A) heart rate
   (B) stroke volume
   (C) the product of stroke volume and heart rate
   (D) stroke volume divided by heart rate

9. Movement of a solute across a biological membrane from an area of low concentration to an area of high concentration occurs via

   (A) osmosis
   (B) diffusion
   (C) active transport
   (D) inertia

10. The right ventricle pumps blood through the ___ valve into the ___.

    (A) atrioventricular; pulmonary veins
    (B) pulmonary semilunar; pulmonary veins
    (C) atrioventricular; pulmonary arteries
    (D) pulmonary semilunar; pulmonary arteries

11. The primary beta-2 catechol amine agonist is

    (A) acetylcholine
    (B) epinephrine
    (C) norepinephrine
    (D) nicotine

12. Action potentials result from an increased membrane permeability to

    (A) calcium
    (B) sodium
    (C) potassium
    (D) chloride

13. Food is prevented from entering the trachea during swallowing by the

(A) glottis
(B) esophageal sphincter
(C) cardiac sphincter
(D) epiglottis

14. Oxygen transported in blood is mainly

(A) dissolved in plasma
(B) combined with hemoglobin
(C) CO_2
(D) carried as bicarbonate

15. Pyramidal tract fibers originate in the

(A) precentral gyrus
(B) postcentral gyrus
(C) thalamus
(D) spinal cord

16. The transmitter substance at the neuromuscular junction is

(A) acetylcholinesterase
(B) norepinephrine
(C) acetylcholine
(D) epinephrine

17. __ dilate or constrict to control the flow of blood into a particular capillary bed.

(A) Arteries
(B) Arterioles
(C) Capillaries
(D) Veins

18. Hormone secretion and neurotransmitter release use the process of ___ to move substances from the cell interior into the extracellular space.

(A) phagocytosis
(B) endocytosis
(C) exocytosis
(D) pinocytosis

19. The area innervated by all the axons in a single dorsal root is a(n)

(A) receptive field
(B) dermatome
(C) sensory unit
(D) motor unit

20. Stratified squamous anatomically describes a form of ___ tissue.

(A) muscle
(B) nerve
(C) connective
(D) epithelial

21. __ forms most of the embryonic skeleton, connects the ribs of the sternum and comprises the solid supportive structures of the nose and trachea.

(A) Bone
(B) Areolar connective tissue
(C) Adipose tissue
(D) Cartilage

22. __ is the fibrous protein found in the stratum corneum that helps give the epidermis its protective properties.

(A) Keratin
(B) Melanin
(C) Carotene
(D) Hemoglobin

23. Pain information is carried by ___ afferents.

(A) A Delta
(B) C
(C) A Alpha
(D) A Delta and C

24. Increased parasympathetic activity will result in

(A) increased heart rate
(B) increased cardiac output
(C) vasoconstriction
(D) decreased heart rate

25. The receptor for the stretch reflex is the

(A) Golgi tendon organ
(B) free nerve ending
(C) hair cell
(D) muscle spindle

26. The glomerular membrane is

(A) more permeable than most other capillaries
(B) less permeable than most other capillaries
(C) highly permeable to proteins
(D) highly permeable to erythrocytes

27. CO_2 transport in blood is mainly
    (A) dissolved in plasma
    (B) as bicarbonate
    (C) dissolved in RBC's
    (D) combined with hemoglobin

28. Glucose is returned in blood in the kidneys by
    (A) glomerular filtration
    (B) tubular reabsorption
    (C) tubular secretion
    (D) reabsorption in the collection duct

29. The outer surface of the diaphysis of a long bone is covered with a double-layered membrane called the ___. The inner layer of that membrane contains bone-forming cells, called ___.
    (A) endosteum; osteoblasts
    (B) endosteum; osteoclasts
    (C) periosteum; osteoclasts
    (D) periosteum; osteoblasts

30. Atrial contraction is
    (A) initiated by the AV node
    (B) most important in a resting subject
    (C) initiated by the SA node
    (D) responsible for most of the ventricular filling

31. The first heart sound is a result of
    (A) closing of the pulmonary valve
    (B) closing of the AV valves
    (C) closing of the aortic valve
    (D) contraction of the atria

32. The portion of the skull overlying the region of the cerebral cortex primarily involved with visual process is the ___ bone.
    (A) frontal
    (B) parietal
    (C) occipital
    (D) temporal

33. Normally, most of the body's total blood is found in the
    (A) veins
    (B) arteries
    (C) capillaries
    (D) heart

34. The kneecap or patella is an example of a(n) ___bone.
    (A) long
    (B) short
    (C) flat
    (D) irregular

35. The normal pacemaker of the heart is the
    (A) SA node
    (B) AV node
    (C) atria
    (D) ventricle

36. Blood pressure is highest in
    (A) arteries
    (B) arterioles
    (C) capillaries
    (D) veins

37. Water permeability is greatest in the ___ of the nephron.
    (A) collecting duct
    (B) distal convoluted tubule
    (C) loop of henle
    (D) proximal convoluted tubule

38. Movement of particles across a biological membrane is enhanced by
    (A) large particle size
    (B) lipid solubility
    (C) particle charge
    (D) lipophobic properties

39. The ___ division of the autonomic nervous system functions during emergencies.
    (A) sympathetic
    (B) parasympathetic
    (C) craniosacral
    (D) somatic

40. Sympathetic preganglionic neurons originate in the
    (A) cervical spinal cord
    (B) thoracic spinal cord
    (C) sacral spinal cord
    (D) coccygeal spinal cord

41. Cellular energy production takes place within
    (A) rough endoplasmic reticulum
    (B) smooth endoplasmic reticulum
    (C) mitochondria
    (D) Golgi apparatus

42. ___ is a bending movement that decreases the angle of a joint and brings two articulating bones closer together.

(A) Retraction
(B) Flexion
(C) Extension
(D) Rotation

43. New epidermal cells are formed in the stratum

(A) germinativum
(B) corneum
(C) spinosum
(D) lucidum

44. Women have a larger percentage of adipose tissue than men; this tissue is mainly found in the ___.

(A) epidermis
(B) dermis
(C) subcutaneous layer
(D) muscle

45. Membranes that line body cavities that open to the outside are

(A) mucous
(B) serous
(C) synovial
(D) cutaneous

46. Epidermal cells are supplied with nutrition from blood vessels located within the

(A) epidermis
(B) dermis
(C) subcutaneous layer
(D) all of the above

47. The terms visceral, nonstriated, and involuntary are descriptive of ___ muscle.

(A) skeletal
(B) smooth
(C) cardiac
(D) postural

48. Blood cell formation is a function of the ___ system.

(A) circulatory
(B) skeletal
(C) endocrine
(D) muscular

49. Blood calcium is elevated by

(A) calcitonin
(B) parathyroid hormone
(C) growth hormone
(D) thyroxine

50. Your 7-year old patient is perspiring freely on the forehead, palms and soles, indicating activity of the ___.

(A) eccrine glands
(B) apocrine glands
(C) sebaceous glands
(D) ceruminous glands

51. Flexion of the elbow results from contraction of the muscle ___ and flexion of the knee involves contraction of the ___ muscle.

(A) biceps brachii; biceps femoris
(B) triceps brachii; triceps femoris
(C) biceps femoris; biceps brachii
(D) triceps femoris; triceps brachii

52. Sweat glands that become functional at puberty are ___ .

(A) apocrine
(B) eccrine
(C) sebaceous
(D) ceruminous

53. An individual with higher than normal blood calcium (hypercalcemia) will compensate by elevating levels of ___.

(A) parathyroid hormone
(B) calcitonin
(C) both a and b
(D) neither a nor b

54. The ___ system carries hormones to their sites of action.

(A) endocrine
(B) cardiovascular
(C) respiratory
(D) skeletal

55. The most rapidly conducting axons within the human nervous system are ___ and ___.

(A) unmyelinated; small diameter
(B) unmyelinated; large diameter
(C) myelinated; small diameter
(D) myelinated; large diameter

56. The basic unit of structure and function within the kidneys is the ___.

 (A) glomerulus
 (B) nephron
 (C) ureter
 (D) urethra

57. The esophagus enters the stomach at the ___ region.

 (A) fundus
 (B) cardiac
 (C) body
 (D) pyloric

58. Release of ___ by the posterior pituitary will lead to contractions of the smooth muscle of the uterus.

 (A) ADH
 (B) ACTH
 (C) oxytocin
 (D) prolactin

59. Inhibition of ADH release will result in

 (A) high blood pressure
 (B) increased urine output
 (C) uterine contractions
 (D) decreased urine output

60. Ovulation occurs in response to

 (A) FSH
 (B) ADH
 (C) prolactin
 (D) LH

61. Heartburn results from reflux of gastric fluids into the esophagus. The structure that normally prevents this is the

 (A) pyloric sphincter
 (B) cardiac spincter
 (C) ileocecal valve
 (D) epiglottis

62. Fat is broken down in the duodenum by ___ from the gall bladder.

 (A) lipase
 (B) amylase
 (C) bile
 (D) HCl

63. Most digestion takes place in the

 (A) stomach
 (B) duodenum
 (C) ileum
 (D) jejunum

64. Visual receptors are located on the

 (A) lens
 (B) cornea
 (C) retina
 (D) optic tract

65. Most food absorption takes place in the

 (A) duodenum
 (B) colon
 (C) ileum
 (D) stomach

66. Centers for cardiovascular and respiratory control, vomiting and coughing are found within the ___, the most inferior part of the brain stem.

 (A) midbrain
 (B) pons
 (C) medulla
 (D) thalamus

67. Bile is manufactured in the

 (A) duodenum
 (B) liver
 (C) gall bladder
 (D) pancreas

68. A patient who is abnormally short and retarded suggests

 (A) hyperthyroidism as an infant
 (B) hypothyroidism as an infant
 (C) adult hyperthyroidism
 (D) adult hypothyroidism

69. Receptors used for color vision are

 (A) hair cells
 (B) rods
 (C) cones
 (D) retinae

70. The inner lining of the digestive system is the ___ layer.

 (A) mucosal
 (B) submucosal
 (C) muscular
 (D) serosal

71. The ___ has both endocrine and exocrine functions.
    (A) adrenal cortex
    (B) pancreas
    (C) parathyroid
    (D) thyroid

72. Lacrimation refers to the production of ___.
    (A) salvia
    (B) mucous
    (C) tears
    (D) urine

73. The sense of smell travels over cranial nerve #___.
    (A) I
    (B) II
    (C) III
    (D) IV

74. The gland adjacent to the urethra which enlarges in older males is the
    (A) testes
    (B) seminal vesicle
    (C) bulbourethral gland
    (D) prostate

75. Linear acceleration of the head is detected by receptors within the ___.
    (A) semicircular canals
    (B) utricles and saccules
    (C) cochlea
    (D) middle ear

76. The most abundant protein in blood is
    (A) alpha globulin
    (B) albumin
    (C) gamma globulin
    (D) fibrin

77. Fertilization normally occurs within the
    (A) fallopian tube
    (B) ovary
    (C) uterus
    (D) vagina

78. Depression is characterized by ___.
    (A) high levels of norepinephrine
    (B) low levels of serotonin
    (C) high levels of serotonin
    (D) high levels of norepinephrine

79. Lymphatic vessels originate at ___.
    (A) vascular capillaries
    (B) lymphatic capillaries
    (C) lymph nodes
    (D) lymphocytes

80. Human chorionic gonadotropin (HCG) is responsible for
    (A) maintaining the corpus luteum
    (B) lowering estrogen levels
    (C) lowering progesterone levels
    (D) initiating menstruation

81. Loss of the sense of sweet and sour tastes from the tongue indicate damage to the ___ nerve.
    (A) first
    (B) fifth
    (C) seventh
    (D) tenth

82. Salivation, lacrimation, urination, and defecation are primarily under control of the ___ division of the autonomic nervous system.
    (A) sympathetic
    (B) parasympathetic
    (C) somatic
    (D) voluntary

83. Sperm cells are stored in the ___ after leaving the seminiferous tubules.
    (A) epididymis
    (B) vas deferens
    (C) seminal vesicle
    (D) prostate

84. The hormone from the pancreas which is responsible for elevating blood glucose levels between meals is ___.
    (A) insulin
    (B) glucagon
    (C) somatostatin
    (D) epinephrine

85. The most abundantly formed elements in blood are
    (A) white blood cells
    (B) red blood cells
    (C) globulins
    (D) albumins

86. The most rapid mechanism of pH adjustment involves

(A) buffers
(B) the respiratory system
(C) the kidneys
(D) the liver

87. Normal pH of blood is

(A) 6
(B) 7.4
(C) 8
(D) 1.0

88. Hematocrit is a measure of ___ levels.

(A) white cell
(B) plasma
(C) blood
(D) erythrocyte

89. Cardiac muscle, because of its constant activity, has a high oxygen demand, which must be met without interruption. Oxygen is supplied to cardiac muscle by ___.

(A) the blood being pumped through the chambers of the heart
(B) coronary arteries
(C) coronary veins
(D) pulmonary arteries

90. Auditory receptors are

(A) rods
(B) hair cells
(C) cones
(D) muscle spindles

91. Blood containing the A antigen and the B antibody is type ___.

(A) A
(B) B
(C) AB
(D) O

92. Hemoglobin forms abnormal long chains in

(A) pernicious anemia
(B) iron deficiency anemia
(C) aplastic anemia
(D) sickle cell anemia

93. Auditory receptors are found within the

(A) outer ear
(B) middle ear
(C) auditory ossicles
(D) cochlea

94. Female menopause is characterized by low levels of

(A) GnRH
(B) LH
(C) FSH
(D) estrogen

95. Hyperventilation resulting from hysteria may cause

(A) respiratory acidosis
(B) respiratory alkalosis
(C) metabolic acidosis
(D) metabolic alkalosis

96. The major component of plasma is

(A) ions
(B) proteins
(C) water
(D) gases

97. ___ acts as a contraceptive agent by inhibiting release of GnRH.

(A) Sperm
(B) Estrogen
(C) Testosterone
(D) LH

98. Coagulation is inhibited by

(A) fibrin
(B) calcium
(C) thrombin
(D) heparin

99. Ovulation is triggered by the release of

(A) FSH
(B) LH
(C) GnRH
(D) estrogen

100. Testosterone is produced by ___ cells.

(A) prostate
(B) seminiferous
(C) epididymis
(D) interstitial

TEST 4: HUMAN ANATOMY AND PHYSIOLOGY ANSWER KEY

1. **D**	26. **A**	51. **B**	76. **B**
2. **A**	27. **B**	52. **A**	77. **A**
3. **A**	28. **B**	53. **B**	78. **B**
4. **B**	29. **D**	54. **B**	79. **B**
5. **B**	30. **C**	55. **D**	80. **A**
6. **D**	31. **B**	56. **B**	81. **C**
7. **C**	32. **C**	57. **B**	82. **B**
8. **C**	33. **A**	58. **C**	83. **A**
9. **B**	34. **B**	59. **B**	84. **B**
10. **D**	35. **A**	60. **D**	85. **B**
11. **B**	36. **A**	61. **B**	86. **A**
12. **B**	37. **D**	62. **C**	87. **B**
13. **D**	38. **B**	63. **B**	88. **B**
14. **B**	39. **A**	64. **C**	89. **A**
15. **A**	40. **B**	65. **C**	90. **B**
16. **C**	41. **C**	66. **C**	91. **A**
17. **B**	42. **B**	67. **B**	92. **D**
18. **C**	43. **A**	68. **B**	93. **D**
19. **B**	44. **C**	69. **C**	94. **D**
20. **D**	45. **A**	70. **A**	95. **B**
21. **D**	46. **B**	71. **B**	96. **C**
22. **A**	47. **B**	72. **C**	97. **B**
23. **D**	48. **B**	73. **A**	98. **D**
24. **D**	49. **B**	74. **D**	99. **B**
25. **D**	50. **A**	75. **B**	100. **D**

TEST 4: HUMAN ANATOMY AND PHYSIOLOGY EXPLANATORY ANSWERS

1. **(D)** Only the lymphatic system is involved in all three of these processes, although the urinary system does receive fluid from blood vessels.

2. **(A)** Internal and abdominal muscles aid expiration. The external intercostal aid inspiration but the diaphragm is the major muscle.

3. **(A)** The integument is comprised of skin, hair, nails and associated structures such as sweat and sebaceous glands.

4. **(B)** Oxytocin and antidiuretic hormone (ADH) are both products of the posterior pituitary. Oxytocin acts on uterine smooth muscle and mammary tissue whereas ADH acts within the kidneys to promote water reabsorption. ADH is also a vasoconstriction and these two actions combine to elevate blood pressure.

5. **(B)** Homeostasis, the tendency to maintain a constant internal environment, most commonly depends upon negative feedback processes which tend to counter the effects of change. Positive feedback mechanisms enhance the effects of change and they generally do not have a beneficial effect on homeostasis.

6. **(D)** Central chemoreceptors respond to changes in CO_2, which is the most important factor in the control of minute-to-minute respiration.

7. **(C)** Sagittal planes divide the body into left and right parts. Frontal (coronal) planes vertically divide the body into anterior and posterior segments. A transverse section divides the body into superior and inferior parts.

8. **(C)** Cardiac output, the volume of blood pumped by the heart per minute, is equal to the product of stroke volume (L./beat) and heart rate (beats/minute).

9. **(B)** Diffusion is the process by which solutes move from an area of high concentration to an area of low concentration. Osmosis is the movement of water down a concentration gradient. Movement of solute against a concentration gradient requires active transport processes and energy.

10. **(D)** Blood exits the right ventricle through the pulmonary semilunar (pulmonic) valve and enters the pulmonary arteries which lead to the lungs. Atrioventricular valves (bicuspid and tricuspid) are situated between atria and ventricles. Pulmonary veins come from the lungs back to the heart.

11. **(B)** While both norepinephrine and epinephrine act at Alpha and Beta-1 receptors, epinephrine is the primary agonist at the Beta-2 sites where it leads to pronounced bronchodilation. Acetylcholine and nicotine are not catechol amines.

12. **(B)** The resting membrane is relative impermeable to sodium which is in a high concentration in the extracellular space relative to the intracellular space. An action potential results from the opening of sodium channels, allowing sodium to diffuse into the intracellular space and making that region positive relative to the outside of the cell.

13. **(D)** During swallowing, the epiglottis covers the trachea to prevent ingested material from entering the respiratory tract.

14. **(B)** The amount of dissolved oxygen in blood is minimal compared to the amount carried as oxyhemoglobin. Carbon dioxide and bicarbonate are not physiologic oxygen transporters.

15. **(A)** Pyramidal tract fibers are motor in function and originate in the primary motor cortex, which is directly anterior to the central sulcus, the precentral gyrus. The postcentral gyrus is part of the somatosensory system.

16. **(C)** Epinephrine and norepinephrine are catechol amine transmitters in the autonomic and central nervous systems. Acetylcholinesterase is the enzyme which metabolizes acetylcholine at autonomic and neuromuscular sites.

17. **(B)** Arterioles are located between arteries and capillaries. Dilation or constriction of arterioles regulates the flow of blood into capillary beds and provides adjustment of arterial blood pressure.

18. **(C)** Exocytosis moves substances from the intracellular space into extracellular fluid. Endocytosis is a mechanism for moving large particles into cells. Phagocytosis is a type of endocytosis by which solid particles are engulfed. Pinocytosis is endocytosis of fluids.

19. **(B)** Dermatomes are body regions innervated by individual dorsal roots and can be related to segmental spinal levels. Receptive fields, sensory units, and motor units related to innervation are characteristics of individual neurons rather than nerve trunks.

20. **(D)** Epithelial tissue is characterized by cell shape (squamous, cuboidal, columnar) and cell layering (simple or compound).

21. **(D)** Cartilage forms the skeleton of the embryo and is subsequently converted to bone. Cartilage also forms the nasal septum and the rings of the trachea. Its flexibility makes it an appropriate material to join the ribs to the sternum.

22. **(A)** Keratin is a protein that waterproofs and adds structural strength to skin. It is formed in the deepest layer of the epidermis and migrates to the surface with time. Melanin, carotene, and hemoglobin are pigments in the skin.

23. **(D)** Sharp "pricking" pain information is carried over the slowly conducting, small, myelinated A delta fibers, while burning and aching pain information is transmitted over the even more slowly conducted unmyelinated C fibers. A alpha fibers, with their high conduction velocity, are involved in other areas such as proprioception.

24. **(D)** Activation of the parasympathetic division will lead directly to a slowing of the heart through activity of the vagus nerve. Vasoconstriction, increased heart rate and cardiac output, and inhibition of digestion are within the domain of the sympathetic division.

25. **(D)** Muscle spindles respond to moderate muscle stretch. The Gogli tendon organ is the receptor for the inverse stretch reflex, free nerve endings are involved in pain reception and hair cells are receptors within the auditory and vestibular systems.

26. **(A)** Although the glomerulus is more permeable than most membranes, it still restricts the passage of proteins, blood cells, and other large particles. Damage to the glomerulus can produce filtration disorders such as glomerulonephritis and substances such as blood and protein may appear in the urine.

27. **(B)** Some CO_2 is carried in a dissolved form obeying Henry's Law, and some is carried by hemoglobin. Most CO_2, however, is carried as bicarbonate.

28. **(B)** Tubular reabsorption is the process by which the kidneys return water and solutes, including glucose, vitamins, and amino acids, to blood. Filtration and secretion involve movement of substances from blood into urine. Glucose is not reabsorbed from the collecting duct.

29. **(D)** Periosteum covers the outer surface of long bones. It contains osteoblasts, cells which form new bone cells. Endosteum lines the hollow inner surface of a long bone. Osteoclasts break down bone cells.

30. **(C)** Activity in the sinoatrial node is responsible for initiating the cardiac cycle, beginning with atrial depolarization and contraction. In a resting subject, the contribution of atrial contraction to ventricular filling is relatively minimal. The AV node is below the atria.

31. **(B)** The first heart sound ("lub") is the atrioventricular valves (tricuspid and bicuspid) closing in response to the ventricles contracting and increasing intraventricular pressure.

32. **(C)** Visual processing occurs within the occipital lobe of the cerebral cortex which is protected by the occipital bone. Frontal bone covers frontal cortex, involved in, among other things, behavioral and motor events. Parietal bone covers parietal cortex, involved in sensory integration processes and temporal bone protects the temporal lobe, involved in audition.

33. **(A)** Veins have large lumens and thin, distensible walls; they contain up to 65% of the body's total blood supply at any time.

34. **(B)** The patella is a sesamoid bone, a special type of short bone.

35. **(A)** The automaticity of the heart is normally a function of the sinoatrial (SA) node which leads to atrial depolarization. The atrioventricular (AV) node may become a pacemaker under certain pathological conditions.

36. **(A)** Arteries are under the greatest pressure due to the force from the contraction of the heart and the elastic properties of arterial walls.

37. **(D)** 99% of the water filtered at the glomerulus is returned by osmosis, most of which occurs within the proximal convoluted tubule.

38. **(B)** Small, uncharged lipid soluble molecules cross biological membranes more readily than other species. Water-soluble molecules cross if they are sufficiently small.

39. **(A)** The sympathetic division of the autonomic nervous system is involved in dealing with emergencies and stress. Parasympathetic (craniosacral) activity is primarily involved with energy conservation and "vegetative" functions.

40. **(B)** The sympathetic division of the autonomic nervous system is anatomically the thoricolumbar division because of its spinal levels of origin. The parasympathetic division is, anatomically, the craniosacral division.

41. **(C)** Cellular respiration, the utilization of oxygen and glucose, occurs within mitochondria. Rough endoplasmic reticulum is involved in protein synthesis and smooth endoplasmic reticulum is involved in synthesis of lipid materials. Golgi apparatus are involved in intracellular packaging and delivery.

42. **(B)** Flexion decreases the angle of a joint, bringing the two bones closer together. Extension increases the angle of a joint, moving the bones farther apart. Retraction and rotation are not joint "bending" in nature.

43. **(A)** Mitosis leading to the formation of new epidermal cells occurs within the stratum germinativum basale, the deepest layer of the epidermis which has the advantage of being near the blood supply of the underlying dermis.

44. **(C)** Compared to males, females have a larger percentage of fat (and a lower content of water) which is deposited within the subcutaneous layer under the influence of estrogen.

45. **(A)** Mucosal membranes line structures such as components of the digestive, respiratory, and reproductive tracts, which access the outside world. Serous membranes line cavities that do not access the external environment, such as the pleural cavities. Synovial membranes line joint cavities and cutaneous membranes comprise the skin.

46. **(B)** The epidermis does not contain blood vessels and depends upon the vascular supply of the underlying dermis for its needs.

47. **(B)** Smooth muscle is found within visceral structures (i.e., digestive, reproductive), does not have a striated histological appearance, and is generally under autonomic (involuntary) control. Skeletal muscle is striated and voluntary. Cardiac muscle is striated but involuntary. Postural muscles are skeletal muscles.

48. **(B)** Although carried by the circulatory system and influenced by the endocrine systems, blood cell formation is largely a function of spongy bone within the skeletal system.

49. **(B)** Parathyroid hormone elevates serum calcium levels by initiating mobilization of calcium from the digestive system. Calcitonin lowers blood calcium and leads to deposition of calcium within bone.

50. **(A)** Eccrine sweat glands of the face, palms and soles are active in children. Apocrine sweat glands become active at puberty. Sebaceous glands produce sebum and are not found on the soles or palms. Ceruminous glands are found within the external auditory meatus.

51. **(B)** The biceps brachii is a flexor of the elbow and the triceps femoris is a flexor of the knee.

52. **(A)** Apocrine sweat glands become active at puberty under the influence of sex hormones. Eccrine, sebaceous, and ceruminous glands are active in children.

53. **(B)** Calcitonin is responsible for lowering an elevated serum calcium, partially by depositing the excess mineral in bone. Parathormone will elevate serum calcium levels.

54. **(B)** Although hormones are produced by endocrine glands, their delivery to target organs is primarily via the cardiovascular system.

55. **(D)** Myelin, an "insulating" substance, is responsible for saltatory conduction in which the impulse "skips" from one Node of Ranvier to the next and is rapidly conducted to the end of the cell. The larger the diameter of an axon, the less resistance present and the faster the axon can conduct. Myelinated, large diameter axons comprise the axons with the fastest conduction velocities.

56. **(B)** The nephron is the basic functional unit of kidneys. Nephrons include Bowman's capsule, the proximal convoluted tubule, the loop of Henle, the distal convoluted tubule and the collecting duct. The glomerulus is part of the circulatory system, the ureters convey urine from the kidneys to the bladder and the urethra carries urine out from the bladder.

57. **(B)** The esophagus enters the stomach below the fundus at the cardiac region, which contains the cardiac sphincter. The body of the stomach is below and the pyloric region marks the most distal portion of the stomach adjacent to the duodenum of the small intestine.

58. **(C)** Oxytocin, produced by the hypothalamus and released by the posterior pituitary, causes contraction of uterine smooth muscle and plays a role in labor and delivery. ADH is also released by the posterior pituitary, but its role is in water conservation within the kidneys.

59. **(B)** ADH, antidiuretic hormone, when released from the posterior pituitary, causes an increased permeability of the collecting duct of the kidneys to water and leads to water reabsorption and conservation. Inhibition of ADH release, produced for example by the ingestion of alcohol, leads to an increase in urine output.

60. **(D)** FSH begins the maturation process of follicles but it is the elevation of LH levels that leads to the release of mature egg cells (ovulation). ADH and prolactin do not participate in the process.

61. **(B)** The cardiac sphincter is located at the junction of the esophagus and the stomach and is responsible for preventing gastric reflux. The pyloric sphincter is at the junction of the stomach and the small intestine, the ileocecal valve is at the junction of the small and large intestines and the epiglottis prevents solids and liquids from entering the trachea.

62. **(C)** Bile, produced in the liver and released from the gall bladder, is involved in fat metabolism in the small intestine. Lipase is also involved in fat metabolism but it is from the pancreas.

63. **(B)** Although some digestion takes place within all of the structures listed, the majority of digestive processes take place within the duodenum.

64. **(C)** Visual receptors, rods and cones, are located at the back of the eye on the retina. The lens and cornea are involved in transmission of light rays from the environment on to the retina; the optic tract is part of the optic neural pathway.

65. **(C)** Food absorption takes place primarily within the ileum and jejunum. Functions of the stomach and duodenum are primarily digestive, while the colon is principally involved in water reabsorption, some digestion, and vitamin synthesis.

66. **(C)** The medulla begins at, and is indistinguishable from, the rostral end of the spinal cord, forming the lowest portion of the brain stem which also includes the pons and the mid-brain both superior. The thalamus, part of the diencephalon, is yet further rostral.

67. **(B)** Although stored and delivered by the gall bladder, bile is manufactured within the liver. The duodenum is the major site of digestion where it receives digestive materials from the pancreas.

68. **(B)** Thyroid hormone contributes to growth and maturation of the nervous system and a hypothyroid infant will show both physical and mental deficits which are not seen in the adult since skeletal and brain development have been completed.

69. **(C)** Rods (which provide vision in black and white) and cones (providing color vision) are located on the retina at the back of the eye. Hair cells are receptors within the auditory and vestibular systems.

70. **(A)** Lining the inside of the digestive system is the epithelial mucosal layer which provides an appropriate setting for absorption of materials into the submucosal layer containing blood vessels, lymphatics and nerves. Serosal membranes surround the digestive tract to form a protective layer.

71. **(B)** The pancreas is classed as an endocrine gland because of its production of insulin and glucagon which are secreted directly into blood. As an exocrine gland, the pancreas produces a series of enzymes contained in pancreatic juice which is carried by the pancreatic duct.

72. **(C)** Lacrimation is the activity of the lacrimal glands, which produce lacrimal fluid or tears.

73. **(A)** Olfaction, the sense of smell, is the domain of the first cranial nerve, the olfactory nerve. Nerves II, III and IV are involved in the sensory and motor functions of the head and face but not the sense of smell.

74. **(D)** Immediately distal to the neck of the bladder is the prostate gland. Its enlargement, common in males beginning at about the age of 40, interferes with urine outflow. Benign hyperplasia prostate (BHP) is a non-malignant enlargement of the gland which is also a common site for cancer in males. Although located in the same general area, the seminal vesicles and bulbourethral (Cowper's) glands do not normally hypertrophy with aging.

75. **(B)** Linear (vertical and horizontal) acceleration is sensed by receptors within the utricles and saccules; the semicircular canals contain receptors activated by rotational movement. Receptors within the cochlea detect sound and the middle ear does not contain auditory or vestibular receptor devices.

76. **(B)** Although the globulins and fibrin are blood proteins, albumin is the protein in the highest plasma concentration.

77. **(A)** Union of sperm and egg normally occurs within the fallopian (uterine) tubes prior to implantation within the uterus. Implantation at non-uterine sites is termed an ectopic pregnancy.

78. **(B)** Depression may result from low levels of serotonin or decreased responsiveness of sertotonergic receptors in the brain and this is the basis for the use of serotonin reuptake inhibitors in the treatment of clinical depression. High levels of catechol amines may contribute to clinical anxiety.

79. **(B)** Lymphatic vessels begin as lymphatic capillaries, blind pouches found in peripheral tissue. Lymph nodes are more proximal structures and lymphocytes are forms of white blood cells.

80. **(A)** HCG rises to detectable levels following egg fertilization and its presence in blood and urine forms the basis of pregnancy testing. The function of HCG is to maintain the corpus luteum which is responsible for maintaining estrogen and progesterone levels, and their effects on the endometrium, during early and middle pregnancy.

81. **(C)** Sweet, sour, and salty taste sensations result from activity in the facial nerve, the seventh cranial nerve. The first cranial nerve is involved in olfaction, the fifth in motor and sensory mechanisms of the head and face. Nerve *x*, the vagus, is not involved in taste from the tongue.

82. **(B)** The parasympathetic division of the autonomic nervous system is primarily involved with energy production and conservation. Its outward effects can be remembered by the acronym, SLUD, salivation, lacrimation, urination, and defecation.

83. **(A)** After their formation within the seminiferous tubules, sperm are stored within the epididymis lying along side the testes. The epididymis leads to the vas deferens, which ultimately empties into the urethra, which receives material from the seminal vesicles.

84. **(B)** Glucagon elevates blood glucose by (1) promoting the breakdown of glycogen to glucose (glycogenolysis), (2) promoting glucose synthesis (gluconeogenesis), and (3) promoting the release of glucose from liver.

85. **(B)** Erythrocytes (red blood cells) are much more numerous than white cells in blood. Globulins and albumin are proteins, not formed elements.

86. **(A)** Although not as powerful as pH regulating mechanisms in the respiratory or renal systems, buffer systems essentially act at the rate of chemical reactions. The liver is not involved in the normal control of blood pH.

87. **(B)** Arterial blood pH is critically maintained between 7.35 and 7.45. Either a decline of pH (acidosis) to a level of 7.0 or an increase in pH (alkalosis) to 8.0 is potentially fatal.

88. **(B)** While the hematocrit reveals the level of plasma, it is intended to evaluate the percentage of erythrocytes (red blood cells) in whole blood and subsequently the oxygen carrying capacity of blood. Normal hematocrit values for females are 37–47%, for males 42–54%. Platelet and white cell enumerations are also useful diagnostics but do not involve the hematocrit.

89. **(A)** Although about 5 liters of blood are pumped through the heart per minute, the myocardial muscle is dependent upon the coronary arteries for delivery of oxygen.

90. **(B)** The term hair cell is applied to receptors within the auditory and vestibular systems. Rods and cones are visual receptors and muscle spindles are the receptors for stretch reflexes.

91. **(A)** Blood typing is based on determining the antigen(s) located on the surfaces of erythrocytes; the "opposite" antibody is located within the individual's plasma. A type A patient therefore has the A antigen and the anti-B antibody. Rh antigens are also located on erythrocyte surfaces leading to an individual being typed as Rh positive (antibody present) or Rh negative (no Rh antigen).

92. **(D)** Sickle cell anemia develops when hemoglobin forms long crystalline chains within erythrocytes, forcing the cells into their bizarre shapes. Pernicious anemia refers to abnormal destruction of red blood cells; iron-deficiency and aplastic anemias involve abnormal blood cell formation.

93. **(D)** Hair cells are the auditory receptors which are located within the cochlea, part of the inner ear. Auditory ossicles are small bones involved in conduction of vibration through the middle ear.

94. **(D)** Female menopause follows aging of the ovaries and is characterized by low estrogen levels which, in turn, result in high levels of GnRH, FSH, and LH, the latter two of which appear to be correlated with the "hot flashes" of menopause.

95. **(B)** Hyperventilation can lead to a decreased arterial CO_2 level, which may result in alkalosis of respiratory origin. Extreme alkalosis may lead to convulsions and may produce seizure activity in epileptic patients.

96. **(C)** Plasma is approximately 90% water with the rest being comprised of numerous solutes including proteins, nutrients, gases, hormones, ions, and products of cell activity.

97. **(B)** Estrogen is involved in a feedback loop to the hypothalamus such that high levels of estrogen inhibit the release of GnRH which reduces levels of LH and prevents ovulation.

98. **(D)** Heparin is an endogenous anticoagulant produced by basophils. Fibrin, calcium and thrombin are all promoters of the coagulation process.

99. **(B)** GnRH from the hypothalamus controls the release of FSH and LH from the anterior pituitary. FSH initiates follicle development and LH leads directly to ovulation, the release of a mature egg.

100. **(D)** Testosterone is produced by interstitial (Leydig) cells under the influence of ICSH, interstitial cell stimulating hormone. The epididymis and prostate gland are not involved in testosterone synthesis.

UNIT VIII: PHYSICAL SCIENCES AND CHEMISTRY

PHYSICAL SCIENCES AND CHEMISTRY TESTS ANSWER SHEET

TEST 1: PHYSICAL SCIENCES

1. Ⓐ Ⓑ Ⓒ Ⓓ	8. Ⓐ Ⓑ Ⓒ Ⓓ	15. Ⓐ Ⓑ Ⓒ Ⓓ
2. Ⓐ Ⓑ Ⓒ Ⓓ	9. Ⓐ Ⓑ Ⓒ Ⓓ	16. Ⓐ Ⓑ Ⓒ Ⓓ
3. Ⓐ Ⓑ Ⓒ Ⓓ	10. Ⓐ Ⓑ Ⓒ Ⓓ	17. Ⓐ Ⓑ Ⓒ Ⓓ
4. Ⓐ Ⓑ Ⓒ Ⓓ	11. Ⓐ Ⓑ Ⓒ Ⓓ	18. Ⓐ Ⓑ Ⓒ Ⓓ
5. Ⓐ Ⓑ Ⓒ Ⓓ	12. Ⓐ Ⓑ Ⓒ Ⓓ	19. Ⓐ Ⓑ Ⓒ Ⓓ
6. Ⓐ Ⓑ Ⓒ Ⓓ	13. Ⓐ Ⓑ Ⓒ Ⓓ	20. Ⓐ Ⓑ Ⓒ Ⓓ
7. Ⓐ Ⓑ Ⓒ Ⓓ	14. Ⓐ Ⓑ Ⓒ Ⓓ	21. Ⓐ Ⓑ Ⓒ Ⓓ

TEST 2: CHEMISTRY

1. Ⓐ Ⓑ Ⓒ Ⓓ	14. Ⓐ Ⓑ Ⓒ Ⓓ	27. Ⓐ Ⓑ Ⓒ Ⓓ	40. Ⓐ Ⓑ Ⓒ Ⓓ
2. Ⓐ Ⓑ Ⓒ Ⓓ	15. Ⓐ Ⓑ Ⓒ Ⓓ	28. Ⓐ Ⓑ Ⓒ Ⓓ	41. Ⓐ Ⓑ Ⓒ Ⓓ
3. Ⓐ Ⓑ Ⓒ Ⓓ	16. Ⓐ Ⓑ Ⓒ Ⓓ	29. Ⓐ Ⓑ Ⓒ Ⓓ	42. Ⓐ Ⓑ Ⓒ Ⓓ
4. Ⓐ Ⓑ Ⓒ Ⓓ	17. Ⓐ Ⓑ Ⓒ Ⓓ	30. Ⓐ Ⓑ Ⓒ Ⓓ	43. Ⓐ Ⓑ Ⓒ Ⓓ
5. Ⓐ Ⓑ Ⓒ Ⓓ	18. Ⓐ Ⓑ Ⓒ Ⓓ	31. Ⓐ Ⓑ Ⓒ Ⓓ	44. Ⓐ Ⓑ Ⓒ Ⓓ
6. Ⓐ Ⓑ Ⓒ Ⓓ	19. Ⓐ Ⓑ Ⓒ Ⓓ	32. Ⓐ Ⓑ Ⓒ Ⓓ	45. Ⓐ Ⓑ Ⓒ Ⓓ
7. Ⓐ Ⓑ Ⓒ Ⓓ	20. Ⓐ Ⓑ Ⓒ Ⓓ	33. Ⓐ Ⓑ Ⓒ Ⓓ	46. Ⓐ Ⓑ Ⓒ Ⓓ
8. Ⓐ Ⓑ Ⓒ Ⓓ	21. Ⓐ Ⓑ Ⓒ Ⓓ	34. Ⓐ Ⓑ Ⓒ Ⓓ	47. Ⓐ Ⓑ Ⓒ Ⓓ
9. Ⓐ Ⓑ Ⓒ Ⓓ	22. Ⓐ Ⓑ Ⓒ Ⓓ	35. Ⓐ Ⓑ Ⓒ Ⓓ	48. Ⓐ Ⓑ Ⓒ Ⓓ
10. Ⓐ Ⓑ Ⓒ Ⓓ	23. Ⓐ Ⓑ Ⓒ Ⓓ	36. Ⓐ Ⓑ Ⓒ Ⓓ	49. Ⓐ Ⓑ Ⓒ Ⓓ
11. Ⓐ Ⓑ Ⓒ Ⓓ	24. Ⓐ Ⓑ Ⓒ Ⓓ	37. Ⓐ Ⓑ Ⓒ Ⓓ	50. Ⓐ Ⓑ Ⓒ Ⓓ
12. Ⓐ Ⓑ Ⓒ Ⓓ	25. Ⓐ Ⓑ Ⓒ Ⓓ	38. Ⓐ Ⓑ Ⓒ Ⓓ	
13. Ⓐ Ⓑ Ⓒ Ⓓ	26. Ⓐ Ⓑ Ⓒ Ⓓ	39. Ⓐ Ⓑ Ⓒ Ⓓ	

PHYSICAL SCIENCES AND CHEMISTRY TESTS

TEST 1: PHYSICAL SCIENCES

21 QUESTIONS • TIME—20 MINUTES

Directions: Read each question carefully and consider all possible answers. When you have decided which choice is best, blacken the corresponding space on your answer sheet. There is only one best answer for each question.

1. A high concentration of H^+ ions is characteristic of

   (A) high pH
   (B) strong acid
   (C) alkaline base
   (D) both A and C

2. Long chains of glucose molecules are involved in the structure of

   (A) proteins
   (B) fats
   (C) cholesterol
   (D) polysaccharides

3. When a solution has a pH of 7, it is

   (A) a strong base
   (B) a strong acid
   (C) a weak base
   (D) neutral

4. Which one of the following is not a carbohydrate?

   (A) maltose
   (B) cellulose
   (C) glycogen
   (D) cholesterol

5. An example of an organic compound is

   (A) water (H_2O)
   (B) ammonia (NH_3)
   (C) salt (NaCl)
   (D) glucose ($C_6H_{12}O_6$)

6. A covalent bond is believed to be caused by

   (A) transfer of electrons
   (B) sharing of electrons
   (C) release of energy
   (D) none of the above

7. An atom has the electron configuration (2-8-8-2). This atom would tend to

   (A) gain electrons
   (B) loose 2 electrons
   (C) be inert
   (D) none of the above

8. Which of the following is a dissaccharide?

   (A) glucose
   (B) maltose
   (C) fructose
   (D) chilin

9. Which one of the following is not a carbohydrate?

   (A) maltose
   (B) cellulose
   (C) glycogen
   (D) wax

10. The basic building blocks of proteins are

    (A) polypeptides
    (B) glucose
    (C) amino acids
    (D) none of the above

11. If the atomic number of magnesium is 12, what will be the number of protons?

    (A) 6
    (B) 10
    (C) 14
    (D) 12

12. Which is **not** an inert element?

    (A) hydrogen
    (B) neon
    (C) oxygen
    (D) nitrogen

13. Atoms are electrically neutral. This means that an atom will contain
    - (A) more protons than neutrons
    - (B) more electrons than protons
    - (C) an equal number of protons and electrons
    - (D) none of the above

14. Which is true of alkaline solutions?
    - (A) more H^+ ion than OH ion
    - (B) same amount of H^+ ion + OH^- ion
    - (C) more OH^- ion than H^+ ion
    - (D) none of the above

15. A common detergent has pH 11.0, so the detergent is
    - (A) neutral
    - (B) acidic
    - (C) alkaline
    - (D) none of these

16. The basic building block of carbohydrate is
    - (A) starch
    - (B) chitin
    - (C) sucrose
    - (D) glucose

17. The number of different amino acids in proteins is
    - (A) 20
    - (B) 26
    - (C) 50
    - (D) 92

18. A nucleotide is
    - (A) phospholipid, sugar, and base
    - (B) phosphate, sugar, and base
    - (C) phosphate, protein, and base
    - (D) phospholipid, sugar, and protein

19. Polar bonds form when
    - (A) electrons are shared unequally between atoms
    - (B) more than one pair of electrons is shared
    - (C) ions are formed
    - (D) an acid and base are combined

20. Which of the following is an example of hydrogen bonding?
    - (A) The bond between O and H in a single molecule of water.
    - (B) The bond between O of one water molecule and H of a second water molecule.
    - (C) The bond between O of one water molecule and O of a second water molecule.
    - (D) The bond between H of one water molecule and H of a second water molecule.

21. The Central Dogma of Information Transfer states that information is passed in what sequence?
    - (A) RNA to proteins to DNA
    - (B) DNA to RNA to proteins
    - (C) Proteins to RNA to DNA
    - (D) RNA to DNA to proteins

TEST 1: PHYSICAL SCIENCES ANSWER KEY

1. **B**
2. **D**
3. **D**
4. **D**
5. **D**
6. **B**
7. **B**
8. **B**
9. **D**
10. **C**
11. **D**
12. **B**
13. **C**
14. **C**
15. **C**
16. **D**
17. **A**
18. **B**
19. **A**
20. **B**
21. **B**

TEST 1: PHYSICAL SCIENCES EXPLANATORY ANSWERS

1. **(B)** Acidic solutions contain hydrogen (H^+) ions, while basic (or alkaline) solution contain a basic ion such as the hydroxyl ion (OH^-).

2. **(D)** Carbohydrates consist of molecules made up of C, H, and O in a ratio of 1:2:1 (e.g. glucose is $C_6H_{12}O_6$). Polysaccharides are chains of three or more simple sugars (e.g., glucose).

3. **(D)** Whether a watery solution is acidic or alkaline depends on its concentration of hydrogen ions (H^+) in relation to hydroxyl ions (OH^-). The ratio is expressed as the solution pH (the letters stand for potential of hydrogen). The pH scale ranges from O (most acidic) to 14 (most alkaline). Pure water is neutral with a pH of 7 because it has equal amounts of hydrogen and hydroxyl ions.

4. **(D)** Carbohydrates consist of molecules made up of C, H, and O in a ratio of 1:2:1, whereas cholesterol is a lipid (steroid) formed of four carbon rings.

5. **(D)** Organic molecules are molecules containing carbon; they are found in living things.

6. **(B)** Covalence is the mutual attraction between two atoms that share a pair of electrons. It is the strongest type of chemical bond.

   $H^+ = H^+ \rightarrow H_2$

7. **(B)** For many atoms, the simplest way to attain a completely filled outer energy level is either to gain or to lose one or two electrons.

8. **(B)** Dissaccharides are double sugar and are formed by linking two simple sugars. For example, glucose and fructose form sucrose, a dissaccharide (table sugar).

9. **(D)** Wax is made of glycerol and fatty acids. It is non-polar and insoluble in water. It is a lipid molecule.

10. **(C)** Proteins are made up of units called amino acids. Amino acids join together by a covalent bond and form polypeptide chains (the primary structure of proteins).

11. **(D)** The nucleus of an atom consists of protons and neutrons. A proton is a subatomic particle with positive electric charge. The number of protons in the nucleus of an atom is equal to the atomic number.

12. **(B)** The chemical activity of an atom is how it reacts with other atoms. Atoms are governed by the number of electrons in their outermost shell. Helium, neon, and other atoms with no electron vacancies in their outermost shell are inert; they tend not to enter into chemical reactions. Hydrogen, oxygen, and other atoms with electron vacancies in their outermost shell tend to interact with other atoms.

13. **(C)** Regardless of the element, atoms have just as many electrons as protons. This means that they carry no net charge, overall. A proton is always positively charged and an electron is negatively charged.

14. **(C)** Basic or alkaline solutions have fewer H^+ than OH^- ions; their pH is above 7.

15. **(C)** Alkaline solutions always have a higher pH and more OH^- ions.

16. **(D)** Glucose is a six carbon simple sugar and serves as a precursor of many complex compounds and as a building block for larger carbohydrates.

17. **(A)** The basic building block of protein is amino acid. Each amino acid is a small organic compound with an amino group, a carboxyl group (an acid), a hydrogen atom, and one or more atoms called its R group. Total amino acids are 20. Examples of amino acids are tryptophane, alanine, glycine, aspartic acid, lysine, proline, etc.

18. **(B)** The small organic compounds called nucleotides have three components, a five-carbon sugar, a phosphate group and a nitrogen-containing base. Nucleotides are the basic building blocks of DNA and RNA.

19. **(A)** In polar covalent bonds, atoms of different elements (which have different number of protons) do not exert the same pull in shared electrons. The more attractive atom ends up with a slight negative charge; the atom is "electronegative." Its effect is balanced out by the other atoms resulting in a slight positive charge. In simple words, a polar covalent bond has no net charge—but the charge is distributed unevenly between the bonds two ends.

20. **(B)** In a hydrogen bond, a small, highly electronegative atom of a molecule interacts weakly with a hydrogen atom that is already participating in a polar covalent bond.

21. **(B)** Genetic information is encoded in the particular order of nucleotides bases which follow one another in DNA. RNA molecules function in the processes by which the genetic information in DNA is used to build proteins.

TEST 2: CHEMISTRY

50 QUESTIONS • TIME—45 MINUTES

Directions: Read each question carefully and consider all possible answers. When you have decided which choice is best, blacken the corresponding space on your answer sheet. There is only one best answer for each question. You may use the periodic table on page 201 if needed.

1. The compound that has the greatest polarity is

   (A) CH_3-CH_2-O-CH_2-CH_3
   (B) CH_3-$CH_2CH_2CH_2$-CH_3
   (C) CH_3-CH_2-CH_2-CH_2-CH_2-Cl
   (D) CH_3-CH_2-CH_2-CH_2-CH_2-OH

2. The formula that represents the strongest acid in the following group is

   (A) HCl
   (B) HCN
   (C) HNO_3
   (D) HCOOH

3. The sugar with the highest molecular weight of those listed is

   (A) fructose
   (B) sucrose
   (C) glucose
   (D) none of the above; all have the same molecular weight

4. A hydride ion and a hydrogen atom both have

   (A) the same number of electrons
   (B) the same charge
   (C) the same number of protons
   (D) equal atomic radii

5. The general formula for an aldehyde is

   (A) RCOOH
   (B) RCOOR
   (C) ROH
   (D) RCHO

6. The compound which will not be acidic when dissolved in water is

   (A) HBr
   (B) N_2O_5
   (C) CaO
   (D) NH_4Cl

7. Atoms that have the same atomic number but different atomic masses

   (A) are from different elements
   (B) are isobars
   (C) have different numbers of electrons
   (D) are isotopes

8. When electrolysis is done with molten NaCl, the substance produced at the anode is

   (A) chlorine
   (B) hydrogen
   (C) sodium
   (D) oxygen

9. The non-electrolyte in the following group is

   (A) acetic acid
   (B) calcium chloride
   (C) sodium bromide
   (D) sugar

10. Rubbing alcohol is

    (A) methyl alcohol
    (B) ethyl alcohol
    (C) phenol
    (D) isopropyl alcohol

11. Which of the following elements is a transition element?

    (A) argon
    (B) copper
    (C) barium
    (D) aluminum

12. When calcium reacts with chlorine to form calcium chloride it

    (A) shares two electrons
    (B) gains two electrons
    (C) loses two electrons
    (D) gains one electron

13. The compound NaClO is called
    (A) sodium perchlorate
    (B) sodium oxychloride
    (C) sodium chlorate
    (D) sodium hypochlorite

14. Reaction kinetics deals with
    (A) equilibrium position
    (B) reaction rates
    (C) molecular reactant size
    (D) none of the above

15. A 1 molar solution of K_3PO_4, potassium phosphate, contains in 1 liter
    (A) one mole of potassium ions
    (B) one mole of oxygen atoms
    (C) one mole of phosphorus atoms
    (D) no ions

16. In the compound propene, $H_2C = CH - CH_3$, the single bond between two carbon atoms is
    (A) stronger than the double bond
    (B) shorter than the double bond
    (C) equal to the double bond in bond strength
    (D) longer than the double bond

17. Of the following groups the least reactive are
    (A) halogen
    (B) the inert gases
    (C) group IIA metals
    (D) precious metals of group IB

18. Per liter, compared to a 3 molar aqueous solution, a 3 molar aqueous solution contains
    (A) the same amount of solute
    (B) more solute
    (C) less solute
    (D) a variable amount of solute

19. For a molecular substance a gram formula weight
    (A) is unrelated to the gram molecular weight
    (B) is always equal to the mass corresponding to its empirical formula
    (C) can always be calculated from its empirical formula alone
    (D) is identical to its gram molecular weight

20. If gas A has a molecular weight four times that of gas B
    (A) the average speed of gas A is about 4 times that of gas B
    (B) the average speed of gas B is about 4 times that of gas A
    (C) the average speed of gas A is about twice that of gas B
    (D) the average speed of gas B is about twice that of gas A

21. Ice can be melted most effectively by the following compound if 1 mole is used.
    (A) sucrose
    (B) calcium chloride
    (C) sodium chloride
    (D) methanol

22. Per atom, an element having an atomic number of 19 contains
    (A) 19 electrons and 19 neutrons
    (B) 19 electrons and 19 protons
    (C) 19 protons and 19 neutrons
    (D) a total of 19 protons and neutrons

23. In a volume of air at one atmosphere pressure at sea level, the partial pressure of nitrogen will be about
    (A) 490 mm of mercury
    (B) 760 mm of mercury
    (C) 106 mm of mercury
    (D) 608 mm of mercury

24. If the stirring of a solution results in precipitation of solute with no change in temperature, the solution must have been
    (A) saturated
    (B) concentrated
    (C) dilute
    (D) supersaturated

25. If the reaction : $A + B \rightarrow C + D$ is designated as first order, the rate depends on
    (A) the concentration of only one reactant
    (B) the concentration of each reactant
    (C) no specific concentration
    (D) the temperature only

26. The loss of an alpha particle from the radioactive atom $^{228}_{88}Ra$ would leave

(A) $^{224}_{86}Rn$
(B) $^{222}_{86}Rn$
(C) $^{224}_{88}Ra$
(D) $^{230}_{90}Th$

27. Which of the following is not a form of radioactive decay?

(A) electron capture
(B) beta emission
(C) alpha emission
(D) proton emission

28. The greatest amount of energy would be produced by the burning of one gram of

(A) fat
(B) carbohydrate
(C) protein
(D) ribonucleic acid

29. For the reaction: $H_2(g) + Br_2(g) \rightarrow 2HBr(g)$, the reaction can be driven to the left by

(A) increasing the pressure
(B) increasing the hydrogen
(C) increasing hydrogen bromide
(D) decreasing hydrogen bromide

30. Carbon-14 has a half life of 5.73 × 10 years. If a sample contained 1 gram of C-14, the time required to decay to only 0.0625 g would be

(A) 11.46 × 10 years
(B) 5.73 × 10 years
(C) 22.92 × 10 years
(D) none of these

31. The oxidation number of Mn in the compound K_2MnO_4 is

(A) +7
(B) +2
(C) 0
(D) +6

32. The element with the highest ionization energy of those below is

(A) Mg
(B) Sr
(C) Ca
(D) Ba

33. The least electronegative of the following elements is

(A) Cl
(B) F
(C) Br
(D) I

34. The element with the smallest atomic radius of the following is

(A) Sr
(B) Mg
(C) Ba
(D) Ra

35. Which of the following salts would be more soluble in 1.0M acid than in pure water?

(A) KCl
(B) $CaCO_3$
(C) $CaCl_2$
(D) KNO_3

36. Which of the following is not an acid/conjugate base pair?

(A) HCN/CN
(B) H_2CO_3/OH^-
(C) H_2SO_4/HSO_4^-
(D) $H_3PO_4/H_2PO_4^-$

37. In a titration of 40.0 ml of 0.20 M NaOH with 0.4 M HCl, what will be the final volume of the solution when the sodium hydroxide is completely neutralized?

(A) 42 ml
(B) 20 ml
(C) 60 ml
(D) 80 ml

38. When dissolved in water to form 0.2 M solutions, which of the following would have the highest pH?

(A) the salt of a strong acid
(B) a weak acid
(C) the ammonium salt of a strong acid
(D) the sodium salt of a weak acid

39. Consider the reaction $N_2(g) + 3H_2(g) \rightarrow 2NH_3(g)$ + heat. Indicate the incorrect statement

    (A) An increase in temperature will shift the equilibrium to the right.
    (B) An increase in pressure applied will shift the equilibrium to the right.
    (C) The addition of ammonia will shift the equilibrium to the left.
    (D) The addition of H_2 will shift the equilibrium to the right.

40. All of the following are colligative properties of solutions except

    (A) vapor pressure
    (B) osmotic pressure
    (C) density
    (D) boiling point elevation

41. What statement is incorrect?

    (A) London dispersion forces are among those binding the units of molecular solids.
    (B) Molten ionic compounds are conductors of electricity.
    (C) Molecular solids have high melting points.
    (D) Molecular solids are non-conductors.

42. Which of the following groups contain no ionic compounds?

    (A) HCN, NO, $Ca(NO_3)_2$
    (B) KOH, CCL_4, SF_6
    (C) NaH, CaF_2, $NaNH_2$
    (D) CH_2O, H_2S, NH_3

43. In a cubic lattice, an atom lying at the corner of a unit cell is shared by how many unit cells?

    (A) 2
    (B) 4
    (C) 8
    (D) 12

44. On the basis of the following boiling point data, which of the following liquids would be expected to have the highest vapor pressure at room temperature?

SUBSTANCE	BOILING POINT
(A) acetone	56.2°C
(B) ethanol	78.5°C
(C) water	100°C
(D) ethylene glycol	198°C

45. $^{34}_{17}$Cl has

    (A) 17 protons, 17 electrons, 17 neutrons
    (B) 17 protons, 19 electrons, 17 neutrons
    (C) 17 protons, 18 electrons, 17 neutrons
    (D) 34 protons, 34 electrons, 17 neutrons

46. Which of the following arrangements gives the correct trend of electronegativitism?

    (A) I < Br < Cl < F
    (B) Sr < Ca < Ra < Mg
    (C) Al > Si > P > S
    (D) Na < K < Li < H

47. The number of unpaired electrons in the outer subshell of a phosphorus atom (atomic number: 15) is

    (A) 2
    (B) 0
    (C) 3
    (D) 1

48. An atom which has five 3 p electrons in its ground state is

    (A) Si
    (B) P
    (C) Cl
    (D) O

49. How many valence electrons are needed to complete the outer valence shell of sulfur?

    (A) 1
    (B) 2
    (C) 3
    (D) 4

50. Consider three 1-liter flasks at STP. Flask A contains NO gas; Flask B contains NH_3 gas; and Flask C contains N_2 gas. Which flask contains the greatest number of atoms?

    (A) Flask A
    (B) Flask B
    (C) Flask C
    (D) all contain the same number of atoms

TEST 2: CHEMISTRY ANSWER KEY

1. **D**	14. **B**	27. **D**	40. **C**
2. **A**	15. **C**	28. **A**	41. **C**
3. **B**	16. **D**	29. **C**	42. **D**
4. **C**	17. **B**	30. **C**	43. **C**
5. **D**	18. **C**	31. **D**	44. **A**
6. **C**	19. **D**	32. **A**	45. **A**
7. **D**	20. **D**	33. **D**	46. **A**
8. **A**	21. **B**	34. **B**	47. **D**
9. **D**	22. **B**	35. **B**	48. **C**
10. **D**	23. **D**	36. **B**	49. **B**
11. **B**	24. **D**	37. **B**	50. **B**
12. **C**	25. **A**	38. **D**	
13. **D**	26. **A**	39. **A**	

TEST 2: CHEMISTRY EXPLANATORY ANSWERS

1. **(D)** Polarity is determined by differences in electronegativities between atoms involved in a bond. The difference in electronegativities between hydrogen and oxygen on a scale devised by Linus Pauling is 1.4 and between carbon and oxygen is 1.0. Carbon and hydrogen differ by only 0.4 and consequently form non-polar bonds.

2. **(A)** Hydrochloric acid has the weakest conjugate base (Cl^-) and therefore dissociates most thoroughly (virtually completely in water) and yields hydrogen ions in high concentration. The other compounds shown dissociate less completely because of their stronger conjugate bases.

3. **(B)** Sucrose is a disaccharide having nearly twice the molar mass of the other two sugars, which are monosaccharides.

4. **(C)** A hydrogen atom must accept an electron in order to form a hydride ion. No other changes occur. The hydride therefore has a single negative charge whereas the hydrogen atom is neutral. An extra negative charge with no change in positive charge expands the radius.

5. **(D)** The functional group contains carbonyl plus a hydrogen linked to the carbon (-C-H). The other connection of the carbonyl group is to another carbon atom. The groups COOH, -OH, and -COOR are found in carboxylic acids, alcohols and esters, respectively.

6. **(C)** Calcium oxide is the only compound in the four which is a metal oxide. Metal oxides form hydroxides (Bases) when dissolved in water, but non-metal oxides form acids.

7. **(D)** The statement given is the definition of isotope, a form of atom of an element which differs from other atoms of the same element by the number of neutrons.

8. **(A)** Oxidation, the loss of electrons, occurs at the anode. Molten sodium chloride has only sodium (Na+) and chloride (Cl-) ions, the latter of which each have a single electron to donate to achieve neutrality. Loss of one electron each yields chlorine atoms, which stabilize by forming diatomic molecules of chlorine gas.

9. **(D)** Sugar alone is the only molecular compound of this group. The others readily dissociate as ions in polar solvents such as water.

10. **(D)** Isopropyl alcohol has a low enough molecular weight to make it volatile and thus capable of giving a noticeable cooling effect during evaporation. It is unsuitable for internal consumption, but relatively inexpensive. There are disadvantages for the use of any of the others as rubbing alcohol. Methyl alcohol is toxic. Phenol causes skin burns, and ethyl alcohol is too valuable for internal consumption and other commercial purposes.

11. **(B)** Argon, barium, and aluminum are in groups VIIIA, IIA, and IIIA respectively. Copper is the only element which is in the transition area of the periodic table (group IB).

12. **(C)** Calcium and the other metals of the group IIA ionize by losing two electrons. It achieves the stable electron structure of argon with eight electrons in the outer shell.

13. **(D)** In the series for the oxyhalogen ions (e.g. ClO_4^-, ClO_3^-, ClO^-) the one with the least amount of oxygen is designated hypochlorite.

14. **(B)** Chemical kinetics is the study of reaction rates and how these change with variation of conditions as well as the various molecular events which transpire during the overall reaction.

15. **(C)** There is one phosphorus in the formula but there are three potassiums and four oxygens. The number of atoms or ions present per formula unit equals the corresponding number of moles of each type in one molecule of the compound (The amount present in a liter of a 1 molar solution). In solution potassium phosphate would separate as potassium ions and phosphate ions.

16. **(D)** Single bonds between carbon atoms are longer but weaker than double bonds between carbon atoms.

17. **(B)** The rare gases have stable electronic structures with eight outer "valence" electrons (2 S and 6 P), and therefore have no compulsion to seek means of donating, accepting or sharing electrons. The halogens need an electron to achieve stability, whereas group IIA need to donate two electrons to form stable ions with eight electrons on the outermost shell. Group IB metals react but show a high resistance to oxidation.

18. **(C)** A molar solution contains one mole of solute per liter of solution. Therefore, one mole of solute is combined with less than one kilogram (one liter) of water. In a one molal solution which contains one mole of solute per kilogram of water the total volume for a solution of one mole exceeds one liter. Therefore one liter of a one molal solution contains less than one mole.

19. **(D)** For a molecular compound the gram formula weight is the same as the gram molecular weight. The empirical formula represents the smallest ratio of the different atoms possible in the compound. The molecular formula may be a multiple of the empirical formulas (e.g., twice).

20. **(D)** The ratio of the rates of effusion of two gases (proportional to the speeds of the gas molecules) is inversely proportional to the square roots of their molecular weights; consequently, rate of effusion of A/rate of effusion of B = $\sqrt{\frac{1}{4}} = \frac{1}{2}$.

21. **(B)** The greater the concentration of soluble particles, the greater the lowering of the freezing point of the solvent. A mole of calcium chloride contains one mole of calcium ions and two moles of chloride ions. A mole of sodium chloride contains only two moles of ions and sucrose and methanol have only one mole of particles each per liter of one molar solution.

22. **(B)** If the atomic mass of an isotope is unknown the number of neutrons cannot be determined. However, if the atomic number is known the number of protons is known. In an atom there is no charge so the number of electrons must equal the number of protons and the atomic number.

23. **(D)** Nitrogen makes up about 80 percent of the air and therefore contributes about 80 percent of the total atmospheric pressure—$0.80 \times 760\text{mm} = 608\text{mm}$.

24. **(D)** A supersaturated solution contains more dissolved solute than is normal at a given temperature. A disturbance will cause the solution to adjust to the normal concentration with the concurrent expulsion of the excess solute. A saturated solution would remain stable.

25. **(A)** A first order reaction has a rate that is proportional to the concentration of only one reactant.

26. **(A)** The loss of an alpha particle reduces the number of positive charges by two and the atomic mass by four.

27. **(D)** Positron (with the mass of an electron) emission can occur, but protons are never expelled from the nucleus during radioactive decay.

28. **(A)** Fat yields the highest amount of energy per gram of any of the foods consumed.

29. **(C)** The total number of moles of reactants and products are equal, therefore a change of pressure has no effect in the equilibrium. Increasing hydrogen or reducing hydrogen bromide drives the reaction to the right. Only increasing hydrogen bromide shifts the equilibrium to the left.

30. **(C)** One gram of carbon-14 must go through four half lives to be reduced to 0.0625 grams. Four $\times$ 5.73 $\times$ 10 years equal 22.92 $\times$ 10 years.

31. **(D)** Since the oxidation number of a compound is O, the total positive values must equal the total negative values. Consequently four times the value for oxygen (–2) must equal the positive values due to potassium (+1 each) and manganese (Mn).

    1 (Oxidation number of Mn) + 2 (Oxidation number of K) + 4

    (Oxidation number of 0) = 0

    Oxidation number of Mn + 2(+1) + 4(–2) = 0

    Oxidation number of Mn = +8 – 2 = +6

32. **(A)** Within a group the element with the lowest atomic number has the highest ionization energy.

33. **(D)** Within a group of nonmetals such as the halogens, the one with the highest atomic number has the least electronegative value.

34. **(B)** The atomic radii of a group of metals increase as the atomic number increases. Therefore, the element with the lowest atomic number has the smallest atomic radius.

35. **(B)** The salt that would yield a weak acid when mixed with acid would dissolve most readily. Calcium carbonate yields carbonic acid (H_2CO_3) when it is acidified. The other salts yield hydrochloric acid (HCl), nitric acid (HNO_3) or phosphoric acid (H_3PO_4) which are both strong acids.

36. **(B)** The conjugate base is obtained when the acid loses a hydrogen ion. Therefore the conjugate base of carbonic acid, H_2CO_3, is the hydrogen carbonate ion (HCO^-_3).

37. **(D)** The number of moles of HCl required for the titration must equal the number of moles of NaOH (40 ml × 0.2 m = 8 moles). Therefore 20 ml of 0.4 ml Cl is required. After titration the total volume of the mixture is 40 + 20 = 60 ml.

38. The salt of a weak acid would hydrolyze in solution to remove hydrogen ions from water and leaving an excess of hydroxide ions. $H_2O + A^- \rightarrow HA + OH^-$. The salt of a strong acid would hydrolyze by removing hydroxide ions from water. $NH_4^+ + H_2O \rightarrow NH_4OH + H^+$.

39. **(A)** Heat is produced by the reaction and according to Le Chatalier's Principle the system will adjust to maintain equilibrium. Heating would force the reaction to the left. A pressure increase shifts the reaction in the direction of smaller volumes (right) and addition of more reactant (N_2 or H_2) also pushes the reaction to the right.

40. **(C)** Colligative properties are based on the number of particles. Vapor pressure, osmotic pressure, boiling point elevation and freezing point lowering all are colligative properties. Density is not.

41. **(C)** Molecular solids are held together by rather weak London forces which increase with molecular weight. The melting points of molecular substances are relatively low since there are no strong forces such as ionic forces to overcome.

42. **(D)** Ionic compounds form readily between nonmetals and metals. The only set that has no such combination is CH_2O, H_2S and NH_3.

43. **(C)** An atom lying at corner of a unit cell will touch four corners of cubes below and four corners of cubes above.

44. **(A)** A higher boiling point for a liquid is seen when more energy is needed to separate the gaseous molecules from the liquid. It shows that for the same amount of energy a higher boiling liquid would expel fewer molecules as vapor at any temperature, resulting in a lower vapor pressure. The lowest boiling substance vaporizes most easily and therefore would have the highest vapor pressure at a specific temperature.

45. **(A)** The mass number of an isotope is the sum of the protons and neutrons in an atom. Seventeen protons and seventeen neutrons are necessary to give a mass number of thirty-four. The number of electrons equals the number of protons in an atom.

46. **(A)** Electronegativism decreases within a group in the periodic table as the atomic number increases. The example of this shown here is the progression from fluorine to iodine.

47. **(D)** Phosphorus has fifteen electrons, all of which are paired except one.

48. **(C)** Chlorine is in the third period and has seven electrons in its outermost shell. Two electrons are in an S orbital leaving five electrons for the P orbitals.

49. **(B)** Sulfur in group VIA needs two electrons added to its six to achieve a stable outer shell of eight electrons.

50. **(B)** Since all three gases are in equal size flasks with the same temperature and pressure, the total number of moles (hence, the total number of molecules) are equal in each case. However a molecule of NH_3 contains four atoms, a molecule of NO contains two and a molecule of N_2 contains two atoms.

UNIT IX: READING COMPREHENSION

READING COMPREHENSION TEST ANSWER SHEET

READING PASSAGE 1

1. Ⓐ Ⓑ Ⓒ Ⓓ
2. Ⓐ Ⓑ Ⓒ Ⓓ
3. Ⓐ Ⓑ Ⓒ Ⓓ
4. Ⓐ Ⓑ Ⓒ Ⓓ

READING PASSAGE 2

1. Ⓐ Ⓑ Ⓒ Ⓓ
2. Ⓐ Ⓑ Ⓒ Ⓓ
3. Ⓐ Ⓑ Ⓒ Ⓓ
4. Ⓐ Ⓑ Ⓒ Ⓓ

READING PASSAGE 3

1. Ⓐ Ⓑ Ⓒ Ⓓ
2. Ⓐ Ⓑ Ⓒ Ⓓ
3. Ⓐ Ⓑ Ⓒ Ⓓ
4. Ⓐ Ⓑ Ⓒ Ⓓ
5. Ⓐ Ⓑ Ⓒ Ⓓ
6. Ⓐ Ⓑ Ⓒ Ⓓ
7. Ⓐ Ⓑ Ⓒ Ⓓ
8. Ⓐ Ⓑ Ⓒ Ⓓ

READING PASSAGE 4

1. Ⓐ Ⓑ Ⓒ Ⓓ
2. Ⓐ Ⓑ Ⓒ Ⓓ
3. Ⓐ Ⓑ Ⓒ Ⓓ
4. Ⓐ Ⓑ Ⓒ Ⓓ
5. Ⓐ Ⓑ Ⓒ Ⓓ
6. Ⓐ Ⓑ Ⓒ Ⓓ
7. Ⓐ Ⓑ Ⓒ Ⓓ
8. Ⓐ Ⓑ Ⓒ Ⓓ
9. Ⓐ Ⓑ Ⓒ Ⓓ

READING COMPREHENSION TEST

READING PASSAGE 1

4 QUESTIONS • TIME—9 MINUTES

Directions: Carefully read the following passage and then answer the accompanying questions, basing your answers on what is stated or implied in the passage. When you have decided which choice is best, blacken the corresponding space on your answer sheet. There is only one best answer for each question.

Communicable means "capable of being transmitted or passed through a medium." A communicable disease is an infection that may be transmitted directly or indirectly from one individual to another. The primary objective of programs for the prevention and control of communicable diseases is to prevent the transmission or spreading of the disease by eliminating conditions supportive to infection. Since communicable diseases are caused by microorganisms, the process of infection can be avoided or reversed by eliminating microbial sources, destroying the infectious organisms, creating conditions unfavorable to the growth of infectious microorganisms, and building up the body defenses against microbial attack.

Any measure designed to control or protect anyone from the hazards of the infectious microbes in the environment is called a barrier. The use of barriers is based upon three factors: time, distance, and shielding. "Time" refers to avoiding prolonged exposure; "distance" refers to keeping away from the infectious source; and "shielding" refers to avoiding bodily contact when exposure cannot be avoided (wearing a mask). The specific plan for selecting barriers in cases where infection exists and for preventing the occurrence of infection is dependent on the characteristics of the causative microorganism(s). All of these microbes have a certain structure, a specific way of digesting foods, a system for utilizing oxygen or the oxidation-reduction processes, and a technique for reproducing. These microbes are classified by similarities in life characteristics. Therefore, the approach to prevention and control of communicable disease is to eliminate environmental sources or to identify the kind of organisms (by characteristics) and alter their life processes, in order to protect human beings from attack.

1. Infectious diseases are "communicable" because they

   (A) attack human beings
   (B) spread from one source to another
   (C) cannot be controlled by barriers
   (D) can cause disease

2. The approach to *controlling* communicable diseases differs from the approach to *prevention* of disease in that

   (A) an infectious source exists and could be spread
   (B) infection has not occurred, and sources are being eliminated
   (C) transmission has occurred, but there is no infection
   (D) transmission cannot occur, because there is no medium

3. A barrier that represents "shielding" would be

   (A) isolating a child with a cold
   (B) using a stick to pick up infected material
   (C) short visits with a friend who has pneumonia
   (D) looking at a baby through a nursery window

4. Having knowledge of the characteristics of an infectious microorganism helps in the prevention and control of communicable disease in that it

   (A) determines how long the infection will last
   (B) identifies which methods should be used to counteract the infection
   (C) establishes whether or not the organism is a hazard
   (D) relates to the severity of the infection

READING PASSAGE 2

4 QUESTIONS • TIME—9 MINUTES

Directions: Carefully read the following passage and then answer the accompanying questions, basing your answers on what is stated or implied in the passage. When you have decided which choice is best, blacken the corresponding space on your answer sheet. There is only one best answer for each question.

The "liberated woman" is a phrase which most of us associate with the sixties and seventies. The ERA and NOW's consciousness-raising and bra-burning blitzed the media with a fury. In reality, the American woman had begun to cast off the restraints of feminine suppression long before the seventies, by snipping the strings of her proverbial apron, if not the straps of her bra. We are referring to both the 1920s and the postwar era.

The flood of labor-saving and timesaving devices pouring from the factories freed women of much of the never-ending drudgery that had been the plight of housewives since the beginning of time.

Women also found new freedom outside the home. The vote was finally rendered to women via the Nineteenth Amendment to the Constitution, and the long awaited dream of political equality between the sexes was fulfilled. Members of what was once known as the "gentle sex" cast down their brooms, cast forth their ballots, and fled their kitchens to take part in a social freedom that catapulted their grandmothers right out of their rocking chairs. Chaperones no longer made the scene at young people's parties. Fashion editors reported "the American woman has lifted her skirt far beyond any modest limitation." The hemline was being hoisted nine inches from the ground and was heading for the knee.

The boyish look was in, and women everywhere invaded the strictly male territory known as the barbershop to have their beautiful and once-treasured tresses "bobbed." Breast implants, no way! Damsels of every social station were binding their chests to acquire that fashionable look of masculinity. In contrast to this trend of fashion, beautiful debutantes took heed to the cliche "powder and paint will make you what you ain't" and plastered their faces doll-style with rouge and lipstick.

Young ladies no longer puffed secretly into the fireplaces of their homes to conceal the damnable sin of which they were partaking. Women were smoking in public for the first time.

Extensive vicissitudes in lifestyle and values placed women in the workplace. The "roaring twenties" were characterized by women finding new opportunities for employment in the booming cities. Though they were limited to a few low-paying jobs such as retail clerking and office typing that were hastily labeled "women's work," they were making an impact on the post-war era. A feisty feminist, Margaret Sanger, led a birth-control movement and openly defended the use of contraceptives. To add insult to injury, the women of the twenties deflated many a male ego with the organization of the National Women's Party in 1923.

"You've Come A Long Way Baby" was putting it mildly in the twenties. In all probability, the women of the 1990s can anticipate recoining the phrase ". . . and you ain't seen nothin' yet!"

1. This passage would suggest that women of the 1920s were
   - (A) docile in their attitudes regarding social change
   - (B) assertive in their views on women's social and political status
   - (C) willing to compromise on political issues concerning women
   - (D) eager to return to life in the kitchen

2. A fitting title for this passage would be
   - (A) "You've Come a Long Way Baby—Twenties Style"
   - (B) "Women in the Workplace"
   - (C) "Women's Political Advancements in the Twenties"
   - (D) "Male Bashing in the Twenties"

3. The tone of this passage would suggest that the author is

   (A) a male chauvinist
   (B) a product of the seventies
   (C) a trendy individual
   (D) an advocate of women's lib

4. This passage reflects that the era known as the "Roaring Twenties" was characterized by

   (A) an increase in women's unemployment
   (B) marked social change
   (C) an industrial slump
   (D) an indifference to fashion and style

READING PASSAGE 3

8 QUESTIONS • TIME—10 MINUTES

Directions: Carefully read the following passage and then answer the accompanying questions, basing your answers on what is stated or implied in the passage. When you have decided which choice is best, blacken the corresponding space on your answer sheet. There is only one best answer for each question.

Every cell in the body is bathed in water. The substances dissolved in the water provide the immediate environment for the cells' existence, that is, for their respiration, digestion, excretion, and reproduction. This water—70% of our body weight and originally from our food and drink—is carried in the blood and is distributed in three places in the body. In terms of body weight,

5% remains in blood
15% goes to tissue spaces
50% goes inside the cell

Of course, more water is needed in the cell than elsewhere in the body because there are more solutes to be dissolved and because ionization must take place for anabolism and catabolism.

All of the substances inside the cell and outside the cell in the tissue spaces were at one time a part of the blood. The blood is the transportation system of the body and, therefore, is the recipient of all substances. Substances are "unloaded" by pushing out those that can filter through the tiny openings of the semipermeable membranes of the capillaries into the tissue spaces. These substances, along with water, are then sucked into the semipermeable membranes of the cells. At the same time, the cell has produced waste substances; it now pushes those out into the tissue fluid so that they can be pushed into the capillaries and thereby excreted by the kidneys, skin, respiratory system, etc.

The pushing and sucking forces are regulated by concentrations. The more concentrated a substance is, the more force it has. What determines whether that force will push or suck is whether the substance is primarily water (solvent) or particles dissolved in water (solute). If water is the primary component of a substance, it will be sucked; that is, it will pass from a lesser to a greater concentration. This is called osmosis. The substance that is sucking in the water has the greater force or pull, called osmotic pressure, because it has the greater concentration. If solutes are the primary component, they can be pushed only by diffusion from a greater to a lesser concentration. The sucking and pushing processes go on simultaneously, and that is why we identify this mechanism as being dynamic. The "equilibrium" of body fluids is explained in terms of a balance of forces. This dynamic factor is controlled by three things:

1. How much of the substance is present (solute/solvent)
2. What kind of substance is present (electrolytes/non-electrolytes)
3. The placement and distribution of the substance (cell/tissue space/blood)

The concentration of a solution is determined by the relationship between the solutes and water. "Solutes" may be electrolytes or non-electrolytes. Nonelectrolytes do not ionize and, therefore, they affect the concentration of a solution and its diffusion processes, but they do not affect the osmolarity of a solution. Osmotic pressure is determined by "tonic" relationships. "Tonic" refers to the comparison of the number of specific ions per unit volume in two given solutions—iso being "the same as," hypo being "less than," and hyper being "more than."

Given two solutions of the same solute, the more concentrated solution contains more solute particles, has a higher potential osmotic pressure, and is hypertonic as compared with the less concentrated solution. Given two solutions of different solutes, the solution containing more particles has the greater concentration, but there are no "tonic" relationships.

1. Why is an adequate intake of water essential to life?

    (A) Solutes will dissolve only in water.
    (B) Water is the medium for exchange of solutes.
    (C) Osmosis will only take place in water.
    (D) Water is necessary for metabolism.

2. The blood is described as "the transportation system of the body" because

    (A) blood has the capacity for osmosis and diffusion
    (B) all nutrients and wastes are received by the blood
    (C) blood has a higher concentration than any other body fluid
    (D) all metabolic processes are controlled by the blood

3. The concentration of a solution is directly determined by

    (A) placement of solutes
    (B) distribution of water
    (C) percentage of solute to solvent
    (D) percentage of electrolytes to non-electrolytes

4. The largest percentage of H_2O in the body is found

    (A) intracellularly
    (B) extracelluarly
    (C) intravascularly
    (D) interstitially

5. In the process of osmosis (sucking), the primary factor is

    (A) water
    (B) solute
    (C) ionization
    (D) force

6. If blood cells were placed in a hypertonic solution of salt, which one of the following blood cell reactions would take place?

    (A) swelling
    (B) shrinkage
    (C) destruction
    (D) no change

7. The primary factor in diffusion (pushing) is

    (A) water
    (B) solute
    (C) ionization
    (D) force

8. If there are two solutions of sodium chloride, which of the following factors will determine which solution has the highest potential for osmosis?

    (A) isotonicity
    (B) hypotonicity
    (C) hypertonicity
    (D) all of the above

READING PASSAGE 4

9 QUESTIONS • TIME—17 MINUTES

Directions: Carefully read the following passage and then answer the accompanying questions, basing your answers on what is stated or implied in the passage. When you have decided which choice is best, blacken the corresponding space on your answer sheet. There is only one best answer for each question.

As the world's population grows, the part played by man in influencing plant life becomes increasingly great. In old and densely populated countries, as in western Europe, man determines almost wholly what shall grow and what shall not grow. In such regions, the influence of man on plant life is in large measure a beneficial one. Laws, often centuries old, protect plants of economic value and preserve soil fertility. In newly settled countries the situation is, unfortunately, quite the reverse. The pioneer's life is too strenuous for him to think of posterity.

Some years ago Mt. Mitchell, the highest summit east of the Mississippi, was covered with a magnificent forest. A lumber company was given full rights to fell the trees. Those not cut down were crushed. The mountain was left a waste area where fire would rage and erosion complete the destruction. There was no stopping the devastating foresting of the company, for the contract had been given. Under a more enlightened civilization, this could not have happened. The denuding of Mt. Mitchell is a minor chapter in the destruction of lands in the United States; and this country is by no means the only sufferer. China, India, Egypt, and East Africa all have their thousands of square miles of wasteland, the result of man's indifference to the future.

Deforestation, grazing, and poor farming techniques are the chief causes of the destruction of land fertility. Wasteful cutting of timer is the first step. Grazing follows lumbering, often bringing about ruin. The Caribbean slopes of northern Venezuela are barren wastes, owing first to ruthless cutting of forests and then to destructive grazing. Hordes of goats roamed these slopes until only a few thorny acacias and cacti remained. Erosion completed the devastation. What is illustrated there on a small scale is the story of vast areas in China and India, countries where famines occur regularly.

Man is not wholly to blame, for nature is often merciless. In parts of India and China, plant life, even when left undisturbed by man, cannot cope with either the disastrous floods of wet seasons or the destructive winds of the dry season. Man has learned much; prudent land management has been the policy of the Chinese people since 2700 B.C., but even they have not learned enough.

When the American forestry service was in its infancy, it met with much opposition from legislators who loudly claimed that the protected land would in one season yield a crop of cabbages of more value than all the timber on it. Herein lay the fallacy, that one season's crop is all that need be thought of. Nature, through the years, adjusts crops to the soil and to the climate. Forests usually occur where precipitation exceeds evaporation. If the reverse is true, grasslands are found; and where evaporation is still greater, desert or scrub vegetation alone survives. The phytogeographic map of a country is very similar to the climatic map based on rainfall, evaporation, and temperature. Man ignores this natural adjustment of crops and strives for one "bumper" crop in a single season; he may produce it, but "year in and year out, the yield of the grassland is certain, that of the planted fields, never."

Man is learning; he sprays his trees with insecticides and fungicides; he imports ladybugs to destroy aphids; he irrigates, fertilizes, and rotates his crops; but he is still indifferent to many of the consequences of his short-sighted policies.

In spite of the evidence from the experience of this country, the people of other countries still in the pioneer stage farm as wastefully as did our own pioneers. In the interiors of Central and South America, natives fell superb forest trees and leave them to rot in order to obtain virgin soil for cultivation. Where the land is hilly, it readily washes, and after one or two seasons it is unfit for crops. So the frontier farmer pushes back into the primeval forest, moving his hut as he goes, and fells more monarchs to lay bare another patch of ground for his plantings to support his family. Valuable timer that will require a century to replace is destroyed and the land laid waste to produce what could be supplied for a pittance.

How badly man can err in his handling of land is shown by the draining of extensive swamp areas, which to the uninformed would seem to be a very good thing to do. One of the first effects of the drainage is the lowering of the watertable, which may bring about the death of the dominant species and leave to another species the possession of the soil, even when the difference in water level is little more than an inch. Bog country will frequently yield marketable crops of cranberries and blueberries but if drained, will grow neither these nor any other economically useful plant on the fallow soil. Swamps and marshes may have their drawbacks, but man should beware of disturbing the ecosphere. When drained; wetlands may leave waste land, the surface of which can erode rapidly and be blown away in dust blizzards disastrous to both man and wild beasts.

1. The best title for this passage might be

   (A) "How to Increase Soil Productivity"
   (B) "Conservation of Natural Resources"
   (C) "Man's Effect on Soil"
   (D) "Soil Conditions and Plant Growth"

2. A policy of good management is sometimes upset by

   (A) the indifference of man
   (B) centuries-old laws
   (C) floods and winds
   (D) grazing animals

3. Areas in which the total amounts of rain and snow falling on the ground are greater than the moisture evaporated will support

 (A) forests
 (B) grasslands
 (C) scrub vegetation
 (D) no plants

4. Pioneers usually do not have a long range view on soil problems, since they

 (A) are not protected by laws
 (B) live under adverse conditions
 (C) use poor methods of farming
 (D) must protect themselves from famine

5. *Phytogeographic* maps are those that show

 (A) areas of grassland
 (B) areas of bumper crops
 (C) areas of similar climate
 (D) areas of similar plants

6. What is meant by, "the yield of the grasslands is certain; that of the planted field, never"?

 (A) It is impossible to get more than one bumper crop from any one cultivated area.
 (B) Crops planted in former grasslands will not give good yields.
 (C) Through the indifference of man, dust blizzards have occurred informer grasslands.
 (D) If man does not interfere, plants will grow in the most suitable environment.

7. The first act of prudent land management might be to

 (A) prohibit drainage of swamps
 (B) use irrigation and crop rotation in planted areas
 (C) increase use of fertilizers
 (D) prohibit excessive forest lumbering

8. The results of good land management may usually be found in

 (A) heavily populated areas
 (B) areas not given over to grazing
 (C) underdeveloped areas
 (D) ancient civilizations

9. Long-range programs of soil management are possible only in

 (A) young nations
 (B) ancient civilizations
 (C) those nations with an agricultural economy
 (D) those nations that want it

READING COMPREHENSION TEST ANSWER KEY

READING PASSAGE 1

1. **B**
2. **A**
3. **D**
4. **B**

READING PASSAGE 2

1. **B**
2. **A**
3. **D**
4. **B**

READING PASSAGE 3

1. **D**
2. **B**
3. **C**
4. **A**
5. **A**
6. **A**
7. **B**
8. **C**

READING PASSAGE 4

1. **C**
2. **C**
3. **A**
4. **B**
5. **D**
6. **D**
7. **D**
8. **A**
9. **C**

Part IV

PRACTICE FOR PRACTICAL/ VOCATIONAL NURSING SCHOOL ENTRANCE EXAMINATIONS

INTRODUCTION

Modern nursing is complex and multifaceted. Nurses practice in a variety of settings that emphasize different roles. Various educational programs are available to provide opportunities for nurses to enter different careers within the same profession of nursing. Nursing has experienced many changes throughout its history, and the changes are not over yet. A major change that has occurred in practical/vocational nursing history is a gradual increase in the required formal knowledge base.

Prior to the Civil War, untrained compassionate women cared for sick relatives and friends using skills that they had learned from their mothers and friends. The practical/vocational nurse became a permanent member of the health team when society needed a trained individual who could render competent and intelligent bedside care to patients. The need for an educational program for practical/vocational nurses was recognized, and in 1893 the first school for practical nurses in the United States was founded in New York. This was the Ballard School, which consisted of a three-month educational program.

Today's practical/vocational nurses are educationally prepared and technically skilled individuals capable of rendering competent, scientific, and personal care to patients. The educational program is approximately one year in length. The emphasis in practical/vocational nursing education is on learning basic skills that can be used in a variety of clinical settings. Care is rendered to patients in hospitals, physicians' offices, extended-care facilities, community health centers, private homes, day camps, industries, nursing homes, hospice facilities, and the armed forces. Men as well as women find this a rewarding vocation.

The practical/vocational nurse works under the supervision and direction of the registered nurse, physician, or other person(s) authorized by law. The practical/vocational nurse participates in assessing the patient's physical and mental health; records and reports; participates in implementing health care plans designed by the registered nurse or other authorized persons; reinforces teaching, and documents the patient's response to nursing care given.

The practical/vocational nurse is a graduate of a state-approved school and is licensed to practice after passing the National Council Licensure Examination (NCLEX-PN), which is a computerized test. Practical/vocational nursing programs may be administered at technical and vocational schools; community and junior colleges: universities; hospitals; and private or government agencies. Knowledge is basic to all occupations. Because nursing is comprehensive, you will be required to take many courses in theory and practice to provide you with the knowledge and information essential to your vocation. The nursing curriculum is based on scientific theory from the natural, social, and health sciences. Basic principles of selected nursing techniques are also included. Clinical experience is provided in such areas as nursing care of mothers and infants, pediatrics, care of the mentally ill, medical and surgical nursing, and care of the aged and chronically ill. Licensed practical/vocational nurses (LPNs or LVNs) have excellent employment opportunities. Many new positions have been created by population growth and the increase in public-health consciousness. Salaries for practical/vocational nurses have increased proportionately, as they have for registered nurses. The salary for the licensed practical nurse or licensed vocational nurse is usually three-fourths that of the registered nurse.

Any career that you choose entails effort, trials, and preserverance. Your nursing program is no exception and will present many exciting challenges to you. A nursing examination is usually required before admission to a practical/vocational nursing program. This section is designed to help you achieve an acceptable score on the examination.

TEST-TAKING STRATEGIES

An important objective in preparing for admission into nursing school is to develop your test-taking skills. Success in test-taking is very important to the majority of us. We learn early on in life that by obtaining certain test scores, we are permitted or denied certain opportunities. With the importance that our society has placed on passing or failing tests, it is understandable that there will be a certain amount of stress before, during, and after a test. This feeling can be termed "test stress."

EFFECTS OF STRESS

Stress is a normal part of everyday life, and it is inherent in health care professions. Stress is the wear and tear put on the body through normal or abnormal events of life. Our reactions to stress may include some painful emotions, such as fear, anxiety, confusion, and humiliation. Minimal stress can be helpful and positive because it keeps us alert and "on our toes." Intense stress is negative because it will interfere with the learning process by elevating your anxiety level until it causes a blockage. For example, a person may be unable to concentrate, may forget, and may make errors in judgement. All in all, the combined effects of stress can be a deciding factor in whether a test-taker will be successful or unsuccessful in passing tests.

REDUCING TEST STRESS

It has been determined that test-takers who anticipate failure will have an increase in their stress level. You must learn to control this source of stress by focusing on positive events that have occurred in your life and by anticipating future successes. Focus on positive thinking!

Relaxation exercises can be very effective in relieving tension and stress. One technique is begun by taking deep, slow, deliberate breaths. Following this, you should tense each major muscle group for ten seconds, then relax. Once you learn how to perform these exercises, you can use them at any time that you feel tense or stressed.

Tests are a fact of life for students. You must be prepared to deal with them. Preparation for tests includes planned study or review sessions. This preparation will help to build your self-confidence. If you study effectively, concentrate, and apply what you have learned, you will reduce stress to a minimum.

Many people experience stress when dealing with the unknown. Try to learn as much as you can about the examination and the condition of testing. Sample tests included in this book will help you to prepare for the unknown.

TEST-TAKING TACTICS

In the following paragraphs, ten tactics for test-taking have been identified for you. These tactics provide solutions to the most common problems faced by test-takers.

Many of the tests that you take will be multiple-choice. How do you successfully take a multiple-choice test? The answer to this question can be complex, but the more practice you have, the better you will become in passing them. Listed below are general tactics for taking multiple-choice tests.

1. Read instructions or directions carefully. Reading may seem like a simple matter, but mistakes can be made when the test-taker does not read the information carefully and completely.

2. Manage your time effectively during test-taking. If you are a slow test-taker, practice reading at a faster pace. Do not spend too much time on one question; leave it if you have to and return to it later. If you progress in a timely fashion, you will feel confident and maintain composure during the testing situation.

3. Do not change answers without good reason or sound rationale. Usually your first answer is the best, unless you are positive that it is wrong. Your first attempt at answering a test item is usually accomplished by a logical and orderly thinking process. If you are uncertain of an answer and you change it, you are most likely doing it impulsively, not because of logical thinking. Do not change your answer unless you have a GOOD reason to do so.

4. Use a process of elimination to weed out unsound, unreasonable options that do not fit. By reducing your choices on a difficult question, you can sharpen your focus and make the question more manageable.

5. Do not become angry or upset with a question. Put the emotion away until after the test.
6. Maintain a positive attitude. You may not know the answer, but try to figure it out.
7. Don't overlook key words or phrases such as "not," "except," "never," "all," "always," and "only." These are only some of these types of words, so be on the lookout. These words may cause you to give an inaccurate response.
8. Attempt every question. Do not avoid questions that seem complicated. After you read them carefully, they may be easier than you think.
9. Do not jump to conclusions. Read the questions slowly and carefully.
10. Do not read too deeply into questions or answers. Answer only what the item writer has asked, not what you think should be asked.

Will these tactics improve your test-taking skills? They should, and when combined with a proper planned review, they should help you to do better on the admission examination and to achieve your goal of becoming a practical/vocational nurse.

UNIT X: VERBAL SKILLS

VERBAL SKILLS TESTS ANSWER SHEET

TEST 1: VERBAL SKILLS ANTONYMS

1. Ⓐ Ⓑ Ⓒ Ⓓ	14. Ⓐ Ⓑ Ⓒ Ⓓ	27. Ⓐ Ⓑ Ⓒ Ⓓ	40. Ⓐ Ⓑ Ⓒ Ⓓ
2. Ⓐ Ⓑ Ⓒ Ⓓ	15. Ⓐ Ⓑ Ⓒ Ⓓ	28. Ⓐ Ⓑ Ⓒ Ⓓ	41. Ⓐ Ⓑ Ⓒ Ⓓ
3. Ⓐ Ⓑ Ⓒ Ⓓ	16. Ⓐ Ⓑ Ⓒ Ⓓ	29. Ⓐ Ⓑ Ⓒ Ⓓ	42. Ⓐ Ⓑ Ⓒ Ⓓ
4. Ⓐ Ⓑ Ⓒ Ⓓ	17. Ⓐ Ⓑ Ⓒ Ⓓ	30. Ⓐ Ⓑ Ⓒ Ⓓ	43. Ⓐ Ⓑ Ⓒ Ⓓ
5. Ⓐ Ⓑ Ⓒ Ⓓ	18. Ⓐ Ⓑ Ⓒ Ⓓ	31. Ⓐ Ⓑ Ⓒ Ⓓ	44. Ⓐ Ⓑ Ⓒ Ⓓ
6. Ⓐ Ⓑ Ⓒ Ⓓ	19. Ⓐ Ⓑ Ⓒ Ⓓ	32. Ⓐ Ⓑ Ⓒ Ⓓ	45. Ⓐ Ⓑ Ⓒ Ⓓ
7. Ⓐ Ⓑ Ⓒ Ⓓ	20. Ⓐ Ⓑ Ⓒ Ⓓ	33. Ⓐ Ⓑ Ⓒ Ⓓ	46. Ⓐ Ⓑ Ⓒ Ⓓ
8. Ⓐ Ⓑ Ⓒ Ⓓ	21. Ⓐ Ⓑ Ⓒ Ⓓ	34. Ⓐ Ⓑ Ⓒ Ⓓ	47. Ⓐ Ⓑ Ⓒ Ⓓ
9. Ⓐ Ⓑ Ⓒ Ⓓ	22. Ⓐ Ⓑ Ⓒ Ⓓ	35. Ⓐ Ⓑ Ⓒ Ⓓ	48. Ⓐ Ⓑ Ⓒ Ⓓ
10. Ⓐ Ⓑ Ⓒ Ⓓ	23. Ⓐ Ⓑ Ⓒ Ⓓ	36. Ⓐ Ⓑ Ⓒ Ⓓ	49. Ⓐ Ⓑ Ⓒ Ⓓ
11. Ⓐ Ⓑ Ⓒ Ⓓ	24. Ⓐ Ⓑ Ⓒ Ⓓ	37. Ⓐ Ⓑ Ⓒ Ⓓ	50. Ⓐ Ⓑ Ⓒ Ⓓ
12. Ⓐ Ⓑ Ⓒ Ⓓ	25. Ⓐ Ⓑ Ⓒ Ⓓ	38. Ⓐ Ⓑ Ⓒ Ⓓ	
13. Ⓐ Ⓑ Ⓒ Ⓓ	26. Ⓐ Ⓑ Ⓒ Ⓓ	39. Ⓐ Ⓑ Ⓒ Ⓓ	

TEST 2: VERBAL SKILLS ANTONYMS

1. Ⓐ Ⓑ Ⓒ Ⓓ	6. Ⓐ Ⓑ Ⓒ Ⓓ	11. Ⓐ Ⓑ Ⓒ Ⓓ	16. Ⓐ Ⓑ Ⓒ Ⓓ
2. Ⓐ Ⓑ Ⓒ Ⓓ	7. Ⓐ Ⓑ Ⓒ Ⓓ	12. Ⓐ Ⓑ Ⓒ Ⓓ	17. Ⓐ Ⓑ Ⓒ Ⓓ
3. Ⓐ Ⓑ Ⓒ Ⓓ	8. Ⓐ Ⓑ Ⓒ Ⓓ	13. Ⓐ Ⓑ Ⓒ Ⓓ	18. Ⓐ Ⓑ Ⓒ Ⓓ
4. Ⓐ Ⓑ Ⓒ Ⓓ	9. Ⓐ Ⓑ Ⓒ Ⓓ	14. Ⓐ Ⓑ Ⓒ Ⓓ	19. Ⓐ Ⓑ Ⓒ Ⓓ
5. Ⓐ Ⓑ Ⓒ Ⓓ	10. Ⓐ Ⓑ Ⓒ Ⓓ	15. Ⓐ Ⓑ Ⓒ Ⓓ	20. Ⓐ Ⓑ Ⓒ Ⓓ

TEST 3: VERBAL SKILLS SYNONYMS

1. Ⓐ Ⓑ Ⓒ Ⓓ	14. Ⓐ Ⓑ Ⓒ Ⓓ	27. Ⓐ Ⓑ Ⓒ Ⓓ	40. Ⓐ Ⓑ Ⓒ Ⓓ
2. Ⓐ Ⓑ Ⓒ Ⓓ	15. Ⓐ Ⓑ Ⓒ Ⓓ	28. Ⓐ Ⓑ Ⓒ Ⓓ	41. Ⓐ Ⓑ Ⓒ Ⓓ
3. Ⓐ Ⓑ Ⓒ Ⓓ	16. Ⓐ Ⓑ Ⓒ Ⓓ	29. Ⓐ Ⓑ Ⓒ Ⓓ	42. Ⓐ Ⓑ Ⓒ Ⓓ
4. Ⓐ Ⓑ Ⓒ Ⓓ	17. Ⓐ Ⓑ Ⓒ Ⓓ	30. Ⓐ Ⓑ Ⓒ Ⓓ	43. Ⓐ Ⓑ Ⓒ Ⓓ
5. Ⓐ Ⓑ Ⓒ Ⓓ	18. Ⓐ Ⓑ Ⓒ Ⓓ	31. Ⓐ Ⓑ Ⓒ Ⓓ	44. Ⓐ Ⓑ Ⓒ Ⓓ
6. Ⓐ Ⓑ Ⓒ Ⓓ	19. Ⓐ Ⓑ Ⓒ Ⓓ	32. Ⓐ Ⓑ Ⓒ Ⓓ	45. Ⓐ Ⓑ Ⓒ Ⓓ
7. Ⓐ Ⓑ Ⓒ Ⓓ	20. Ⓐ Ⓑ Ⓒ Ⓓ	33. Ⓐ Ⓑ Ⓒ Ⓓ	46. Ⓐ Ⓑ Ⓒ Ⓓ
8. Ⓐ Ⓑ Ⓒ Ⓓ	21. Ⓐ Ⓑ Ⓒ Ⓓ	34. Ⓐ Ⓑ Ⓒ Ⓓ	47. Ⓐ Ⓑ Ⓒ Ⓓ
9. Ⓐ Ⓑ Ⓒ Ⓓ	22. Ⓐ Ⓑ Ⓒ Ⓓ	35. Ⓐ Ⓑ Ⓒ Ⓓ	48. Ⓐ Ⓑ Ⓒ Ⓓ
10. Ⓐ Ⓑ Ⓒ Ⓓ	23. Ⓐ Ⓑ Ⓒ Ⓓ	36. Ⓐ Ⓑ Ⓒ Ⓓ	49. Ⓐ Ⓑ Ⓒ Ⓓ
11. Ⓐ Ⓑ Ⓒ Ⓓ	24. Ⓐ Ⓑ Ⓒ Ⓓ	37. Ⓐ Ⓑ Ⓒ Ⓓ	50. Ⓐ Ⓑ Ⓒ Ⓓ
12. Ⓐ Ⓑ Ⓒ Ⓓ	25. Ⓐ Ⓑ Ⓒ Ⓓ	38. Ⓐ Ⓑ Ⓒ Ⓓ	
13. Ⓐ Ⓑ Ⓒ Ⓓ	26. Ⓐ Ⓑ Ⓒ Ⓓ	39. Ⓐ Ⓑ Ⓒ Ⓓ	

TEST 4: VERBAL SKILLS SYNONYMS

1. Ⓐ Ⓑ Ⓒ Ⓓ	6. Ⓐ Ⓑ Ⓒ Ⓓ	11. Ⓐ Ⓑ Ⓒ Ⓓ	16. Ⓐ Ⓑ Ⓒ Ⓓ
2. Ⓐ Ⓑ Ⓒ Ⓓ	7. Ⓐ Ⓑ Ⓒ Ⓓ	12. Ⓐ Ⓑ Ⓒ Ⓓ	17. Ⓐ Ⓑ Ⓒ Ⓓ
3. Ⓐ Ⓑ Ⓒ Ⓓ	8. Ⓐ Ⓑ Ⓒ Ⓓ	13. Ⓐ Ⓑ Ⓒ Ⓓ	18. Ⓐ Ⓑ Ⓒ Ⓓ
4. Ⓐ Ⓑ Ⓒ Ⓓ	9. Ⓐ Ⓑ Ⓒ Ⓓ	14. Ⓐ Ⓑ Ⓒ Ⓓ	19. Ⓐ Ⓑ Ⓒ Ⓓ
5. Ⓐ Ⓑ Ⓒ Ⓓ	10. Ⓐ Ⓑ Ⓒ Ⓓ	15. Ⓐ Ⓑ Ⓒ Ⓓ	20. Ⓐ Ⓑ Ⓒ Ⓓ

TEST 5: SPELLING USAGE

1. Ⓐ Ⓑ Ⓒ Ⓓ	10. Ⓐ Ⓑ Ⓒ Ⓓ	19. Ⓐ Ⓑ Ⓒ Ⓓ	28. Ⓐ Ⓑ Ⓒ Ⓓ
2. Ⓐ Ⓑ Ⓒ Ⓓ	11. Ⓐ Ⓑ Ⓒ Ⓓ	20. Ⓐ Ⓑ Ⓒ Ⓓ	29. Ⓐ Ⓑ Ⓒ Ⓓ
3. Ⓐ Ⓑ Ⓒ Ⓓ	12. Ⓐ Ⓑ Ⓒ Ⓓ	21. Ⓐ Ⓑ Ⓒ Ⓓ	30. Ⓐ Ⓑ Ⓒ Ⓓ
4. Ⓐ Ⓑ Ⓒ Ⓓ	13. Ⓐ Ⓑ Ⓒ Ⓓ	22. Ⓐ Ⓑ Ⓒ Ⓓ	31. Ⓐ Ⓑ Ⓒ Ⓓ
5. Ⓐ Ⓑ Ⓒ Ⓓ	14. Ⓐ Ⓑ Ⓒ Ⓓ	23. Ⓐ Ⓑ Ⓒ Ⓓ	32. Ⓐ Ⓑ Ⓒ Ⓓ
6. Ⓐ Ⓑ Ⓒ Ⓓ	15. Ⓐ Ⓑ Ⓒ Ⓓ	24. Ⓐ Ⓑ Ⓒ Ⓓ	33. Ⓐ Ⓑ Ⓒ Ⓓ
7. Ⓐ Ⓑ Ⓒ Ⓓ	16. Ⓐ Ⓑ Ⓒ Ⓓ	25. Ⓐ Ⓑ Ⓒ Ⓓ	34. Ⓐ Ⓑ Ⓒ Ⓓ
8. Ⓐ Ⓑ Ⓒ Ⓓ	17. Ⓐ Ⓑ Ⓒ Ⓓ	26. Ⓐ Ⓑ Ⓒ Ⓓ	35. Ⓐ Ⓑ Ⓒ Ⓓ
9. Ⓐ Ⓑ Ⓒ Ⓓ	18. Ⓐ Ⓑ Ⓒ Ⓓ	27. Ⓐ Ⓑ Ⓒ Ⓓ	

VERBAL SKILLS TESTS

Please Refer to Unit I, Pages 21–78, for Review Before Doing This Section.

TEST 1: VERBAL SKILLS ANTONYMS

50 QUESTIONS • TIME—30 MINUTES

Directions: For each question in this test, select the word that is opposite in meaning to the capitalized word. Blacken the corresponding space on your answer sheet.

1. GARRULOUS
   (A) talkative
   (B) reserved
   (C) unruly
   (D) fraternal

2. TRANSLUCENT
   (A) patent
   (B) transitory
   (C) transparent
   (D) opaque

3. BENEVOLENT
   (A) generous
   (B) charitable
   (C) malevolent
   (D) good

4. LETHARGIC
   (A) energetic
   (B) sluggish
   (C) apathetic
   (D) fatal

5. AMICABLE
   (A) lonely
   (B) reactionary
   (C) hostile
   (D) laconic

6. TRANQUILITY
   (A) complacency
   (B) tumult
   (C) plagiarism
   (D) prophecy

7. PROCRASTINATE
   (A) elegiac
   (B) mediate
   (C) expedite
   (D) investiture

8. QUIESCENT
   (A) restless
   (B) lethargic
   (C) mendicant
   (D) malignant

9. DELETERIOUS
   (A) fractious
   (B) pathetic
   (C) salubrious
   (D) gullible

10. COGNIZANCE
    (A) ignorance
    (B) abeyance
    (C) anecdote
    (D) idiom

11. CLEMENCY
    (A) mercy
    (B) indulgence
    (C) kindness
    (D) vindictiveness

12. IGNOBLE
    (A) honorable
    (B) shameful
    (C) disgraceful
    (D) humble

13. CURSORY
  (A) hasty
  (B) superficial
  (C) awful
  (D) thorough

14. ADMONISH
  (A) warn
  (B) praise
  (C) advise
  (D) reprove

15. PHLEGMATIC
  (A) energetic
  (B) dull
  (C) extraordinary
  (D) morbid

16. LAMENTABLE
  (A) laughable
  (B) generous
  (C) emotional
  (D) doleful

17. PERILOUS
  (A) vivacious
  (B) fatal
  (C) safe
  (D) hazardous

18. INIQUITOUS
  (A) unequaled
  (B) unfriendly
  (C) righteous
  (D) injurious

19. ASSIDUOUS
  (A) cooperative
  (B) indifferent
  (C) active
  (D) satisfactory

20. CORROBORATE
  (A) fascinate
  (B) corrupt
  (C) confirm
  (D) dispute

21. CONFLUENCE
  (A) convention
  (B) sympathy
  (C) divergence
  (D) concurrence

22. DASTARDLY
  (A) cowardly
  (B) bravely
  (C) friendly
  (D) sinfully

23. ABSTRUSE
  (A) understandable
  (B) hidden
  (C) absurd
  (D) religious

24. ILLUSION
  (A) delusion
  (B) conception
  (C) reality
  (D) dramatization

25. AVARICIOUS
  (A) greedy
  (B) persuasive
  (C) generous
  (D) gracious

26. COERCE
  (A) enforce
  (B) cohere
  (C) forestall
  (D) coax

27. TEMERITY
  (A) recklessness
  (B) prudence
  (C) support
  (D) sanity

28. LACONIC
  (A) verbose
  (B) concise
  (C) serene
  (D) interesting

29. CREDULOUS
    (A) exuberant
    (B) skeptical
    (C) dangerous
    (D) legible

30. INCARCERATE
    (A) immunize
    (B) anesthetize
    (C) transport
    (D) release

31. OBTUSE
    (A) oblique
    (B) obese
    (C) perpendicular
    (D) acute

32. MUNIFICENT
    (A) political
    (B) miserly
    (C) liberal
    (D) educational

33. DERANGED
    (A) unsettled
    (B) paralyzed
    (C) sane
    (D) awkward

34. LEVITY
    (A) flippancy
    (B) peace
    (C) gravity
    (D) trickery

35. EQUANIMITY
    (A) peace
    (B) inflation
    (C) agitation
    (D) tranquility

36. MARAUD
    (A) purchase
    (B) plunder
    (C) masticate
    (D) elevate

37. ENCOMIUM
    (A) immorality
    (B) praise
    (C) egotism
    (D) defamation

38. ABOMINABLE
    (A) delightful
    (B) horrible
    (C) meaningful
    (D) insane

39. ABSTEMIOUS
    (A) frugal
    (B) happy
    (C) greedy
    (D) radiant

40. ADVERTENT
    (A) retentive
    (B) inconsiderate
    (C) empathetic
    (D) abnormal

41. ENIGMATIC
    (A) perplexing
    (B) explicit
    (C) persistent
    (D) officious

42. EXECRABLE
    (A) unusual
    (B) detestable
    (C) fallible
    (D) respectable

43. IGNOMINIOUS
    (A) reputable
    (B) shameful
    (C) intangible
    (D) irascible

44. SAGACITY
    (A) sorrowfulness
    (B) support
    (C) satisfaction
    (D) stupidity

45. PROVERBIAL

(A) innovative
(B) current
(C) wise
(D) cautious

46. ANNIHILATE

(A) advertise
(B) destroy
(C) preserve
(D) announce

47. AFFABLE

(A) discourteous
(B) beloved
(C) sociable
(D) debonair

48. CAPRICIOUS

(A) logical
(B) agreeable
(C) awkward
(D) constant

49. CONTINGENT

(A) conditional
(B) independent
(C) confinable
(D) familiar

50. OFFICIOUS

(A) meddling
(B) modest
(C) emaciated
(D) authentic

TEST 1: VERBAL SKILLS ANTONYMS ANSWER KEY

1. **B**
2. **D**
3. **C**
4. **A**
5. **C**
6. **B**
7. **C**
8. **A**
9. **C**
10. **A**
11. **D**
12. **A**
13. **D**
14. **B**
15. **A**
16. **A**
17. **C**
18. **C**
19. **B**
20. **D**
21. **C**
22. **B**
23. **A**
24. **C**
25. **C**
26. **D**
27. **B**
28. **A**
29. **B**
30. **D**
31. **D**
32. **B**
33. **C**
34. **C**
35. **C**
36. **A**
37. **D**
38. **A**
39. **C**
40. **B**
41. **B**
42. **D**
43. **A**
44. **D**
45. **A**
46. **C**
47. **A**
48. **D**
49. **B**
50. **B**

TEST 2: VERBAL SKILLS ANTONYMS

20 QUESTIONS • TIME—10 MINUTES

Directions: For each question in this test, select the word that is opposite in meaning to the capitalized word. Blacken the corresponding space on your answer sheet.

1. DECEIT
   (A) fraud
   (B) truthfulness
   (C) treachery
   (D) imposition
2. DOCILE
   (A) teachable
   (B) compliant
   (C) tame
   (D) inflexible
3. HARMLESS
   (A) safe
   (B) hurtful
   (C) innocent
   (D) innocuous
4. MELANCHOLY
   (A) jolly
   (B) low-spirited
   (C) dreamy
   (D) sad
5. IMPETUOUS
   (A) violent
   (B) furious
   (C) calm
   (D) vehement
6. JOY
   (A) gladness
   (B) grief
   (C) mirth
   (D) delight
7. LUNACY
   (A) sanity
   (B) madness
   (C) derangement
   (D) mania
8. MOIST
   (A) dank
   (B) dry
   (C) damp
   (D) humid
9. PUERILE
   (A) youthful
   (B) weak
   (C) silly
   (D) mature
10. WEIGHT
    (A) gravity
    (B) heaviness
    (C) lightness
    (D) burden
11. SUPERFLUOUS
    (A) necessary
    (B) excessive
    (C) unnecessary
    (D) expanded
12. REFORM
    (A) amend
    (B) correct
    (C) better
    (D) corrupt
13. SCANTY
    (A) bare
    (B) ample
    (C) insufficient
    (D) meager
14. MISERY
    (A) happiness
    (B) woe
    (C) privation
    (D) penury

15. PROPER

    (A) honest
    (B) appropriate
    (C) wrong
    (D) pertinent

16. INCONGRUOUS

    (A) compatible
    (B) absurd
    (C) contrary
    (D) incoherent

17. FATIGUE

    (A) lassitude
    (B) weariness
    (C) malaise
    (D) vigor

18. HASTEN

    (A) delay
    (B) accelerate
    (C) dispatch
    (D) expedite

19. ABSORB

    (A) emit
    (B) engulf
    (C) engross
    (D) consume

20. ABUSE

    (A) ribaldry
    (B) protection
    (C) contumely
    (D) obloquy

TEST 2: VERBAL SKILLS ANTONYMS ANSWER KEY

1. **B**
2. **D**
3. **B**
4. **A**
5. **C**
6. **B**
7. **A**
8. **B**
9. **D**
10. **C**
11. **A**
12. **D**
13. **B**
14. **A**
15. **C**
16. **A**
17. **D**
18. **A**
19. **A**
20. **B**

TEST 3: VERBAL SKILLS SYNONYMS

50 QUESTIONS • TIME—30 MINUTES

Directions: In each of the following sentences, one word is in italics. Below each sentence are words lettered A, B, C, D. For each sentence choose the word that best corresponds in meaning to the italicized word. Blacken the corresponding space on your answer sheet.

1. Her efforts to revive the child were *futile*.

    (A) strong
    (B) clumsy
    (C) useless
    (D) sincere

2. The supply of pamphlets has been *depleted*.

    (A) exhausted
    (B) delivered
    (C) included
    (D) rejected

3. The *gist* of his speech was that we should strike.

    (A) end
    (B) essence
    (C) strength
    (D) spirit

4. The soldier was decorated for his *valor* in battle in Korea.

    (A) injury
    (B) ability
    (C) cooperation
    (D) courage

5. When Mary arrived in California, her future seemed *auspicious*.

    (A) bleak
    (B) uncertain
    (C) promising
    (D) somber

6. To our *consternation*, the child's bicycle rolled into the busy street.

    (A) dismay
    (B) amazement
    (C) incompetence
    (D) annoyance

7. *Indolence* is a habit that cannot be excused.

    (A) incompetency
    (B) snoring
    (C) carelessness
    (D) idleness

8. The political candidate made *cogent* remarks.

    (A) pleasing
    (B) convincing
    (C) flattering
    (D) slandering

9. A *prolific* writer is one who is

    (A) productive
    (B) popular
    (C) frank
    (D) effective

10. He was *meticulous* when performing his work.

    (A) careless
    (B) patient
    (C) scrupulous
    (D) nervous

11. There were *sporadic* outbreaks of food poisoning at the camp.

    (A) epidemic
    (B) widespread
    (C) serious
    (D) scattered

12. The motion passed even though there were three *dissenting* votes.

    (A) annoying
    (B) disagreeing
    (C) abstaining
    (D) approving

13. It is *traditional* for the bride to wear a white gown.

    (A) normal
    (B) customary
    (C) ordinary
    (D) gracious

14. The company has *rescinded* the order.

    (A) canceled
    (B) revised
    (C) confirmed
    (D) misinterpreted

15. Although the prisoner was released early, he was *vindictive* toward society.

    (A) prejudiced
    (B) impatient
    (C) revengeful
    (D) unreasonable

16. The *sedulous* student worked many hours in the laboratory.

    (A) eager
    (B) persistent
    (C) intelligent
    (D) inexperienced

17. The neighbors were *interrogated* by the police.

    (A) arrested
    (B) detained
    (C) investigated
    (D) questioned

18. The lifeguard *disparaged* his brave rescue of the child.

    (A) explained
    (B) belittled
    (C) demonstrated
    (D) elucidated

19. The water could not *permeate* the rubber apron.

    (A) saturate
    (B) wet
    (C) harm
    (D) discolor

20. The *docile* dog waited at the gate.

    (A) mongrel
    (B) hungry
    (C) intractable
    (D) obedient

21. The two hospitals in our town will *amalgamate* next year.

    (A) close
    (B) expand
    (C) relocate
    (D) merge

22. She wasted her money on *frivolous* things.

    (A) sweet
    (B) expensive
    (C) unimportant
    (D) cheap

23. The teacher *divulged* the test grades.

    (A) whispered
    (B) disregarded
    (C) revealed
    (D) averaged

24. *Remuneration* to the shareholders was ten percent higher than last year.

    (A) shares
    (B) payment
    (C) liquidation
    (D) speculation

25. The art dealer *scrutinized* the painting to verify its authenticity.

    (A) touched
    (B) bought
    (C) inspected
    (D) measured

26. The bridge was closed because it was *decrepit*.

    (A) slippery
    (B) weak
    (C) swaying
    (D) flooded

27. The driver *conceded* that he was at fault.

    (A) denied
    (B) explained
    (C) complained
    (D) admitted

28. The machinery in the vocational classroom was *obsolete*.

    (A) out of date
    (B) new
    (C) reliable
    (D) complicated

29. The speaker made *candid* remarks about the candidate's record.
    (A) biased
    (B) confidential
    (C) frank
    (D) insulting

30. When the hostage was released, he was speaking *incoherently.*
    (A) disconnectedly
    (B) cohesively
    (C) prolifically
    (D) sluggishly

31. The mother tried to *pacify* the child.
    (A) detain
    (B) restrain
    (C) accompany
    (D) calm

32. The head nurse on 2 West was young and *vivacious.*
    (A) kind
    (B) lively
    (C) short
    (D) talkative

33. The town was *devastated* after the earthquake.
    (A) rebuilt
    (B) deserted
    (C) destroyed
    (D) saved

34. The teacher *digressed* from her custom and didn't give any homework.
    (A) deviated
    (B) reposed
    (C) alighted
    (D) moored

35. The Colonel was a *gallant* man.
    (A) rude
    (B) fastidious
    (C) cowardly
    (D) chivalrous

36. The family gathering was a *melancholic* scene.
    (A) happy
    (B) sad
    (C) heart-warming
    (D) ardent

37. When I visited her in the nursing home, she was *querulous* and unhappy.
    (A) satisfied
    (B) cheerful
    (C) complaining
    (D) painful

38. The FBI agent kept a *vigilant* guard on the suspect.
    (A) careful
    (B) continuous
    (C) observant
    (D) reciprocal

39. The play treated current social issues *satirically.*
    (A) frankly
    (B) interminably
    (C) musically
    (D) ironically

40. She felt an *antipathy* for lizards.
    (A) aversion
    (B) fondness
    (C) interest
    (D) fear

41. The hiker had a *premonition* of danger.
    (A) vision
    (B) forewarning
    (C) recurrence
    (D) apprehension

42. The policeman *confiscated* the illegal drugs
    (A) stored
    (B) distributed
    (C) destroyed
    (D) appropriated

43. John was asked to resign because of his *improbity.*
    (A) age
    (B) tardiness
    (C) dishonesty
    (D) absenteeism

44. There is no *tangible* evidence of damage.
    (A) concrete
    (B) theoretical
    (C) verified
    (D) scientific

45. Her *blithe* spirit made her popular.

(A) free
(B) cheerful
(C) kind
(D) insolent

46. The jury *deliberated* for eight hours.

(A) met
(B) convened
(C) considered
(D) summarized

47. He had a *sinister* motive for entering the building.

(A) practical
(B) wrong
(C) important
(D) honest

48. The requirements for admission to the school were *stringent*.

(A) unusual
(B) numerous
(C) rigid
(D) lax

49. The students refused to give up their *prerogatives*.

(A) demands
(B) rights
(C) ideals
(D) duties

50. The widow and her children were *destitute*.

(A) impoverished
(B) detained
(C) loathed
(D) ill

TEST 3: VERBAL SKILLS SYNONYMS ANSWER KEY

1. **C**
2. **A**
3. **B**
4. **D**
5. **C**
6. **A**
7. **D**
8. **B**
9. **A**
10. **C**
11. **D**
12. **B**
13. **B**
14. **A**
15. **C**
16. **B**
17. **D**
18. **B**
19. **A**
20. **D**
21. **D**
22. **C**
23. **C**
24. **B**
25. **C**
26. **B**
27. **D**
28. **A**
29. **C**
30. **A**
31. **D**
32. **B**
33. **C**
34. **A**
35. **D**
36. **B**
37. **C**
38. **C**
39. **D**
40. **A**
41. **B**
42. **D**
43. **C**
44. **A**
45. **B**
46. **C**
47. **B**
48. **C**
49. **B**
50. **A**

TEST 4: VERBAL SKILLS SYNONYMS

20 QUESTIONS • TIME—10 MINUTES

Directions: For each question in this test, select the word that corresponds in meaning to the capitalized word. Blacken the corresponding space on your answer sheet.

1. COMPETENT
   (A) agreeable
   (B) inept
   (C) vigorous
   (D) capable
2. OMNIBUS
   (A) threatening
   (B) all-embracing
   (C) rotund
   (D) slow-moving
3. INGENUITY
   (A) deceitfulness
   (B) appeal
   (C) cleverness
   (D) innocence
4. CONCAVE
   (A) curving inward
   (B) curving outward
   (C) oval-shaped
   (D) rounded
5. CANON
   (A) barrier
   (B) noisy place
   (C) guiding principle
   (D) vigorous
6. AUSPICIOUS
   (A) questionable
   (B) well-known
   (C) free
   (D) favorable
7. VACILLATING
   (A) changeable
   (B) decisive
   (C) equalizing
   (D) progressing
8. FORFEIT
   (A) exchange
   (B) relinquish
   (C) protect
   (D) withdraw
9. QUERY
   (A) question
   (B) look over carefully
   (C) follow through
   (D) act peculiarly
10. STEADFAST
   (A) gradual
   (B) strong
   (C) friendly
   (D) unwavering
11. ACCESS
   (A) too much
   (B) extra
   (C) admittance
   (D) arrival
12. PERMUTATION
   (A) alteration
   (B) permission
   (C) combination
   (D) seepage
13. SPRITZ
   (A) spray
   (B) bubble
   (C) protrude
   (D) sail
14. PERSONABLE
   (A) intimate
   (B) cheerful
   (C) attractive
   (D) superficial

15. EXPEDITE
    (A) dismiss
    (B) advise
    (C) accelerate
    (D) demolish

16. COMPULSORY
    (A) imperative
    (B) impossible
    (C) imminent
    (D) logical

17. PRACTICABLE
    (A) lenient
    (B) feasible
    (C) simple
    (D) visible

18. AGREE
    (A) inquire
    (B) acquiesce
    (C) discharge
    (D) endeavor

19. FLORID
    (A) overflowing
    (B) ruddy
    (C) seedy
    (D) flowery

20. NEARNESS
    (A) adherence
    (B) declivity
    (C) worldliness
    (D) proximity

TEST 4: VERBAL SKILLS SYNONYMS ANSWER KEY

1. **D**
2. **B**
3. **C**
4. **A**
5. **C**
6. **D**
7. **A**
8. **B**
9. **A**
10. **D**
11. **C**
12. **A**
13. **A**
14. **C**
15. **C**
16. **A**
17. **B**
18. **B**
19. **B**
20. **D**

TEST 5: SPELLING USAGE

35 QUESTIONS • TIME—20 MINUTES

Directions: Select the letter that belongs in the blank space in the sentence.

1. The demonstrators were ____ from the property.

   (A) band
   (B) banned

2. The nurse had to ____ the baby.

   (A) weigh
   (B) way

3. She looked on the ____ for the date of the meeting.

   (A) calendar
   (B) calender

4. The perfume had a ____ of roses.

   (A) sent
   (B) scent

5. The injury caused a ____ on her arm.

   (A) bruise
   (B) brews

6. The student received a ____ for passing the test.

   (A) complement
   (B) compliment

7. The ___ gave the faculty their assignments.

   (A) principal
   (B) principle

8. The ulcer on the patient's foot did not ___.

   (A) heel
   (B) heal

9. A tiny opening in the skin is called a ___.

   (A) pour
   (B) pore

10. The ____ after surgery caused the child to cry.

    (A) pain
    (B) pane

11. A ____ is a sour berry.

    (A) current
    (B) currant

12. It is important to ____ in order to strengthen muscles.

    (A) exercise
    (B) exorcise

13. The secretary purchased new ____ on which to type letters.

    (A) stationery
    (B) stationary

14. They wanted ____ food right away.

    (A) there
    (B) their

15. He was too ____ to climb the stairs.

    (A) week
    (B) weak

16. The ____ is a timid animal.

    (A) dear
    (B) deer

17. I want to ____ the president.

    (A) meat
    (B) meet

18. She wanted a ____ of candy.

    (A) piece
    (B) peace

19. The child did not ____ the vase.

    (A) brake
    (B) break

20. To ____ means to stop living.

    (A) dye
    (B) die

21. She wanted to purchase two ____ of milk.

    (A) quartz
    (B) quarts

22. He could not ____ his book.

    (A) find
    (B) fined

23. The ____ led to a dead-end street.

    (A) rode
    (B) road

24. The telephone was ____.

    (A) ringing
    (B) wringing

25. The ____ was chocolate cake.

    (A) dessert
    (B) desert

26. The thief was going to ____ the money.

    (A) steel
    (B) steal

27. She placed an ____ in the local newspaper.

    (A) ad
    (B) add

28. He turned ____ because he was so afraid.

    (A) pale
    (B) pail

29. The man wanted the bank to ____ him some money.

    (A) lone
    (B) loan

30. The area around the incision was ____.

    (A) sore
    (B) soar

31. The ____ in the paragraph was not clear.

    (A) clause
    (B) claws

32. The passenger had to pay a ____ to ride the bus.

    (A) fair
    (B) fare

33. When her blood pressure dropped, she started to ____.

    (A) feint
    (B) faint

34. He ____ a loud sound.

    (A) heard
    (B) herd

35. We will go ____ it rains or not.

    (A) weather
    (B) whether

TEST 5: SPELLING USAGE ANSWER KEY

1. **B**
2. **A**
3. **A**
4. **B**
5. **A**
6. **B**
7. **A**
8. **B**
9. **B**
10. **A**
11. **B**
12. **A**
13. **A**
14. **B**
15. **B**
16. **B**
17. **B**
18. **A**
19. **B**
20. **B**
21. **B**
22. **A**
23. **B**
24. **A**
25. **A**
26. **B**
27. **A**
28. **A**
29. **B**
30. **A**
31. **A**
32. **B**
33. **B**
34. **A**
35. **B**

UNIT XI: ARITHMETIC AND MATHEMATICS

Arithmetic is an important part of the study of pharmacology and the related sciences. In this section practice problems on fractions, decimals, ratio, proportion, and percent are included with a review of the appropriate processes. The problem solutions are presented after each set of exercises. If you have made errors, go back to the explanation for that kind of problem. After you have completed all practice tests, take the final test.

REVIEW OF BASIC OPERATION

FRACTIONS

Reduction of Fractions

To reduce fractions to lowest terms, divide both the numerator and the denominator by the same number.

Example: $\frac{4}{8} = \frac{4 \div 4}{8 \div 4} \div 4 = \frac{1}{2}$

Practice Exercise A

Reduce the following fractions to their lowest terms.

1. $\frac{8}{16}$ = ____
2. $\frac{3}{12}$ = ____
3. $\frac{5}{10}$ = ____
4. $\frac{25}{100}$ = ____
5. $\frac{18}{72}$ = ____
6. $\frac{50}{60}$ = ____
7. $\frac{27}{54}$ = ____
8. $\frac{4}{64}$ = ____
9. $\frac{12}{144}$ = ____
10. $\frac{25}{150}$ = ____

Improper Fractions

To change an improper fraction to a mixed number, divide the numerator by the denominator and show the remainder, if any, over the denominator. Reduce to the lowest terms.

Example:

$$\frac{21}{7} = 7\overline{)21} \quad \begin{array}{r} 3 \\ 21 \\ \underline{21} \\ 0 \end{array}$$

$$\frac{15}{9} = 9\overline{)15} = 1\frac{2}{3} \quad \begin{array}{r} 1\frac{6}{9} \\ 15 \\ \underline{9} \\ 6 \end{array}$$

To change a mixed number to an improper fraction, add the numerator of the fraction to the product of the whole number and the denominator of the fraction. Show the total over the denominator of the fraction.

Example: $4\frac{3}{8} = \frac{(4 \times 8) + 3}{8} = \frac{32 + 3}{8} = \frac{35}{8}$

Practice Exercise B

Change the following improper fractions to mixed numbers.

1. $\frac{15}{4}$ = ____
2. $\frac{13}{6}$ = ____
3. $\frac{27}{5}$ = ____
4. $\frac{17}{3}$ = ____
5. $\frac{99}{10}$ = ____
6. $2\frac{1}{9}$ = ____
7. $6\frac{4}{5}$ = ____
8. $8\frac{3}{4}$ = ____
9. $3\frac{7}{8}$ = ____
10. $2\frac{1}{6}$ = ____

Addition of Fractions

To add two or more fractions, the denominators must be the same. Rewrite each fraction as an equivalent fraction with the Least (smallest) Common Multiple (LCM) as the common denominator. Then add the numerators and reduce the answer to lowest terms.

Example: Add $\frac{2}{3} + \frac{3}{4}$

Multiples of 3 = 3, 6, 9, 12, 15, 18, 21, 24, . . .
Multiples of 4 = 4, 8, 12, 16, 20, 24, . . .
Common multiples are 12 and 24
LCM = 12 (the common denominator)

To make an equivalent fraction, divide the common denominator by the original denominator and multiply the original numerator by the result.

$12 \div 3 = 4; 2 \times 4 = 8$
$12 \div 4 = 3; 3 \times 3 = 9$

Add and reduce to lowest terms.

$\frac{2}{3} + \frac{3}{4} = \frac{8}{12} + \frac{9}{12} = \frac{17}{12} = 1\frac{5}{12}$

Practice Exercise C

1. $\frac{1}{2}$
   $\frac{1}{3}$
   $\frac{1}{6}$

2. $\frac{3}{4}$
   $\frac{1}{12}$
   $\frac{2}{3}$

3. $7\frac{2}{3}$
   $3\frac{5}{24}$
   $\frac{5}{12}$

4. $1\frac{1}{4}$
   $5\frac{3}{16}$
   $2\frac{5}{12}$

5. $26\frac{3}{5}$
   $14\frac{1}{5}$
   $5\frac{7}{8}$

6. $7\frac{5}{8}$
   $\frac{1}{32}$
   $3\frac{1}{10}$

7. $4\frac{1}{2}$
   $3\frac{1}{4}$
   $9\frac{3}{8}$

8. $7\frac{11}{12}$
   $16\frac{3}{4}$
   $2\frac{4}{8}$

9. $1\frac{3}{24}$
   $8\frac{1}{3}$
   $3\frac{5}{6}$

10. $5\frac{5}{6}$
    $7\frac{3}{8}$
    $2\frac{3}{10}$

Subtraction of Fractions

Rewrite each fraction as an equivalent fraction with the LCM as the common denominator as shown above. If the fraction of the mixed number to be subtracted is larger than the one from which it is to be subtracted, you must borrow 1 from the whole number of the larger mixed number. Add the numerator and denominator of the larger mixed number to make a new numerator. Subtract and reduce to lowest terms.

Example:

$$\begin{array}{rcrcr} 9\frac{1}{2} & = & 9\frac{3}{6} & = & 8\frac{9}{6} \\ -1\frac{2}{3} & = & 1\frac{4}{6} & = & 1\frac{4}{6} \\ \hline & & & & 7\frac{5}{6} \end{array}$$

Find the common denominator and make equivalent fractions.
Borrow from the whole number of the larger mixed number (9 –1 = 8).
Add the numerator and denominator to make a new numerator (3 + 6 =9).
Subtract and reduce to lowest terms.

Practice Exercise D

1. $\frac{5}{8} - \frac{3}{16}$

2. $7\frac{5}{12} - 3\frac{1}{4}$

3. $\frac{1}{2} - \frac{1}{8}$

4. $3\frac{1}{8} - 1\frac{3}{4}$

5. $\frac{7}{9} - \frac{1}{6}$

6. $\frac{17}{20} - \frac{3}{4}$

7. $5\frac{3}{8} - 1\frac{7}{16}$

8. $\frac{2}{5} - \frac{2}{9}$

9. $4\frac{3}{4} - 2\frac{2}{3}$

10. $11\frac{7}{8} - 1\frac{3}{4}$

Multiplication of Fractions

To multiply fractions, multiply the numerators, then multiply the denominators. You may be able to simplify the fractions before multiplying, which allows you to work with smaller numbers. To simplify, divide the numerator of one fraction and the denominator of another fraction by the same number. Multiply and reduce to lowest terms.

Example: $\frac{12}{25} \times \frac{5}{9} = \frac{\cancel{12}^{4}}{\cancel{25}_{5}} \times \frac{\cancel{5}^{1}}{\cancel{9}_{3}} = \frac{4}{15}$

To multiply a fraction by a whole number, change the whole number to a fraction by placing the whole number over one. Multiply, simplify, if possible, and reduce to lowest terms.

Example: $4 \times \frac{1}{12} = \frac{4}{1} \times \frac{1}{12} = \frac{\cancel{4}^{1}}{1} \times \frac{1}{\cancel{12}_{3}} = \frac{1}{3}$

To multiply mixed numbers, change the mixed number to an improper fraction. Simplify, if possible, and then multiply as above. Reduce answer to lowest terms.

Example: $3\frac{1}{2} \times \frac{6}{21} = \frac{7}{2} \times \frac{6}{21} = \frac{\cancel{7}^{1}}{\cancel{2}_{1}} \times \frac{\cancel{6}^{3}}{\cancel{21}_{3}} = \frac{3}{3} = 1$

Practice Exercise E

1. $\frac{2}{3} \times \frac{1}{8} =$ ____
2. $\frac{2}{5} \times \frac{5}{12} =$ ____
3. $\frac{4}{21} \times \frac{7}{8} =$ ____
4. $\frac{15}{16} \times \frac{9}{10} =$ ____
5. $\frac{4}{6} \times \frac{2}{4} =$ ____
6. $3\frac{3}{8} \times \frac{27}{8} =$ ____
7. $\frac{1}{2} \times 8 =$ ____
8. $6\frac{1}{2} \times 5\frac{4}{8} =$ ____
9. $3\frac{2}{3} \times \frac{3}{4} =$ ____
10. $9 \times 3\frac{1}{3} =$ ____

Division of Fractions

To divide fractions, invert the divisor (the second fraction) and change the sign from division (÷) to multiplication (×) and then follow the rules for multiplication. Whole numbers are written as fractions with denominator of one. Mixed numbers are written as improper fractions.

Example: $\frac{2}{3} \div \frac{3}{4} = \frac{2}{3} \times \frac{4}{3} = \frac{8}{9}$

$5 \div 6\frac{2}{3} = \frac{5}{1} \div \frac{20}{3} = \frac{\cancel{5}^{1}}{1} \times \frac{3}{\cancel{20}_{4}} = \frac{3}{4}$

Practice Exercise F

1. $2\frac{1}{5} \div 11 =$ ____
2. $\frac{1}{50} \div \frac{1}{200} =$ ____
3. $6\frac{3}{5} \div 8\frac{3}{10} =$ ____
4. $\frac{3}{4} \div \frac{1}{8} =$ ____
5. $\frac{5}{12} \div \frac{5}{60} =$ ____
6. $10\frac{1}{2} \div \frac{1}{3} =$ ____
7. $\frac{1}{60} \div \frac{1}{2} =$ ____
8. $8 \div \frac{2}{3} =$ ____
9. $\frac{1}{6} \div \frac{1}{3} =$ ____
10. $\frac{7}{8} \div \frac{3}{4} =$ ____

DECIMALS, RATIOS AND PROPORTIONS, PERCENT DECIMALS

The decimal system is based on the number ten. All numbers to the right of the decimal point are decimal fractions whose denominator is ten or a multiple of ten. *Tenths* are directly after the decimal point, *hundredths* two places after, *thousandths* three places after, *ten-thousandths* four places, etc. Whole numbers are written to the left of the decimal point and the decimal point is read as "and."

Millions	Hundred-thousands	Ten-thousands	Thousands	Hundreds	Tens	Ones		Tenths	Hundreths	Thousandths	Ten-Thousandths	Hundred-Thousandths	Millionths

Changing Fractions to Decimals

To change a fraction to a decimal, divide the numerator by the denominator. Write a decimal after the numerator and add as many zeros as needed. The division ends when the remainder is zero.

Example:

$$\frac{3}{4} = 4\overline{)3.00} = .75$$

```
        .75
3/4 = 4)3.00
        28
         20
         20
          0
```

Sometimes the division is not exact and a remainder may repeat itself. Draw a bar over the number in the answer that repeats.

$$\frac{1}{12} = 12\overline{)1.0000} = .08\bar{3}$$

```
       .0833
12 ) 1.0000
      96
      --
       40
       36
       --
        40
        36
        --
         4
```

Practice Exercise G

Change the following fractions to decimals

1. $\frac{1}{4}$ = ____
2. $\frac{7}{8}$ = ____
3. $\frac{5}{6}$ = ____
4. $\frac{5}{125}$ = ____
5. $\frac{5}{16}$ = ____
6. $\frac{3}{25}$ = ____
7. $\frac{9}{20}$ = ____
8. $\frac{1}{75}$ = ____
9. $\frac{3}{8}$ = ____
10. $\frac{3}{10}$ = ____

Changing Decimals to Fractions

Decimals may be changed to fractions by dropping the decimal point and using the proper denominator. The number of decimal places to the right of the decimal point represents the number of zeros to be used in the denominator preceded by the number one. Remove the decimal point from the number that you are converting and this becomes the numerator.

0.025

Example: There are three places to the right of the decimal point. Therefore, the denominator is one followed by three zeros (1000). Next, remove the decimal point from 0.025; this number (25) becomes the numerator.

$0.025 = \frac{25}{1000}$

Practice Exercise H

Change the following decimals to fractions and reduce to lowest terms.

1. 0.16 = ____
2. 0.04 = ____
3. 0.125 = ____
4. 0.06 = ____
5. 0.257 = ____
6. 0.75 = ____
7. 0.250 = ____
8. 0.525 = ____
9. 0.2 = ____
10. 4.75 = ____

Adding Decimals

To add decimals, place the numbers in columns so that the decimal points are directly under each other. Then add in the same manner that you would add columns of whole numbers. Place a decimal point in your answer directly under the others.

Example: Add 22.05 + 1.375 + 10.2.

```
 22.05
  1.375
 10.2
 33.625
```

Practice Exercise I

Add the following decimals.

1. 7.2 + 3.57 + 10.8 = ____
2. 48.3 + 18.25 + 4.002 = ____
3. 6.3 + 0.005 + 2.67 = ____
4. 25.4 + 37.06 + 41 = ____
5. 8.50 + 19.625 + 0.17 = ____
6. 29.042 + 2.6 + 3.120 = ____
7. 5.4 + 8.62 + 0.95 = ____
8. 2.246 + 16.8 + 4.26 = ____
9. 16.1 + 1.12 + 3.525 = ____
10. 30.7 + 4.05 + 20.5 = ____

Subtracting Decimals

To subtract decimals, use the same rule as for adding decimals[md]place decimal points directly under one another. Then subtract in the same manner you would subtract whole numbers, placing the decimal point in your answer directly under the others.

Example:

```
  50.789
– 24.19
  26.599
```

Practice Exercise J

Subtract the following decimals.

1. 5.67 – 3.9 = ____
2. 37.2 – 25.37 = ____
3. 17.4 – 13.262 = ____
4. 58.94 – 27.363 = ____
5. 2.425 – 0.675 = ____
6. 15 – 7.82 = ____
7. 205.6 – 105.23 = ____
8. 246.52 – 107.988 = ____
9. 35.25 – 17.0 = ____
10. 1725.5 – 50.6325 = ____

Multiplying Decimals

To multiply decimals, multiply the numbers as if they were whole numbers. Then place the decimal point in the answer by counting from the right the number of decimal places in the multiplier and the multiplicand.

Example:

```
 2.56   (2 decimal places)
× 0.6   (1 decimal place)
 1.536  (2 + 1 or 3 decimal places)
```

Practice Exercise K

Multiply the following decimals.

1. 5.64 × 1.2 = ____
2. 4.25 × 12 = ____
3. 35.6 × 2.5 = ____
4. 4.92 × 9.5 = ____
5. 51. × 0.92 = ____
6. 28.6 × 8.16 = ____
7. 50.06 × 2.15 = ____
8. 32.2 × 3.15 = ____
9. 21.0 × 41.6 = ____
10. 8.06 × 3.654 = ____

Dividing Decimals

To divide decimals, the divisor must always be a whole number. If the divisor is a decimal, move the decimal to the right as many places as necessary to make the decimal a whole number. Then move the decimal point in the dividend the same number of places to the right to avoid changing the value of the quotient. The decimal point in the quotient is placed directly above the decimal point in the dividend.

Example:

```
                    112
.25)28  =  .25)28.00
               25
                30
                25
                 50
                 50
                  0
```

Practice Exercise L

1. 100 ÷ 2.5 = ____
2. 0.9 ÷ 0.3 = ____
3. 38.6 ÷ 1.7 = ____
4. 115 ÷ 1.5 = ____
5. 5.5 ÷ 2.5 = ____
6. 3.22 ÷ 0.46 = ____
7. 4.65 ÷ 1.5 = ____
8. 15 ÷ 7.5 = ____
9. 0.042 ÷ 0.3 = ____
10. 0.006 ÷ 0.05 = ____

RATIOS AND PROPORTIONS

Ratio

A ratio is the comparison of two numbers by division. A ratio can be written using the symbol (:) or can be written as a fraction. The ratio 1:8 shows the relationship between one and eight. The ratio 1:8 can be written as the fraction 1/8.

Example: 2 : 50 = 1 : 25

Practice Exercise M

Write the following fractions as ratios and reduce to lowest terms:

1. $\frac{4}{5}$ = ____
2. $\frac{1}{3}$ = ____
3. $\frac{3}{4}$ = ____
4. $\frac{3}{8}$ = ____
5. $\frac{1}{10}$ = ____
6. $\frac{2}{3}$ = ____
7. $\frac{1}{2}$ = ____
8. $\frac{25}{50}$ = ____
9. $\frac{3}{9}$ = ____
10. $\frac{2}{5}$ = ____

Proportion

A proportion states that two ratios are equal. Proportions may be expressed in two ways:

Example: $\frac{1}{2} = \frac{50}{100}$ or 1 : 2 :: 50 : 100

Both are read: *One is to two as fifty is to one hundred.* The product of the means equals the product of the extremes.

Example:

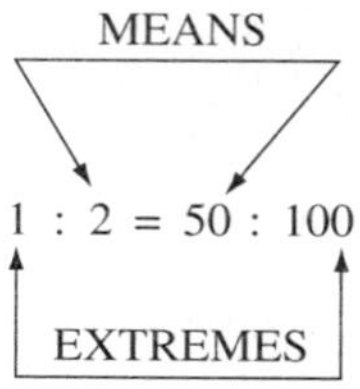

$\frac{1}{2} = \frac{50}{100}$ $\quad$ $1 \times 100 = 2 \times 50$

If one number is not known, substitute an alphabet letter and solve for the unknown number by multiplying the means and the extremes, or multiplying the diagonals.

Example: $5 : y = 25 : 125$ $\quad \frac{5}{y} \boxtimes \frac{25}{125}$

Example: $25 \times y = 5 \times 125$ $\quad$ $25y = 625$

$25y = 625$ $\quad$ $y = 5$

$y = 25$

Practice Exercise N

Solve for x in the following proportions.

1. $8 : 10 = x : 30$
2. $\frac{9}{15} = \frac{x}{5}$
3. $x : 80 = 3 : 12$
4. $\frac{3}{x} = \frac{8}{24}$
5. $2 : 3 = x : 63$
6. $5 : 15 = x : 60$
7. $\frac{7}{x} = \frac{4}{28}$
8. $0.2 : 8 = 25 : x$
9. $\frac{5}{7} = \frac{4}{28}$
10. $\frac{1}{10}x : 2000 = 1 : 100$

PERCENTAGES

To change a decimal to percent, multiply the decimal by 100 (move the decimal point two places to the right), and then add the percent sign.

Example: $0.25 = .25$

$= 25\%$

To find the percent of a number, change the percent to its decimal equivalent, or to a fraction, and multiply.

Find 7% of 40. (Note: "of" means multiply)

Example:

$$\begin{array}{r} 40 \\ \times .07 \\ \hline \end{array}$$

2.80 or $\frac{7}{\cancel{100}\ 10} \times \frac{\cancel{40}\ 4}{1} = \frac{28}{10} = 2.8$

To find the percent one number is of another, use the is/of method. The "is" number is the numerator and the "of" number is the denominator.

18 is what percent of 24?

Example:

$$\frac{18}{24} = \frac{3}{4} = 4\overset{.75}{\overline{)3.00}} = 25\%$$

```
  .75
4)3.00
  28
  --
   20
   20
   --
    0
```

What percent of 500 is 125?

Example:

$$\frac{125}{500} = \frac{1}{4} = 4\overset{.25}{\overline{)1.00}} = 25\%$$

```
  .25
4)1.00
   8
  --
   20
   20
   --
    0
```

To find the percent of change, subtract to find the amount of change. Then find what percent is of the original amount using the is/of method.

A sweater is on sale for $42.00. The original price was $56.00. What is the percent of change?

Example:

```
  $56
 – 42
 ----
  $14
```

$$\frac{14}{56} = \frac{1}{4} = 4\overset{.25}{\overline{)1.00}} = 25\%$$

```
  .25
4)1.00
   8
  --
   20
   20
   --
    0
```

Practice Exercise O

Change the following decimals to percents.

1. 0.225 = ____
2. 3.45 = ____
3. 0.7 = ____
4. 0.14 = ____
5. 4.5 = ____
6. 24 percent of 72 = ____
7. 5 percent of 12 = ____
8. 225 is what percent of 300?
9. What percent of 60 is 24?
10. What percent of 45 is 135?

ROMAN NUMERALS

Roman numerals are written using letters of the alphabet. The letters used to designate arabic numbers are:

Roman	Arabic Equivalent
I	1
V	5
X	10
L	50
C	100
D	500
M	1000

Rules Governing the Use of Roman Numerals

Addition—Placing one or more Roman numerals after the basic numeral adds to its value.

VII = 7

The same numeral cannot be repeated more than three times in succession. If this seems necessary the rule for subtraction is used.

XXX = 30 XXXX—not allowed XL = 40.

Subtraction—Placing one or more Roman numerals in front of the basic numeral removes value from it.

IV = 4

The symbols, V, D, and L are never used in subtraction.

Practice Exercise P

Write the proper Roman numerals:

1. 8 ____
2. 15 ____
3. 50 ____
4. 4 ____
5. 23 ____
6. 44 ____
7. 93 ____
8. 36 ____
9. 56 ____
10. 19 ____
11. 25 ____
12. 100 ____
13. 37 ____
14. 7 ____
15. 18 ____
16. 526 ____
17. 94 ____
18. 39 ____
19. 62 ____
20. 1980 ____

Write the proper Arabic numbers:

1. XXIV ____
2. XVII ____
3. L ____
4. XL ____
5. V ____
6. III ____
7. M ____
8. XIX ____
9. XXX ____
10. XXIX ____
11. VI ____
12. LXX ____
13. C ____
14. XCII ____
15. LXIX ____
16. XVII ____
17. XXII ____
18. XI ____
19. CCIV ____
20. MCXV ____

SOLUTIONS TO PRACTICE EXERCISES

Practice Exercise A

1. $\frac{8}{16} = \frac{1}{2}$
2. $\frac{3}{12} = \frac{1}{4}$
3. $\frac{5}{10} = \frac{1}{2}$
4. $\frac{25}{100} = \frac{1}{4}$
5. $\frac{18}{72} = \frac{1}{4}$
6. $\frac{50}{60} = \frac{5}{6}$
7. $\frac{27}{54} = \frac{1}{2}$
8. $\frac{4}{64} = \frac{1}{16}$
9. $\frac{12}{144} = \frac{1}{12}$
10. $\frac{25}{150} = \frac{1}{6}$

Practice Exercise B

1. $\frac{15}{4} = 3\frac{3}{4}$
2. $\frac{13}{6} = 2\frac{1}{6}$
3. $\frac{27}{5} = 5\frac{2}{5}$
4. $\frac{17}{3} = 5\frac{2}{3}$
5. $\frac{99}{10} = 9\frac{9}{10}$
6. $2\frac{1}{9} = \frac{19}{2}$
7. $6\frac{4}{5} = \frac{34}{5}$
8. $8\frac{3}{4} = \frac{35}{4}$
9. $3\frac{7}{8} = \frac{31}{8}$
10. $2\frac{1}{6} = \frac{13}{6}$

Practice Exercise C

1.
$$\begin{aligned} \tfrac{1}{2} &= \tfrac{3}{6} \\ \tfrac{1}{3} &= \tfrac{2}{6} \\ \tfrac{1}{6} &= \tfrac{1}{6} \\ \hline & \tfrac{6}{6} = 1 \end{aligned}$$

2.
$$\begin{aligned} \tfrac{3}{4} &= \tfrac{9}{12} \\ \tfrac{1}{12} &= \tfrac{1}{12} \\ \tfrac{2}{3} &= \tfrac{8}{12} \\ \hline & \tfrac{18}{12} = 1\tfrac{6}{12} = 1\tfrac{1}{2} \end{aligned}$$

3.
$$\begin{aligned} 7\tfrac{2}{3} &= 7\tfrac{16}{24} \\ 3\tfrac{5}{24} &= 3\tfrac{5}{24} \\ \tfrac{5}{12} &= \tfrac{10}{24} \\ \hline & 10\tfrac{31}{24} = 11\tfrac{7}{24} \end{aligned}$$

4.
$$\begin{aligned} 1\tfrac{1}{4} &= 1\tfrac{12}{48} \\ 5\tfrac{3}{16} &= 5\tfrac{9}{8} \\ 2\tfrac{5}{12} &= 2\tfrac{20}{48} \\ \hline & 8\tfrac{41}{48} \end{aligned}$$

5.
$$\begin{aligned} 26\tfrac{3}{5} &= 26\tfrac{72}{120} \\ 14\tfrac{1}{5} &= 14\tfrac{20}{120} \\ 5\tfrac{7}{8} &= 5\tfrac{105}{120} \\ \hline & 45\tfrac{197}{120} = 46\tfrac{77}{120} \end{aligned}$$

6.
$$\begin{aligned} 7\tfrac{5}{8} &= 7\tfrac{100}{160} \\ \tfrac{1}{32} &= \tfrac{5}{160} \\ 3\tfrac{1}{10} &= 3\tfrac{16}{160} \\ \hline & 10\tfrac{121}{160} \end{aligned}$$

7.
$$\begin{array}{rcl} 4\frac{1}{2} &=& 4\frac{4}{8} \\ 3\frac{1}{4} &=& 3\frac{2}{8} \\ 9\frac{3}{8} &=& 9\frac{3}{8} \\ \hline & & 16\frac{9}{8} = 17\frac{1}{8} \end{array}$$

8.
$$\begin{array}{rcl} 7\frac{11}{12} &=& 7\frac{33}{36} \\ 16\frac{3}{4} &=& 16\frac{27}{36} \\ 2\frac{4}{18} &=& 2\frac{8}{36} \\ \hline & & 25\frac{68}{36} = 26\frac{32}{36} = 26\frac{8}{9} \end{array}$$

9.
$$\begin{array}{rcl} 1\frac{3}{24} &=& 1\frac{3}{24} \\ 8\frac{1}{3} &=& 8\frac{8}{24} \\ 3\frac{5}{6} &=& 3\frac{20}{24} \\ \hline & & 12\frac{31}{24} = 13\frac{7}{24} \end{array}$$

10.
$$\begin{array}{rcl} 5\frac{5}{6} &=& 5\frac{100}{120} \\ 7\frac{3}{8} &=& 7\frac{45}{120} \\ 2\frac{3}{10} &=& 2\frac{36}{120} \\ \hline & & 14\frac{181}{120} = 15\frac{61}{120} \end{array}$$

Practice Exercise D

1.
$$\begin{array}{rcl} \frac{5}{8} &=& \frac{10}{16} \\ -\frac{3}{16} &=& \frac{3}{16} \\ \hline & & \frac{7}{16} \end{array}$$

2.
$$\begin{array}{rcl} 7\frac{5}{12} &=& 7\frac{5}{12} \\ -3\frac{1}{4} &=& \frac{3}{16} \\ \hline & & 4\frac{2}{12} = 4\frac{1}{6} \end{array}$$

3.
$$\begin{array}{rcl} \frac{1}{2} &=& \frac{4}{8} \\ -\frac{1}{8} &=& \frac{1}{8} \\ \hline & & \frac{3}{8} \end{array}$$

4.
$$\begin{array}{rcl} 3\frac{1}{8} &=& 3\frac{1}{8} = 2\frac{9}{8} \\ -1\frac{3}{4} &=& 1\frac{6}{8} = 1\frac{6}{8} \\ \hline & & 1\frac{3}{8} \end{array}$$

5.
$$\begin{array}{rcl} \frac{7}{9} &=& \frac{14}{18} \\ -\frac{1}{6} &=& \frac{3}{18} \\ \hline & & \frac{11}{18} \end{array}$$

6.
$$\begin{array}{rcl} \frac{17}{20} &=& \frac{17}{20} \\ -\frac{3}{4} &=& \frac{15}{20} \\ \hline & & \frac{2}{20} = \frac{1}{10} \end{array}$$

7.
$$\begin{array}{rcl} 5\frac{3}{8} &=& 5\frac{6}{16} = 4\frac{22}{16} \\ -1\frac{7}{16} &=& 1\frac{7}{16} = 1\frac{7}{16} \\ \hline & & 3\frac{15}{16} \end{array}$$

8.
$$\begin{array}{rcl} \frac{2}{5} &=& \frac{18}{45} \\ -\frac{2}{9} &=& -\frac{10}{45} \\ \hline & & \frac{8}{45} \end{array}$$

9.
$$\begin{array}{rcl} 4\frac{3}{4} &=& 4\frac{9}{12} \\ -2\frac{2}{3} &=& -2\frac{8}{12} \\ \hline & & 2\frac{1}{12} \end{array}$$

10.
$$\begin{array}{rcl} 11\frac{7}{8} &=& 11\frac{7}{8} \\ -1\frac{3}{4} &=& -1\frac{6}{8} \\ \hline & & 10\frac{1}{8} \end{array}$$

Practice Exercise E

1. $\frac{{}^{1}\cancel{2}}{3} \times \frac{1}{\cancel{8}_{4}} = \frac{1}{12}$

2. $\frac{{}^{1}\cancel{2}}{\cancel{3}_{1}} \times \frac{{}^{1}\cancel{3}}{\cancel{12}_{6}} = \frac{1}{6}$

3. $\frac{{}^{1}\cancel{4}}{\cancel{21}_{3}} \times \frac{{}^{1}\cancel{7}}{\cancel{8}_{2}} = \frac{1}{6}$

4. $\frac{{}^{3}\cancel{15}}{16} \times \frac{9}{\cancel{10}_{2}} = \frac{27}{32}$

5. $\frac{{}^{1}\cancel{4}}{\cancel{6}_{3}} \times \frac{{}^{1}\cancel{2}}{\cancel{4}_{1}} = \frac{1}{3}$

6. $3\frac{3}{8} \times \frac{27}{8} = \frac{27}{8} \times \frac{27}{8} = \frac{729}{64} = 11\frac{25}{64}$

7. $\frac{1}{2} \times 8 = \frac{1}{\cancel{2}_{1}} \times \frac{{}^{4}\cancel{8}}{1} = 4$

8. $6\frac{1}{2} \times 5\frac{4}{8} = \frac{13}{2} \times \frac{{}^{11}\cancel{44}}{\cancel{8}_{2}} = \frac{143}{4} = 35\frac{3}{4}$

9. $3\frac{2}{3} \times \frac{3}{4} = \frac{11}{\cancel{3}_{1}} \times \frac{{}^{1}\cancel{3}}{4} = \frac{11}{4} = 2\frac{3}{4}$

10. $9 \times 3\frac{1}{3} = \frac{{}^{3}\cancel{9}}{1} \times \frac{10}{\cancel{3}_{1}} = 30$

Practice Exercise F

1. $2\frac{1}{5} \div 11 = \frac{11}{5} \div \frac{11}{1} = \frac{{}^{1}\cancel{11}}{5} \times \frac{1}{\cancel{11}_{1}} = \frac{1}{5}$

2. $\frac{1}{50} \div \frac{1}{200} = \frac{1}{\cancel{50}_{1}} \times \frac{{}^{4}\cancel{200}}{1} = \frac{4}{1} = 4$

3. $6\frac{3}{5} \div 8\frac{3}{10} = \frac{33}{5} \div \frac{83}{10} = \frac{33}{\cancel{5}_{1}} \times \frac{{}^{2}\cancel{10}}{83} = \frac{66}{83}$

4. $\frac{3}{4} \div \frac{1}{8} = \frac{3}{\cancel{4}_{1}} \times \frac{{}^{2}\cancel{8}}{1} = \frac{6}{1} = 6$

5. $\frac{5}{12} \div \frac{5}{60} = \frac{{}^{1}\cancel{5}}{\cancel{12}_{1}} \times \frac{{}^{5}\cancel{60}}{\cancel{5}_{1}} = \frac{5}{1} = 5$

6. $10\frac{1}{2} \div \frac{1}{3} = \frac{21}{2} \times \frac{3}{1} = \frac{63}{2} = 31\frac{1}{2}$

7. $\frac{1}{60} \div \frac{1}{2} = \frac{1}{\cancel{60}_{30}} \times \frac{{}^{1}\cancel{2}}{1} = \frac{1}{30}$

8. $8 \div \frac{2}{3} = \frac{{}^{4}\cancel{8}}{1} \times \frac{3}{\cancel{2}_{1}} = \frac{12}{1} = 12$

9. $\frac{1}{6} \div \frac{1}{3} = \frac{1}{\cancel{6}_{2}} \times \frac{{}^{1}\cancel{3}}{1} = \frac{1}{2}$

10. $\frac{7}{8} \div \frac{3}{4} = \frac{7}{\cancel{8}_{2}} \times \frac{{}^{1}\cancel{4}}{3} = \frac{7}{6} = 1\frac{1}{6}$

Practice Exercise G

1. $\frac{1}{4} = 4\overline{)1.00}$ = .25

Answer: 0.25

2. $\frac{7}{8} = 8\overline{)7.000}$ = .875

```
   64
   60
   56
   40
   40
    0
```

Answer: 0.87

3. $\frac{5}{6} = 6\overline{)5.00}$ = $.8\bar{3}$

```
   48
   20
   18
    2
```

Answer: 0.83

4. $\frac{5}{125} = 125\overline{)5.00}$ = .04

```
   5 00
     00
```

Answer: 0.04

5.

$$\frac{5}{16} = 16\overline{)5.000}^{\;.3125}$$

$$\begin{array}{r} \underline{48} \\ 20 \\ \underline{18} \\ 2 \end{array}$$

Answer: 0.31

6.

$$\frac{3}{25} = 25\overline{)3.00}^{\;.12}$$

$$\begin{array}{r} \underline{25} \\ 50 \\ \underline{50} \\ 0 \end{array}$$

Answer: 0.12

7.

$$\frac{9}{20} = 20\overline{)9.00}^{\;.45}$$

$$\begin{array}{r} \underline{80} \\ 100 \\ \underline{100} \\ 0 \end{array}$$

Answer: 0.45

8.

$$\frac{1}{75} = 75\overline{)1.000}^{\;.01\bar{3}}$$

$$\begin{array}{r} \underline{75} \\ 250 \\ \underline{225} \\ 0 \end{array}$$

Answer: 0.013

9.

$$\frac{3}{8} = 8\overline{)3.000}^{\;.375}$$

$$\begin{array}{r} \underline{24} \\ 60 \\ \underline{56} \\ 40 \\ \underline{40} \\ \underline{0} \end{array}$$

Answer: 0.37

10.

$$\frac{3}{10} = 10\overline{)3.00}^{\;.30}$$

$$\begin{array}{r} \underline{30} \\ 00 \end{array}$$

Answer: 0.3

Practice Exercise H

1. $0.16 = \frac{16}{100} = \frac{4}{25}$
2. $0.04 = \frac{4}{100} = \frac{1}{25}$
3. $0.125 = \frac{125}{1000} = \frac{1}{8}$
4. $0.06 = \frac{6}{100} = \frac{3}{50}$
5. $0.257 = \frac{257}{1000}$
6. $0.75 = \frac{75}{100} = \frac{3}{4}$
7. $0.250 = \frac{250}{1000} = \frac{1}{4}$
8. $0.525 = \frac{525}{1000} = \frac{21}{40}$
9. $0.2 = \frac{2}{10} = \frac{1}{5}$
10. $4.75 = 4\frac{75}{100} = 4\frac{3}{4}$

Practice Exercise I

1. $\begin{array}{r} 7.2 \\ 3.57 \\ +\ 10.8 \\ \hline 21.57 \end{array}$

2. $\begin{array}{r} 48.3 \\ 18.25 \\ +\ 4.002 \\ \hline 70.522 \end{array}$

3. $\begin{array}{r} 6.3 \\ 0.005 \\ +\ 2.67 \\ \hline 8.975 \end{array}$

4. $\begin{array}{r} 25.4 \\ 37.06 \\ +\ 41.0 \\ \hline 103.46 \end{array}$

5. $\begin{array}{r} 8.50 \\ 19.625 \\ +\ 0.17 \\ \hline 28.295 \end{array}$

6. $\begin{array}{r} 29.042 \\ 2.6 \\ +\ 3.12 \\ \hline 34.762 \end{array}$

7. $\begin{array}{r} 5.4 \\ 8.62 \\ +\ 0.95 \\ \hline 14.97 \end{array}$

8. $\begin{array}{r} 2.246 \\ 16.8 \\ +\ 4.26 \\ \hline 23.306 \end{array}$

9. $\begin{array}{r} 16.1 \\ 1.12 \\ +\ 3.525 \\ \hline 20.745 \end{array}$

10. $\begin{array}{r} 30.7 \\ 4.05 \\ +\ 20.5 \\ \hline 55.25 \end{array}$

Practice Exercise J

1. $\begin{array}{r} 5.67 \\ -\ 3.90 \\ \hline 1.77 \end{array}$

2. $\begin{array}{r} 37.20 \\ -\ 25.37 \\ \hline 11.83 \end{array}$

3. $\begin{array}{r} 17.400 \\ -\ 13.262 \\ \hline 4.138 \end{array}$

4. $\begin{array}{r} 58.940 \\ -\ 27.363 \\ \hline 31.577 \end{array}$

5. $\begin{array}{r} 2.425 \\ -\ 0.675 \\ \hline 1.750 \end{array}$

6. $\begin{array}{r} 15.00 \\ -\ 7.82 \\ \hline 7.18 \end{array}$

7. $\begin{array}{r} 205.60 \\ -\ 105.23 \\ \hline 100.37 \end{array}$

8. $\begin{array}{r} 246.520 \\ -\ 107.988 \\ \hline 138.532 \end{array}$

9. $\begin{array}{r} 35.25 \\ -\ 17.00 \\ \hline 18.25 \end{array}$

10. $\begin{array}{r} 1725.5000 \\ -\ 50.6325 \\ \hline 1674.8675 \end{array}$

Practice Exercise K

1.
$$\begin{array}{r} 5.64 \\ \underline{\times 1.2} \\ 1128 \\ \underline{564} \\ 6.768 \end{array}$$

2.
$$\begin{array}{r} 4.25 \\ \underline{\times 12} \\ 850 \\ \underline{425} \\ 51.00 \end{array}$$

3.
$$\begin{array}{r} 35.6 \\ \underline{\times 2.5} \\ 1780 \\ \underline{712} \\ 89.00 \end{array}$$

4.
$$\begin{array}{r} 4.92 \\ \underline{\times 9.5} \\ 2460 \\ \underline{4428} \\ 46.740 \end{array}$$

5.
$$\begin{array}{r} 51 \\ \underline{\times .92} \\ 102 \\ \underline{459} \\ 46.92 \end{array}$$

6.
$$\begin{array}{r} 28.6 \\ \underline{\times 8.16} \\ 1716 \\ 286 \\ \underline{2288} \\ 233.376 \end{array}$$

7.
$$\begin{array}{r} 50.06 \\ \underline{\times 2.15} \\ 25030 \\ 5006 \\ \underline{10012} \\ 107.6290 \end{array}$$

8.
$$\begin{array}{r} 32.2 \\ \underline{\times 3.15} \\ 1610 \\ 322 \\ \underline{966} \\ 101.430 \end{array}$$

9.
$$\begin{array}{r} 21.0 \\ \underline{\times 41.6} \\ 1260 \\ 210 \\ \underline{840} \\ 873.60 \end{array}$$

10.
$$\begin{array}{r} 8.06 \\ \underline{\times 3.654} \\ 3224 \\ 4030 \\ 4836 \\ \underline{2418} \\ 29.45124 \end{array}$$

Practice Exercise L

1.
$$\begin{array}{r} 40. \\ 2.5\overline{)100.0} \end{array}$$

Answer: 40

2.
$$\begin{array}{r} 3. \\ .3\overline{).9} \end{array}$$

Answer: 3

3.
$$\begin{array}{r} 22.7 \\ 1.7\overline{)38.6} \\ \underline{34} \\ 46 \\ \underline{34} \\ 120 \\ \underline{119} \end{array}$$

Answer: 22.7

4.
```
         76.66
   1.5 )115.000
        105
        100
         90
        100
         90
         100
```

Answer: 76.66

5.
```
        2.2
  2.5 )5.50
       50
        50
        50
```

Answer: 2.2

6.
```
          7.
  4.6 )3.22
       322
         0
```

Answer: 7

7.
```
        3.1
  1.5 )4.65
       4.5
        15
        15
```

Answer: 3.1

8.
```
          2.
  7.5 )15.0
       15 0
          0
```

Answer: 2

9.
```
       .14
  .3 ).042
        3
       12
       12
```

Answer: 0.14

10.
```
         .12
  .05 ).0060
          5
         10
```

Answer: 0.12

Practice Exercise M

1. $\frac{4}{5} = 4 : 5$
2. $\frac{1}{3} = 1 : 3$
3. $\frac{3}{4} = 3 : 4$
4. $\frac{3}{8} = 3 : 8$
5. $\frac{1}{10} = 1 : 10$
6. $\frac{2}{3} = 2 : 3$
7. $\frac{1}{2} = 1 : 2$
8. $\frac{25}{50} = 25 : 50 = 1 : 2$
9. $\frac{3}{9} = 3{:}9 = 1 : 3$
10. $\frac{2}{5} = 2 : 5$

Practice Exercise N

1. $8 : 10 = x : 30$
   $10x = 240$
   $x = 24$
2. $9 : 15 = x : 5$
   $15x = 45$
   $x = 3$
3. $x : 80 = 3 : 12$
   $12x = 240$
   $x = 20$
4. $3 : x = 8 : 24$
   $8x = 72$
   $x = 9$
5. $2 : 3 = x = 63$
   $3x = 126$
   $x = 42$
6. $5 : 15 = x : 60$
   $15x = 300$
   $x = 20$
7. $7 : x = 4 : 28$
   $4x = 196$
   $x = 49$
8. $0.2 : 8 = 25 : x$
   $0.2x = 200$
   $x = 1000$
9. $5 : 7 = x : 28$
   $7x = 140$
   $x = 20$
10. $\frac{1}{10} x : 2000 = 1 : 100$
    $10x = 2000$
    $x = 200$

Practice Exercise O

1. 0.225 = 22.5%
2. 3.45 = 345%
3. 0.7 = 70%
4. 0.14 = 14%
5. 4.5 = 450%
6. $\begin{array}{r} 72 \\ \times .24 \\ \hline 17.28 \end{array}$
7. $\begin{array}{r} 12 \\ \times .05 \\ \hline .60 \end{array}$
8. $\frac{\cancel{225}\,3}{\cancel{300}\,4} = \frac{3}{4} = 4\overline{)3.00} = 75\%$ (quotient .75)
   $\begin{array}{r} 28 \\ \hline 20 \\ 20 \\ \hline 0 \end{array}$
9. $\frac{24}{60} = \frac{2}{5} = 5\overline{)2.0} = 40\%$ (quotient .4)
   $\begin{array}{r} 20 \\ \hline 0 \end{array}$
10. $\frac{135}{45} = 3. = 300\%$

Practice Exercise P

Roman Numerals

1. VIII
2. XV
3. L
4. IV
5. XXIII
6. XLIV
7. XCIII
8. XXXVI
9. LVI
10. XIX
11. XXV
12. C
13. XXXVII
14. VII
15. XVIII
16. DXXVI
17. XCIV
18. XXXIX
19. LXII
20. MCMLXXX

Arabic Numbers

1. 24
2. 17
3. 50
4. 40
5. 5
6. 3
7. 1000
8. 19
9. 30
10. 29
11. 6
12. 70
13. 100
14. 92
15. 69
16. 17
17. 22
18. 11
19. 204
20. 1115

ARITHMETIC TESTS

TEST 1: ARITHMETIC

30 QUESTIONS • TIME—30 MINUTES

Directions: Work out each problem and fill in your answer in the space provided.

Reduce to lowest terms:

1. $\frac{3}{6}$ = ____

2. $\frac{10}{12}$ = ____

3. $\frac{40}{1000}$ = ____

4. $\frac{15}{50}$ = ____

5. $\frac{75}{90}$ = ____

Change to improper fractions:

6. $2\frac{3}{5}$ = ____

7. $10\frac{3}{5}$ = ____

8. $6\frac{5}{6}$ = ____

9. $17\frac{1}{2}$ = ____

10. $9\frac{1}{3}$ = ____

Add:

11. $\frac{2}{3}$
 $\frac{1}{4}$
 $+\ \frac{5}{6}$

12. $\frac{5}{9}$
 $\frac{3}{8}$
 $+\ \frac{1}{4}$

13. $\frac{4}{5}$
 $\frac{3}{8}$
 $+\ \frac{1}{20}$

14. $17\frac{2}{3}$
 $\frac{8}{9}$
 $+\ 2\frac{1}{12}$

15. $1\frac{9}{10}$
 $8\frac{4}{5}$
 $+\ 9\frac{2}{3}$

Subtract:

16. $\frac{7}{8}$
 $-\ \frac{1}{3}$

17. $\frac{11}{18}$
 $-\ \frac{2}{9}$

18. $7\frac{1}{3}$
 $-\ 2\frac{3}{4}$

19. $2\frac{5}{6}$
$- \frac{8}{9}$
____

20. $17\frac{1}{3}$
$- 8\frac{5}{15}$
____

Multiply:

21. $\frac{1}{5} \times \frac{25}{50} =$ ____

22. $\frac{1}{3} \times \frac{3}{4} =$ ____

23. $\frac{7}{10} \times \frac{5}{6} =$ ____

24. $15 \times 2\frac{1}{3} =$ ____

25. $\frac{2}{3} \times \frac{9}{16} =$ ____

Divide:

26. $\frac{1}{2} \div \frac{1}{50} =$ ____

27. $\frac{1}{2} \div 6 =$ ____

28. $2\frac{1}{4} \div 3\frac{1}{2} =$ ____

29. $2\frac{4}{5} \div 7 =$ ____

30. $\frac{1}{2} \div \frac{3}{50} =$ ____

TEST 1: ARITHMETIC ANSWER KEY

1. $\frac{1}{2}$
2. $\frac{5}{6}$
3. $\frac{1}{25}$
4. $\frac{3}{10}$
5. $\frac{5}{6}$
6. $\frac{13}{5}$
7. $\frac{53}{5}$
8. $\frac{41}{6}$
9. $\frac{35}{2}$
10. $\frac{28}{3}$
11. $1\frac{3}{4}$
12. $1\frac{13}{72}$
13. $1\frac{9}{40}$
14. $20\frac{23}{36}$
15. $20\frac{11}{30}$
16. $\frac{13}{24}$
17. $\frac{7}{18}$
18. $4\frac{7}{12}$
19. $1\frac{17}{18}$
20. 9
21. $\frac{1}{10}$
22. $\frac{1}{4}$
23. $\frac{7}{12}$
24. 35
25. $\frac{3}{8}$
26. 25
27. $\frac{1}{12}$
28. $\frac{9}{14}$
29. $\frac{2}{5}$
30. $8\frac{1}{3}$

SOLUTIONS FOR TEST 1: ARITHMETIC

1. $\frac{3}{6} = \frac{1}{2}$

2. $\frac{10}{12} = \frac{5}{6}$

3. $\frac{40}{1000} = \frac{1}{25}$

4. $\frac{15}{50} = \frac{3}{10}$

5. $\frac{75}{90} = \frac{5}{6}$

6. $2\frac{3}{5} = \frac{13}{5}$

7. $10\frac{3}{5} = \frac{53}{5}$

8. $6\frac{5}{6} = \frac{41}{6}$

9. $17\frac{1}{2} = \frac{35}{2}$

10. $9\frac{1}{3} = \frac{28}{3}$

11.
$$\begin{array}{r}
\frac{2}{3} = \frac{8}{12} \\
\frac{1}{4} = \frac{3}{12} \\
\frac{5}{6} = \frac{10}{12} \\
\hline
\frac{21}{12} = 1\frac{9}{12} = 1\frac{3}{4}
\end{array}$$

12.
$$\begin{array}{r}
\frac{5}{9} = \frac{40}{72} \\
\frac{3}{8} = \frac{27}{72} \\
\frac{1}{4} = \frac{85}{72} \\
\hline
\frac{85}{72} = 1\frac{13}{72}
\end{array}$$

13.
$$\begin{array}{r}
\frac{4}{5} = \frac{32}{40} \\
\frac{3}{8} = \frac{15}{40} \\
\frac{1}{20} = \frac{2}{40} \\
\hline
\frac{49}{40} = 1\frac{9}{40}
\end{array}$$

14.
$$\begin{array}{r}
17\frac{2}{3} = 17\frac{24}{36} \\
\frac{8}{9} = \frac{32}{36} \\
2\frac{1}{12} = 2\frac{3}{36} \\
\hline
19\frac{59}{36} = 20\frac{23}{36}
\end{array}$$

15.
$$\begin{array}{r}
1\frac{9}{10} = 1\frac{27}{30} \\
8\frac{4}{5} = 8\frac{24}{30} \\
9\frac{2}{3} = 9\frac{20}{30} \\
\hline
18\frac{71}{30} = 20\frac{11}{30}
\end{array}$$

16.
$$\begin{array}{r}
\frac{7}{8} = \frac{21}{24} \\
-\frac{1}{3} = \frac{8}{24} \\
\hline
\frac{13}{24}
\end{array}$$

17.
$$\begin{array}{r}
\frac{11}{18} = \frac{11}{18} \\
-\frac{2}{9} = \frac{4}{18} \\
\hline
\frac{7}{18}
\end{array}$$

18.
$$\begin{array}{r}
7\frac{1}{3} = 7\frac{4}{12} = 6\frac{16}{12} \\
2\frac{3}{4} = 2\frac{9}{12} = 2\frac{9}{12} \\
\hline
4\frac{7}{12}
\end{array}$$

19.
$$\begin{array}{r}
2\frac{5}{6} = 2\frac{15}{18} = 1\frac{33}{18} \\
\frac{8}{9} = \frac{16}{18} = \frac{16}{18} \\
\hline
1\frac{17}{18}
\end{array}$$

20.
$$\begin{array}{r}
17\frac{1}{3} = 17\frac{5}{15} \\
8\frac{5}{15} = 8\frac{5}{15} \\
\hline
9
\end{array}$$

21. $\frac{1}{5} \times \frac{^{1}\cancel{25}}{\cancel{50}_{2}} = \frac{1}{10}$

22. $\frac{1}{\cancel{3}_{1}} \times \frac{^{1}\cancel{3}}{4} = \frac{1}{4}$

23. $\frac{7}{\cancel{10}_{2}} \times \frac{^{1}\cancel{5}}{6} = \frac{7}{12}$

24. $15 \times 2\frac{1}{3} = \cancel{15}^{5} \times \frac{7}{\cancel{3}_{1}} = \frac{35}{1}$

25. $\frac{^{1}\cancel{2}}{\cancel{3}_{1}} \times \frac{^{3}\cancel{9}}{\cancel{16}_{8}} = \frac{3}{8}$

26. $\frac{1}{2} \div \frac{1}{50} = \frac{1}{_{1}\cancel{2}} \frac{^{25}\cancel{50}}{1} = \frac{25}{1} = 25$

27. $\frac{1}{2} \div 6 = \frac{1}{2} \times \frac{1}{6} = \frac{1}{12}$

28. $2\frac{1}{4} \div 3\frac{1}{2} = \frac{9}{4} \div \frac{7}{2} = \frac{9}{\cancel{4}_{2}} \times \frac{^{1}\cancel{2}}{7} = \frac{9}{14}$

29. $2\frac{4}{5} \div 7 = \frac{14}{5} \div \frac{7}{1} = \frac{^{2}\cancel{14}}{5} \times \frac{1}{\cancel{7}_{1}} = \frac{2}{5}$

30. $\frac{1}{2} \div \frac{3}{50} = \frac{1}{\cancel{2}_{1}} \times \frac{^{25}\cancel{50}}{3} = \frac{25}{3} = 8\frac{1}{3}$

ARITHMETIC TESTS ANSWER SHEET

TEST 2: ARITHMETIC

1. Ⓐ Ⓑ Ⓒ Ⓓ	6. Ⓐ Ⓑ Ⓒ Ⓓ	11. Ⓐ Ⓑ Ⓒ Ⓓ	16. Ⓐ Ⓑ Ⓒ Ⓓ
2. Ⓐ Ⓑ Ⓒ Ⓓ	7. Ⓐ Ⓑ Ⓒ Ⓓ	12. Ⓐ Ⓑ Ⓒ Ⓓ	17. Ⓐ Ⓑ Ⓒ Ⓓ
3. Ⓐ Ⓑ Ⓒ Ⓓ	8. Ⓐ Ⓑ Ⓒ Ⓓ	13. Ⓐ Ⓑ Ⓒ Ⓓ	18. Ⓐ Ⓑ Ⓒ Ⓓ
4. Ⓐ Ⓑ Ⓒ Ⓓ	9. Ⓐ Ⓑ Ⓒ Ⓓ	14. Ⓐ Ⓑ Ⓒ Ⓓ	19. Ⓐ Ⓑ Ⓒ Ⓓ
5. Ⓐ Ⓑ Ⓒ Ⓓ	10. Ⓐ Ⓑ Ⓒ Ⓓ	15. Ⓐ Ⓑ Ⓒ Ⓓ	20. Ⓐ Ⓑ Ⓒ Ⓓ

FINAL ARITHMETIC AND MATHEMATICS TEST

1. Ⓐ Ⓑ Ⓒ Ⓓ	6. Ⓐ Ⓑ Ⓒ Ⓓ	11. Ⓐ Ⓑ Ⓒ Ⓓ	16. Ⓐ Ⓑ Ⓒ Ⓓ
2. Ⓐ Ⓑ Ⓒ Ⓓ	7. Ⓐ Ⓑ Ⓒ Ⓓ	12. Ⓐ Ⓑ Ⓒ Ⓓ	17. Ⓐ Ⓑ Ⓒ Ⓓ
3. Ⓐ Ⓑ Ⓒ Ⓓ	8. Ⓐ Ⓑ Ⓒ Ⓓ	13. Ⓐ Ⓑ Ⓒ Ⓓ	18. Ⓐ Ⓑ Ⓒ Ⓓ
4. Ⓐ Ⓑ Ⓒ Ⓓ	9. Ⓐ Ⓑ Ⓒ Ⓓ	14. Ⓐ Ⓑ Ⓒ Ⓓ	19. Ⓐ Ⓑ Ⓒ Ⓓ
5. Ⓐ Ⓑ Ⓒ Ⓓ	10. Ⓐ Ⓑ Ⓒ Ⓓ	15. Ⓐ Ⓑ Ⓒ Ⓓ	20. Ⓐ Ⓑ Ⓒ Ⓓ

TEST 2: ARITHMETIC

20 QUESTIONS • TIME—20 MINUTES

Directions: Read each question carefully, then decide which choice is the best. Blacken the corresponding space on your answer sheet.

1. $23 + 4.67 + 19.2 + 0.365 =$

   (A) 1047.0
   (B) 47.235
   (C) 1172.4
   (D) 46.235

2. $2.37 \times 0.6 =$

   (A) 14.22
   (B) 1.282
   (C) 1.422
   (D) 12.82

3. The freshman nursing class consists of 40 students. Seven-eighths of the class are women. How many women are in the class?

   (A) 35
   (B) 38
   (C) 21
   (D) 24

4. What percentage of 20 is 12?

   (A) 12 percent
   (B) 60 percent
   (C) 14 percent
   (D) 8 percent

5. What is the value of x in the proportion $1 : 5 : : x : 1500$?

   (A) 5
   (B) $\frac{1}{3}$
   (C) 750,000
   (D) 300

6. Three percent of the 900 students in a school went on a trip. How many students remained in school?

   (A) 27
   (B) 30
   (C) 873
   (D) 773

7. The fraction $\frac{7}{16}$ expressed as a decimal is

   (A) .1120
   (B) .2286
   (C) .4850
   (D) .4375

8. If 30 is divided by .06, the result is

   (A) 5
   (B) 50
   (C) 500
   (D) 5000

9. The sum of 637.894, 8352.16, 4.8673, and 301.5 is, most nearly

   (A) 8989.5
   (B) 9021.35
   (C) 9294.9
   (D) 9296.4

10. The sum of \$82.79, \$103.06, and \$697.85 is

    (A) \$883.70
    (B) \$1628
    (C) \$791
    (D) \$873

11. One percent of \$23,000 is

    (A) \$23
    (B) \$2.30
    (C) \$230
    (D) \$2300

12. If one and one-half pounds of candy are required to fill an Easter basket, how many baskets can be filled with ten and one-half pounds of candy?

    (A) 7.5
    (B) 2.5
    (C) $5\frac{1}{2}$
    (D) 7

13. If one tee shirt costs \$5.60, how many tee shirts can be bought for \$61.60?

    (A) $8\frac{1}{2}$
    (B) 10
    (C) 9
    (D) 11

14. The decimal 410.07 less 38.49 equals

(A) 372.58
(B) 371.58
(C) 381.58
(D) 382.68

15. The fraction $\frac{3}{10}$ written as a decimal is

(A) 0.3
(B) 0.03
(C) 0.003
(D) 0.0003

16. The decimal 12.5 written as a fraction is

(A) $\frac{1}{25}$
(B) $12\frac{1}{2}$
(C) $1\frac{1}{2}$
(D) $\frac{125}{100}$

17. The product of 8.3×80 is

(A) 6.64
(B) 66.4
(C) 664
(D) 6640

18. The fraction equal to 0.0625 is

(A) $\frac{1}{16}$
(B) $\frac{1}{15}$
(C) $\frac{1}{14}$
(D) $\frac{1}{13}$

19. The number 0.03125 equals

(A) $\frac{3}{64}$
(B) $\frac{1}{16}$
(C) $\frac{1}{64}$
(D) $\frac{1}{32}$

20. The quantity 21.70 divided by 1.75 equals

(A) 124
(B) 12.4
(C) 1.24
(D) .124

TEST 2: ARITHMETIC ANSWER KEY

1. **B**	11. **C**
2. **C**	12. **D**
3. **A**	13. **D**
4. **B**	14. **B**
5. **D**	15. **A**
6. **C**	16. **B**
7. **D**	17. **C**
8. **C**	18. **A**
9. **D**	19. **D**
10. **A**	20. **B**

SOLUTIONS FOR TEST 2: ARITHMETIC

1. **(B)**
$$\begin{array}{r} 23.0 \\ 4.67 \\ 19.2 \\ \underline{+\,0.365} \\ 47.235 \end{array}$$

2. **(C)**
$$\begin{array}{r} 2.37 \\ \underline{\times\,0.6} \\ 1.422 \end{array}$$

3. **(A)** $\frac{7}{\cancel{8}_{1}} - \frac{{}^{5}\cancel{40}}{1} = 35$

4. **(B)** $\frac{12}{20} = \frac{3}{5} = .6 = 60\%$
$5x = 355$
$x = 60\%$

5. **(D)** $1{:}5 :: x{:}1500$
$5x = 1500$
$x = 300$

6. **(C)**
$$\begin{array}{r} 900 \\ \underline{\times\,.03} \\ 27.00 \end{array} \qquad \begin{array}{r} 900 \\ \underline{-\,27} \\ 87 \end{array}$$

7. **(D)**
$$\frac{7}{16} = 16\,\overline{)7.0000}^{\;.4375}$$
$$\begin{array}{r} \underline{64} \\ 60 \\ \underline{48} \\ 120 \\ \underline{112} \\ 80 \\ \underline{80} \end{array}$$

8. **(C)**
$$.06\,\overline{)30.00}^{\;500.}$$
$$\begin{array}{r} \underline{30} \\ 00 \end{array}$$

9. **(D)**
$$\begin{array}{r} 637.894 \\ 8352.16 \\ 4.8673 \\ \underline{301.5} \\ 9296.4213 \end{array}$$

10. **(A)**
$$\begin{array}{r} \$\,82.79 \\ 103.06 \\ \underline{+\,697.85} \\ \$883.70 \end{array}$$

11. **(C)** $\begin{array}{r} \$\,23{,}000 \\ \underline{\times\, 0.01} \\ \$230.00 \end{array}$

12. **(D)** $\frac{1.5}{1} = \frac{10.5}{x}$

$1.5x = 10.5$

$x = 7$

13. **(D)** $\begin{array}{r} 11. \\ 5.60\overline{)61.60} \\ \underline{560} \\ 560 \end{array}$

14. **(B)** $\begin{array}{r} 410.07 \\ \underline{-\,38.49} \\ 371.58 \end{array}$

15. **(A)** $\frac{3}{10} = 0.3$

16. **(B)** $12.5 = 12\frac{5}{10} = 12\frac{1}{2}$

17. **(C)** $\begin{array}{r} 8.3 \\ \underline{\times\, 80} \\ 00 \\ \underline{664} \\ 664.0 \end{array}$

18. **(A)** $.0625 = \frac{625}{10{,}000} = \frac{1}{16}$

19. **(D)** $0.03125 = \frac{3125}{100{,}000} = \frac{1}{32}$

20. **(B)** $\begin{array}{r} 12.4 \\ 1.75\overline{)21.700} \\ \underline{17.5} \\ 4.20 \\ \underline{3.50} \\ 700 \\ \underline{700} \end{array}$

B

$\frac{1^{\times 4}}{4^{\times 4}}$ $\frac{4}{16}$

$\frac{3^{\times 2}}{8^{\times 2}}$ $\frac{6}{16}$

$+$ $\frac{7^{\times 1}}{16^{\times 1}}$ $\frac{7}{16}$

16 | 17
16
1

$\frac{17}{16} = 1\frac{1}{16}$

D

25.50
× 0.326
15300
1.5100
7650
8.31300

D

307.401
− 25.246
282.155

14.7560
15.1256
+ 0.07
29.9456

$\frac{\overset{1}{\cancel{15}}}{\underset{1}{\cancel{75}}} = \frac{1}{5}$

15
x3
45

15
x5
75

5X1
5X3

$\frac{5}{15} = 1/3$

FINAL ARITHMETIC AND MATHEMATICS TEST

20 QUESTIONS • TIME—30 MINUTES

Directions: Work out each of the following problems. Blacken the corresponding space on your answer sheet.

1. Add $\frac{1}{4}$, $\frac{3}{8}$, and $\frac{7}{16}$.

   (A) $\frac{11}{16}$
   (B) $1\frac{1}{16}$
   (C) $\frac{11}{28}$
   (D) $\frac{18}{16}$

2. Multiply 25.5 by 0.326.

   (A) 83.13
   (B) 25.826
   (C) 0.2805
   (D) 8.313

3. Subtract 25.246 from 307.401.

   (A) 282.155
   (B) 54.941
   (C) 549.41
   (D) 28.2155

4. 14.75 + 15.1256 + 0.07 =

   (A) 299.46
   (B) 36.8756
   (C) 29.946
   (D) 268.756

5. Divide 36.36 by 0.0606.

   (A) .06
   (B) 0.6
   (C) 60
   (D) 600

6. Write the fraction $\frac{1}{8}$ as a ratio.

   (A) 8:1
   (B) 0.18
   (C) 1:8
   (D) 0.125

7. Solve for x in $2:8 = 11:x$

   (A) 44
   (B) $2\frac{3}{4}$
   (C) $\frac{11}{16}$
   (D) 4.4

8. Change 85 percent to a fraction and reduce to lowest terms.

   (A) $\frac{85}{100}$
   (B) $\frac{17}{20}$
   (C) $\frac{100}{85}$
   (D) $\frac{20}{17}$

9. Change 0.12 to a percent.

   (A) 0.12 percent
   (B) 0.0012 percent
   (C) .12 percent
   (D) 12 percent

10. Subtract $\frac{1}{8}$ from $\frac{1}{6}$.

    (A) $\frac{2}{8}$
    (B) $\frac{3}{24}$
    (C) $\frac{1}{24}$
    (D) $\frac{1}{12}$

11. How many grains of codeine are there in one and one-half tablets of one-eighth grain each?

    (A) $\frac{2}{8}$
    (B) $\frac{3}{16}$
    (C) $\frac{3}{8}$
    (D) $\frac{5}{8}$

12. Mary drank eight ounces of milk from a quart containing 32 ounces of milk. What part of the quart had she consumed?

    (A) $\frac{1}{4}$
    (B) $\frac{1}{8}$
    (C) $\frac{1}{3}$
    (D) $\frac{1}{2}$

13. There are 75 nursing students in the freshman class and 15 are men. What is the ratio of women students to men students?

(A) $\frac{1}{4}$

(B) $\frac{1}{5}$

(C) $\frac{4}{1}$

(D) $\frac{5}{1}$

14. If a recipe calls for five ounces of sugar for every 15 ounces of flour, what part of the mixture will be sugar?

(A) $\frac{1}{2}$

(B) $\frac{1}{5}$

(C) $\frac{1}{3}$

(D) $\frac{1}{4}$

15. If a suit is on sale for $120.00, and the original cost was $150.00, what percentage would you save by buying it on sale?

(A) 40 percent
(B) 30 percent
(C) 10 percent
(D) 20 percent

16. A seamstress bought two and two-thirds yards of wool material and one and three-fourths yards of crepe material. How many yards of material did she buy?

(A) $4\frac{5}{12}$

(B) $4\frac{2}{3}$

(C) $5\frac{1}{4}$

(D) $4\frac{1}{3}$

17. A sack contained ten pounds of potatoes. Mrs. Brown used one and three-fourths pounds for french fries yesterday and two and one-third pounds for a casserole today. How many pounds of potatoes does she have left?

(A) $5\frac{1}{2}$

(B) $5\frac{11}{12}$

(C) $6\frac{2}{3}$

(D) $6\frac{11}{12}$

18. How many ounces is three-eighths of a pound if a pound equals 16 ounces?

(A) 6 ounces
(B) 12 ounces
(C) 8 ounces
(D) 10 ounces

19. If John receives two-fifths of $10.00, how much does he receive?

(A) $2.00
(B) $4.00
(C) $5.00
(D) $3.00

20. If there are 3000 registered voters in Center City and three-fifths of them are Democrats, how many Democrats are there in Center City?

(A) 500
(B) 600
(C) 1800
(D) 1500

FINAL ARITHMETIC AND MATHEMATICS TEST ANSWER KEY

1. **B**
2. **D**
3. **A**
4. **C**
5. **D**
6. **C**
7. **A**
8. **B**
9. **D**
10. **C**
11. **B**
12. **A**
13. **C**
14. **D**
15. **D**
16. **A**
17. **B**
18. **A**
19. **B**
20. **C**

SOLUTIONS FOR FINAL ARITHMETIC AND MATHEMATICS TEST

1. **(B)** $\frac{1}{4} = \frac{4}{16}$

   $\frac{3}{8} = \frac{6}{16}$

   $\frac{7}{16} = \frac{7}{16}$

   $\frac{17}{16} = 1\frac{1}{16}$

2. **(D)**
$$\begin{array}{r} 25.5 \\ \underline{\times .326} \\ 1530 \\ 510 \\ \underline{765} \\ 8.3130 \end{array}$$

3. **(A)**
$$\begin{array}{r} 307.401 \\ \underline{-\ 25.246} \\ 282.155 \end{array}$$

4. **(C)**
$$\begin{array}{l} 14.75 \\ 15.1256 \\ \underline{\ 0.07} \\ 29.9456 = 29.946 \end{array}$$

5. **(D)**
$$\begin{array}{r} 600. \\ 0.0606\overline{)36.3600} \\ \underline{36.36} \\ 00 \end{array}$$

6. **(C)** $\frac{1}{8} = 1 : 8$

7. **(A)** $2 : 8 = 11 : x$

   $2x = 88$

   $x = 44$

8. **(B)** $85\% = 0.85 = \frac{85}{100} = \frac{17}{20}$

9. **(D)** $0.12 = 12\%$

10. **(C)** $\frac{1}{6} = \frac{4}{24}$

    $-\frac{1}{8} = \frac{3}{24}$

    $\frac{1}{24}$

11. **(B)** $1\frac{1}{2} \times \frac{1}{8} = \frac{3}{2} \times \frac{1}{8} = \frac{3}{16}$

12. **(A)** $\frac{8}{32} = \frac{1}{4}$

13. **(C)** $\frac{60 \text{ women}}{15 \text{ men}} = \frac{4}{1}$

14. **(D)** $\frac{5 \text{ oz. sugar}}{20 \text{ oz. total mixture}} = \frac{1}{4}$

15. **(D)**

$$\frac{30}{150} = 150\overline{)30.00} = 20\%$$

$$\begin{array}{r} .20 \\ 150\overline{)30.00} \\ \underline{30\,0} \\ 0\,0 \end{array}$$

16. **(A)**

$$\begin{array}{r} 2\frac{2}{3} = 2\frac{8}{12} \\ \underline{1\frac{3}{4} = 1\frac{9}{12}} \\ 3\frac{17}{12} = 4\frac{5}{12} \end{array}$$

17. **(B)**

$$\begin{array}{r} 1\frac{3}{4} = 1\frac{9}{12} \\ \underline{+\,2\frac{1}{3} = 2\frac{4}{12}} \\ 3\frac{13}{12} = 4\frac{1}{12} \end{array}$$

$$\begin{array}{r} 10 \text{ lbs} \\ \underline{-\,4\frac{1}{12} \text{ lbs}} \\ 5\frac{11}{12} \text{ lbs} \end{array}$$

18. **(A)** $\frac{3}{\cancel{8}_1} \times \frac{^2\cancel{16}}{1} = 6$ ounces

19. **(B)** $\frac{2}{\cancel{5}_1} \times \frac{^2\cancel{10}}{1} = \$4.00$

20. **(C)** $\frac{3}{\cancel{5}_1} \times \frac{^{600}\cancel{3000}}{1} = 1800$ Democrats

UNIT XII: HEALTH AND SCIENCE

The Practical Nurse needs a comprehensive knowledge of the basic concepts of the biological and physical sciences in order to understand normal body structure and functions and to recognize deviations from the normal. In order for the practical nurse to function as a competent health care provider, basic principles of chemistry, physics, microbiology, and pathology must be included in the nursing curriculum. The questions in this section include facts and principles related to:

1. knowledge of the body structure
2. understanding of how the body functions
3. knowledge of principles of nutrition
4. knowledge of factors affecting health

HEALTH AND SCIENCE GLOSSARY

The purpose of this glossary is to acquaint the reader with some of the common terms that are used in body structure and functions.

A

abductor	A muscle that draws a part of the body away from the median line or normal position.
acetabulum	The socket of the hip bone.
adductor	A muscle that pulls a part of the body toward the median line.
adrenal glands	The two small glands that are on the upper part of the kidneys.
adrenalin	A hormone produced by the adrenal glands; a drug containing this hormone used to raise blood pressure.
alimentary canal	The passageway in the body extending from the mouth to the anus.
alveolus	An air cell of a lung; a tooth socket.
anatomy	The science of the structure of plants and animals.
aorta	The main artery of the body.
artery	A blood vessel carrying blood away from the heart to all parts of the body.
atrium	A chamber of the heart.
atrophy	A wasting away or failure of an organ to grow.
auditory	A term referring to the sense of hearing.
axilla	The armpit.

B

backbone	The column of bones (vertebrae) along the center of the back.
bile	A substance produced by the liver and stored in the gallbladder.
brachial	A term referring to the upper part of the forelimb of the vertebrae.
bronchus	Either of the two main branches or tubes extending from the trachea (windpipe).
bursa	A sac or cavity, especially between joints.

C

cardiac	Of or near the heart.
caudal	Near the tail.
cell	The basic unit of protoplasm.
cephalic	Of the head, skull, or cranium.
clavicle	The collarbone.
clonus	A series of muscle spasms.
colon	That part of the large intestine extending from the cecum to the rectum.
conjunctiva	The mucous membrane lining the inner surface of the eyelids and covering the front part of the eyeball.
cornea	The transparent outer coating of the eyeball.
cranium	The skull; especially that part containing the brain.
cutaneous	Of or on the skin; affecting the skin.

D

dactyl	A finger or toe.
dermis	The layer of skin just below the epidermis.
digit	A finger or toe.
duct	A tube through which secretions or excretions pass through the body.
duodenum	The first section of the small intestine, below the stomach.

E

enamel	The hard, white coating of the crowns of teeth.
endothelium	A membrane that lines the heart, blood vessels, and lymphatic vessels.
epidermis	The outermost layer of the skin.
esophagus	The passage for food from the pharynx to the stomach; gullet.
eviscerate	To remove the entrails from; disembowel.
extensor	A muscle that straightens some part of the body.

F

fascia	A thin layer of connective tissue.
femur	The thighbone.
fibrin	A protein formed in the clotting of blood.
flexor	A muscle that bends a part of the body.
foramen	A small opening.

G

ganglion	A mass of nerve cells serving as a center from which nerve impulses are transmitted.
gastric	In or near the stomach.
genitals	The sexual organs.
glottis	The opening between the vocal cords in the larynx.
gullet	The esophagus.

H

hemoglobin The red coloring matter of the red blood cells.

humerus The bone of the upper arm or forelimb, extending from the shoulder to the elbow.

hyoid A U-shaped bone at the base of the tongue.

hypophysis The pituitary gland.

I

ileum The lowest part of the small intestine.

ilium The uppermost part of the three sections of the hipbone.

insulin A secretion of the pancreas that helps the body use sugar.

intestines The lower part of the alimentary canal, extending from the stomach to the anus.

J

jejunum The middle part of the small intestine.

jugular Two large veins in the neck carrying blood from the head to the heart.

K

kidney Either of a pair of organs that separate water and products from the blood and excrete them as urine through the bladder.

L

lacrimal Of, for, or producing tears.

larynx A structure serving as an organ of the voice.

ligament A band of tough tissue connecting bones or holding organs in place.

lumbar Pertaining to the small of the back.

lymph A clear, yellowish fluid found in the lymphatic system of the body.

lymphatic system A system of vessels and nodes that leads from the tissue spaces to large veins entering the heart.

M

mastication The act of chewing.

maxilla The upper jawbone.

membrane A thin, soft layer of tissue that covers or lines an organ or part.

meninges The three membranes that enclose the brain and spinal cord.

meningitis Inflammation of the meninges.

metacarpals The bones in the hand between the wrist and the fingers.

metatarsals The bones in the foot between the ankle and toes.

mucous A membrane lining cavities leading to the outside of the body, such as to the mouth, membrane anus, etc.

mucus The slimy secretion that moistens and protects the mucous membrane.

N

neural Pertaining to the nerves or the nervous system.

nutrition The series or processes by which an organism takes in and assimilates food for promoting growth and repairing tissues.

O

occiput	The back of the skull or head.
ocular	Pertaining to the eye.
olfactory	A term referring to the sense of smell.
ophthalmic	Of or connected with the eyes.
optic nerve	The nerve running from the brain to the eye.
orbit	The eye socket.
osteology	The study of bones.

P

pancreas	The gland that secretes insulin and other digestive juices.
parathyroid	Four small glands embedded in the thyroid gland; their secretions increase the calcium content in the blood.
pathogenic	Disease-producing.
pepsin	An enzyme secreted in the stomach, aiding in the digestion of proteins.
pharynx	The cavity extending from the mouth and nasal passages to the larynx and esophagus; throat.
placenta	The structure through which the fetus is nourished.
protoplasm	The essential living matter of animal and plant cells.
protozoa	A one-celled microscopic animal.
pubis	The bone that makes up the front part of the pelvis.

Q

quadrant	A term referring to four or part of four.
quadruped	A mammal or animal with four feet.

R

radius	The bone of the forearm on the same side as the thumb.
rectum	The lowest segment of the large intestine, ending at the anus.
retina	The innermost coating of the back part of the eyeball.
riboflavin	A factor of the vitamin B complex, found in milk, eggs, liver, fruits, leafy vegetables, etc.

S

scapula	The shoulder blade.
semen	The fluid secreted by the male reproductive organs containing sperm.
sphincter	A round muscle that can open or close a natural opening in the body by expanding and contracting.
sternum	The breastbone.
striated	Streaked with fine lines.

T

tarsals	The bones of the ankle.
tendons	The connective tissue that joins muscles to bones.
thrombin	A substance that aids in the clotting of blood.
thyroid gland	A large ductless gland near the trachea that produces thyroxine, which regulates metabolism.

tibia The inner bone of the leg below the knee; shinbone.

trachea The windpipe; the tube that conveys air from the larynx to the bronchi.

U

ulna The bone of the forearm on the side opposite the thumb.

urea A soluble, crystalline solid, found in urine.

urine A yellowish fluid in mammals, containing urea and other waste products.

V

vagina In female mammals, the canal leading from the vulva to the uterus.

vermiform A small saclike appendage of the large intestine.

viscera The internal organs of the body, such as the heart, lungs, stomach, etc.

vomer A bone forming part of the nasal septum.

Z

zoology The branch of biology dealing with the classification of animals and the study of animal life.

HEALTH AND SCIENCE TESTS ANSWER SHEET

Test 1: Health and Science

1. Ⓐ Ⓑ Ⓒ Ⓓ	11. Ⓐ Ⓑ Ⓒ Ⓓ	21. Ⓐ Ⓑ Ⓒ Ⓓ	31. Ⓐ Ⓑ Ⓒ Ⓓ
2. Ⓐ Ⓑ Ⓒ Ⓓ	12. Ⓐ Ⓑ Ⓒ Ⓓ	22. Ⓐ Ⓑ Ⓒ Ⓓ	32. Ⓐ Ⓑ Ⓒ Ⓓ
3. Ⓐ Ⓑ Ⓒ Ⓓ	13. Ⓐ Ⓑ Ⓒ Ⓓ	23. Ⓐ Ⓑ Ⓒ Ⓓ	33. Ⓐ Ⓑ Ⓒ Ⓓ
4. Ⓐ Ⓑ Ⓒ Ⓓ	14. Ⓐ Ⓑ Ⓒ Ⓓ	24. Ⓐ Ⓑ Ⓒ Ⓓ	34. Ⓐ Ⓑ Ⓒ Ⓓ
5. Ⓐ Ⓑ Ⓒ Ⓓ	15. Ⓐ Ⓑ Ⓒ Ⓓ	25. Ⓐ Ⓑ Ⓒ Ⓓ	35. Ⓐ Ⓑ Ⓒ Ⓓ
6. Ⓐ Ⓑ Ⓒ Ⓓ	16. Ⓐ Ⓑ Ⓒ Ⓓ	26. Ⓐ Ⓑ Ⓒ Ⓓ	36. Ⓐ Ⓑ Ⓒ Ⓓ
7. Ⓐ Ⓑ Ⓒ Ⓓ	17. Ⓐ Ⓑ Ⓒ Ⓓ	27. Ⓐ Ⓑ Ⓒ Ⓓ	37. Ⓐ Ⓑ Ⓒ Ⓓ
8. Ⓐ Ⓑ Ⓒ Ⓓ	18. Ⓐ Ⓑ Ⓒ Ⓓ	28. Ⓐ Ⓑ Ⓒ Ⓓ	38. Ⓐ Ⓑ Ⓒ Ⓓ
9. Ⓐ Ⓑ Ⓒ Ⓓ	19. Ⓐ Ⓑ Ⓒ Ⓓ	29. Ⓐ Ⓑ Ⓒ Ⓓ	39. Ⓐ Ⓑ Ⓒ Ⓓ
10. Ⓐ Ⓑ Ⓒ Ⓓ	20. Ⓐ Ⓑ Ⓒ Ⓓ	30. Ⓐ Ⓑ Ⓒ Ⓓ	40. Ⓐ Ⓑ Ⓒ Ⓓ

Test 2: Health and Science

1. Ⓐ Ⓑ Ⓒ Ⓓ	9. Ⓐ Ⓑ Ⓒ Ⓓ	17. Ⓐ Ⓑ Ⓒ Ⓓ	25. Ⓐ Ⓑ Ⓒ Ⓓ
2. Ⓐ Ⓑ Ⓒ Ⓓ	10. Ⓐ Ⓑ Ⓒ Ⓓ	18. Ⓐ Ⓑ Ⓒ Ⓓ	26. Ⓐ Ⓑ Ⓒ Ⓓ
3. Ⓐ Ⓑ Ⓒ Ⓓ	11. Ⓐ Ⓑ Ⓒ Ⓓ	19. Ⓐ Ⓑ Ⓒ Ⓓ	27. Ⓐ Ⓑ Ⓒ Ⓓ
4. Ⓐ Ⓑ Ⓒ Ⓓ	12. Ⓐ Ⓑ Ⓒ Ⓓ	20. Ⓐ Ⓑ Ⓒ Ⓓ	28. Ⓐ Ⓑ Ⓒ Ⓓ
5. Ⓐ Ⓑ Ⓒ Ⓓ	13. Ⓐ Ⓑ Ⓒ Ⓓ	21. Ⓐ Ⓑ Ⓒ Ⓓ	29. Ⓐ Ⓑ Ⓒ Ⓓ
6. Ⓐ Ⓑ Ⓒ Ⓓ	14. Ⓐ Ⓑ Ⓒ Ⓓ	22. Ⓐ Ⓑ Ⓒ Ⓓ	30. Ⓐ Ⓑ Ⓒ Ⓓ
7. Ⓐ Ⓑ Ⓒ Ⓓ	15. Ⓐ Ⓑ Ⓒ Ⓓ	23. Ⓐ Ⓑ Ⓒ Ⓓ	
8. Ⓐ Ⓑ Ⓒ Ⓓ	16. Ⓐ Ⓑ Ⓒ Ⓓ	24. Ⓐ Ⓑ Ⓒ Ⓓ	

Test 3: Health and Science

1. Ⓐ Ⓑ Ⓒ Ⓓ	9. Ⓐ Ⓑ Ⓒ Ⓓ	17. Ⓐ Ⓑ Ⓒ Ⓓ	25. Ⓐ Ⓑ Ⓒ Ⓓ
2. Ⓐ Ⓑ Ⓒ Ⓓ	10. Ⓐ Ⓑ Ⓒ Ⓓ	18. Ⓐ Ⓑ Ⓒ Ⓓ	26. Ⓐ Ⓑ Ⓒ Ⓓ
3. Ⓐ Ⓑ Ⓒ Ⓓ	11. Ⓐ Ⓑ Ⓒ Ⓓ	19. Ⓐ Ⓑ Ⓒ Ⓓ	27. Ⓐ Ⓑ Ⓒ Ⓓ
4. Ⓐ Ⓑ Ⓒ Ⓓ	12. Ⓐ Ⓑ Ⓒ Ⓓ	20. Ⓐ Ⓑ Ⓒ Ⓓ	28. Ⓐ Ⓑ Ⓒ Ⓓ
5. Ⓐ Ⓑ Ⓒ Ⓓ	13. Ⓐ Ⓑ Ⓒ Ⓓ	21. Ⓐ Ⓑ Ⓒ Ⓓ	29. Ⓐ Ⓑ Ⓒ Ⓓ
6. Ⓐ Ⓑ Ⓒ Ⓓ	14. Ⓐ Ⓑ Ⓒ Ⓓ	22. Ⓐ Ⓑ Ⓒ Ⓓ	30. Ⓐ Ⓑ Ⓒ Ⓓ
7. Ⓐ Ⓑ Ⓒ Ⓓ	15. Ⓐ Ⓑ Ⓒ Ⓓ	23. Ⓐ Ⓑ Ⓒ Ⓓ	
8. Ⓐ Ⓑ Ⓒ Ⓓ	16. Ⓐ Ⓑ Ⓒ Ⓓ	24. Ⓐ Ⓑ Ⓒ Ⓓ	

HEALTH AND SCIENCE TESTS

TEST 1: HEALTH AND SCIENCE

40 QUESTIONS • TIME—35 MINUTES

Directions: Each question or incomplete statement below is followed by four suggested answers or completions, lettered A, B, C, and D. For each question select the best of the four choices and blacken the corresponding space on your answer sheet.

1. Muscles whose functions are to close off body openings are

   (A) flexors
   (B) sphincters
   (C) extensors
   (D) adductors

2. Bile aids in the digestion of

   (A) amino acids
   (B) fats
   (C) starches
   (D) carbohydrates

3. Urea is removed from the blood as it goes through the

   (A) bladder
   (B) pancreas
   (C) spleen
   (D) kidney

4. The blood group of a universal recipient is

   (A) AB
   (B) B
   (C) O
   (D) A

5. The stimulant in coffee is

   (A) tannic acid
   (B) theobromine
   (C) theophylline
   (D) caffeine

6. Which of the following foods is the most economical source of proteins?

   (A) dried milk
   (B) green leafy vegetables
   (C) meats
   (D) eggs

7. Connective tissue that attaches muscles to the bones is called

   (A) tendons
   (B) ligaments
   (C) cartilage
   (D) osseous

8. The hormone produced by the testes is

   (A) progesterone
   (B) estrogen
   (C) testosterone
   (D) aldosterone

9. The elbow joint is an example of

   (A) ball-and-socket joint
   (B) hinge joint
   (C) pivot joint
   (D) saddle joint

10. The movement that propels food down the digestive tract is called

    (A) pyloraspasm
    (B) rugae
    (C) mastication
    (D) peristalsis

11. In mumps, the gland affected is the

    (A) parathyroid
    (B) pituitary
    (C) parotid
    (D) pineal

12. The negative charged particle found within the atom is the

    (A) proton
    (B) electron
    (C) nucleus
    (D) neutron

13. The exchange of nutrients and waste products occurs in the

    (A) venules
    (B) capillaries
    (C) arterioles
    (D) arteries

14. Hemoglobin is found in

    (A) basophils
    (B) neutrophils
    (C) monocytes
    (D) erythrocytes

15. Organic substances made up of several amino acids bound together are

    (A) carbohydrates
    (B) fats
    (C) proteins
    (D) fatty acids

16. The exchange of carbon dioxide and oxygen in the lungs occurs in the

    (A) venules
    (B) alveoli
    (C) bronchi
    (D) bronchioles

17. The pacemaker of the heart is the

    (A) Bundle of His
    (B) AV node
    (C) purkinje fibers
    (D) SA node

18. Mitral stenosis involves the

    (A) aortic valve
    (B) pulmonary valve
    (C) bicuspid valve
    (D) tricuspid valve

19. The smallest known microorganisms are

    (A) bacteria
    (B) viruses
    (C) fungi
    (D) protozoa

20. Which one of the following arteries carries deoxygenated blood?

    (A) pulmonary
    (B) coronary
    (C) vena cava
    (D) aorta

21. Electrolyte balance is maintained primarily by the action of the

    (A) testes
    (B) kidney
    (C) bladder
    (D) liver

22. The mineral that is necessary for the proper functioning of the thyroid gland is

    (A) sodium
    (B) iodine
    (C) calcium
    (D) iron

23. Vitamin C prevents

    (A) beriberi
    (B) rickets
    (C) pellagra
    (D) scurvy

24. The function of leukocytes is to

    (A) carry oxygen
    (B) destroy bacteria
    (C) carry food
    (D) regulate metabolism

25. Insulin is produced in the

    (A) pituitary gland
    (B) thymus
    (C) pancreas
    (D) pineal gland

26. The end product of protein metabolism is

    (A) amino acids
    (B) glucose
    (C) glycogen
    (D) fatty acids

27. Carbohydrates are absorbed into the blood as

    (A) glycogen
    (B) amino acids
    (C) glucose
    (D) fatty acids

28. When one muscle of a pair contracts, the opposing muscle must

    (A) also contract
    (B) relax
    (C) produce more energy
    (D) remain in the same position

29. The respiratory center is located in the part of the brain known as the

    (A) thalamus
    (B) cerebrum
    (C) pons
    (D) medulla oblongata

30. Rays pass through various parts of the eye in a process of bending called

    (A) refraction
    (B) reflexion
    (C) retraction
    (D) retroversion

31. The part of the eye commonly called the "window" is

    (A) retina
    (B) cornea
    (C) lens
    (D) pupil

32. A calorie is a form of

    (A) light
    (B) heat
    (C) darkness
    (D) sound

33. The vitamin known as the "sunshine" vitamin is

    (A) vitamin E
    (B) vitamin B
    (C) vitamin K
    (D) vitamin D

34. The process by which the body changes food into substances that can be readily used by the body is

    (A) digestion
    (B) deglutition
    (C) micturition
    (D) absorption

35. The thyroid gland cannot function properly without

    (A) chloride
    (B) iodine
    (C) phosphorous
    (D) iron

36. The vitamin that is necessary for coagulation of the blood is

    (A) vitamin K
    (B) vitamin C
    (C) vitamin A
    (D) vitamin E

37. Another name for vitamin B1 is

    (A) niacin
    (B) thiamin
    (C) riboflavin
    (D) pyridoxine

38. Food is moved through the alimentary canal by wave-like motions called

    (A) excretions
    (B) mastication
    (C) contractions
    (D) peristalsis

39. The femur is a bone located in the

    (A) forearm
    (B) upper arm
    (C) thigh
    (D) lower leg

40. The liquid portion of the blood is called

    (A) serum
    (B) gamma globulin
    (C) plasma
    (D) lymph

TEST 1: HEALTH AND SCIENCE ANSWER KEY

1. **B**	11. **C**	21. **B**	31. **B**
2. **B**	12. **B**	22. **B**	32. **B**
3. **D**	13. **B**	23. **D**	33. **D**
4. **A**	14. **D**	24. **B**	34. **A**
5. **D**	15. **C**	25. **C**	35. **B**
6. **A**	16. **B**	26. **A**	36. **A**
7. **A**	17. **D**	27. **C**	37. **B**
8. **C**	18. **C**	28. **B**	38. **D**
9. **B**	19. **B**	29. **D**	39. **C**
10. **D**	20. **A**	30. **A**	40. **C**

TEST 1: HEALTH AND SCIENCE EXPLANATORY ANSWERS

1. **(B)** Sphincters are circular muscles that contract when stimulated, closing an opening.
2. **(B)** Bile is released into the duodenum and breaks down the undigested fats into small droplets.
3. **(D)** Urea is filtered from the blood by the kidneys and excreted in urine.
4. **(A)** Group AB blood contains both group A and B antigens and neither A nor B antibodies; therefore, it cannot clump any donor red cells containing A and B antigens.
5. **(D)** Caffeine is a stimulant found in coffee.
6. **(A)** Dried milk is an inexpensive but good source of protein.
7. **(A)** Tendons are connective tissue made of dense fibers in the shape of a cord and have great strength.
8. **(C)** Testosterone is the hormone that regulates male sex characteristics.
9. **(B)** Hinge joints allow movement in two directions only.
10. **(D)** Peristalsis is the progressive, wavelike movement that occurs involuntarily to force food forward.
11. **(C)** The parotid gland is a large salivary gland and is affected by mumps.
12. **(B)** The electron is the unit of negative electricity.
13. **(B)** Capillaries connect arterioles with venules and function as exchange vessels.
14. **(D)** Erythrocytes (red blood cells) contain hemoglobin.
15. **(C)** Proteins are nutrients essential for growth and repair of tissue.
16. **(B)** The diffusion of gas occurs across the thin, squamous epithelium lining of the alveoli.
17. **(D)** The SA node, located in the right atrium, starts each heart beat.
18. **(C)** The mitral valve located between the left atrium and left ventricle of the heart is also called the bicuspid valve.
19. **(B)** Viruses are so small that they can be seen only through special electron microscopes.
20. **(A)** The pulmonary artery carries deoxygenated blood from the heart.
21. **(B)** When water intake is excessive, the kidneys excrete generous amounts of urine; if water intake is lost, they produce less urine; the process is regulated by hormones.
22. **(B)** Iodine makes up about 65 percent of thyroxine, a hormone secreted by the thyroid gland.
23. **(D)** Scurvy is a disease caused by a deficiency of vitamin C.
24. **(B)** Leukocytes (white blood cells) destroy bacteria when there is an infection in the body.
25. **(C)** The islets of Langerhans are located in the pancreas and produce insulin.
26. **(A)** Gastric and intestinal enzymes gradually break down the protein molecule into its separate amino acids.
27. **(C)** Glucose is the end product of carbohydrate digestion.
28. **(B)** When one muscle contracts, the opposing muscle must relax; in this way movements are coordinated and normal functions are carried out.
29. **(D)** The medulla oblongata is located between the pons and the spinal cord, and the vital centers are located in it.
30. **(A)** Rays pass through a series of transparent colorless eye parts. On the way, they undergo a process of bending called refraction which makes it possible for light from a large area to focus on the retina.
31. **(B)** The cornea is referred to frequently as the "window" of the eye.

32. **(B)** A calorie is the unit of measure of heat[md]the amount of heat required to raise the temperature of one kilogram of water by 1°C.

33. **(D)** Vitamin D is referred to as the "sunshine" vitamin because it is formed in the body by the action of the sunshine on the cholesterol products in the skin.

34. **(A)** Digestion is the process whereby the enzymes in the body change food into simple substances that can be readily used by the body.

35. **(B)** The thyroid gland needs iodine for the formation of thyroxine.

36. **(A)** Vitamin K helps the liver to produce substances necessary for the clotting of blood.

37. **(B)** Thiamine is another name for vitamin B_1.

38. **(D)** Peristalsis is a wave-like progression of muscular contractions that moves food through the alimentary canal.

39. **(C)** The thigh bone is the femur. It is the longest and strongest bone in the body.

40. **(C)** Plasma is the liquid portion of the blood in which corpuscles are suspended.

TEST 2: HEALTH AND SCIENCE

30 QUESTIONS • TIME—25 MINUTES

Directions: For each question in this test, choose the answer that you consider correct or most nearly correct. Blacken the appropriate space on your answer sheet.

1. The force of the blood exerted against the wall of the blood vessel is called

   (A) pulse deficit
   (B) apical pulse
   (C) blood pressure
   (D) pulse pressure

2. The relative amount of moisture in the air is the

   (A) evaporation factor
   (B) temperature
   (C) dew
   (D) humidity

3. A laboratory sample is called a(n)

   (A) collection
   (B) agar
   (C) specimen
   (D) symptom

4. Defecation means

   (A) swallowing
   (B) eliminating solid waste
   (C) irrigating the colon
   (D) relieving flatus

5. An object completely free of all microorganisms is

   (A) sterile
   (B) clean
   (C) septic
   (D) contaminated

6. Carbon dioxide is a

   (A) respiratory depressant
   (B) circulatory stimulant
   (C) respiratory stimulant
   (D) circulatory depressant

7. The presence of protein in the urine is called

   (A) polyuria
   (B) anuria
   (C) albuminuria
   (D) hematuria

8. The substance basic to life is

   (A) carbohydrates
   (B) proteins
   (C) starches
   (D) fats

9. In diseases of the gallbladder, which of the following nutrients is limited?

   (A) starches
   (B) proteins
   (C) fats
   (D) carbohydrates

10. Water soluble vitamins include

    (A) vitamin A
    (B) vitamin C
    (C) vitamin D
    (D) vitamin K

11. Diets in the United States are most often deficient in

    (A) iron and calcium
    (B) calcium and potassium
    (C) iodine and sodium
    (D) phosphorous and iron

12. Tetany may be corrected by increasing the amount of

    (A) iron
    (B) iodine
    (C) calcium
    (D) thiamine

13. Which helps conserve body heat?

    (A) increased sweat production
    (B) increased respiratory activity
    (C) dilation of the capillaries of the skin
    (D) constriction of the capillaries of the skin

14. Milk is not a "perfect food" because it lacks

    (A) iron
    (B) calcium
    (C) phosphorous
    (D) carbohydrates

15. The body obtains most of its nitrogen from

(A) carbohydrates
(B) proteins
(C) fats
(D) cellulose

16. An ion is

(A) one molecule of water
(B) one particle of hydrogen
(C) the same as a neutron
(D) an atom with an electric charge

17. The basic unit of the living organism is

(A) the brain
(B) the cell
(C) a tissue
(D) the nervous system

18. The diffusion of water through a semipermeable membrane is known as

(A) anabolism
(B) synthesis
(C) mitosis
(D) osmosis

19. A physician who specializes in diseases of the heart is known as a

(A) dermatologist
(B) cardiologist
(C) pediatrician
(D) neurologist

20. A fracture that occurs without breaking through the skin is called

(A) complex
(B) compound
(C) greenstick
(D) comminuted

21. Smoking and pollution have a deadly effect upon the lungs and pulmonary function. These are classified as

(A) environmental factors
(B) biological factors
(C) sociological factors
(D) physiological factors

22. In the digestive process, almost all of the water is reabsorbed by the

(A) sigmoid
(B) cecum
(C) colon
(D) rectum

23. In what structure does fertilization normally occur?

(A) vagina
(B) cervix
(C) ovary
(D) fallopian tube

24. The process in which carbon dioxide and water is combined under the influence of light in green plants is called

(A) respiration
(B) fermentation
(C) assimilation
(D) photosynthesis

25. The most abundant gas in the atmosphere is

(A) oxygen
(B) nitrogen
(C) carbon dioxide
(D) chlorine

26. A protein substance that initiates and accelerates a chemical reaction is called a(n)

(A) gene
(B) enzyme
(C) hormone
(D) base

27. Amino acids that cannot be manufactured by the body are called

(A) essential amino acids
(B) synthetic amino acids
(C) basic amino acids
(D) dependent amino acids

28. The instrument used to measure air pressure is called a

(A) thermometer
(B) hydrometer
(C) barometer
(D) sphygmomanometer

29. An elevation above normal body temperature is called

    (A) hypothermia
    (B) pyrexia
    (C) intermittent
    (D) remittent

30. The instrument used to examine the ears is called the

    (A) ophthalmoscope
    (B) stethoscope
    (C) cystoscope
    (D) otoscope

TEST 2: HEALTH AND SCIENCE ANSWER KEY

1. **C**
2. **D**
3. **C**
4. **B**
5. **A**
6. **C**
7. **C**
8. **B**
9. **C**
10. **B**
11. **A**
12. **C**
13. **D**
14. **A**
15. **B**
16. **D**
17. **B**
18. **D**
19. **B**
20. **C**
21. **A**
22. **C**
23. **D**
24. **D**
25. **B**
26. **B**
27. **A**
28. **C**
29. **B**
30. **D**

TEST 2: HEALTH AND SCIENCE EXPLANATORY ANSWERS

1. **(C)** Blood pressure is the force of the blood exerted against the wall of the blood vessel.
2. **(D)** Relative humidity refers to the amount of moisture in the air in relation to the temperature.
3. **(C)** Specimen is a laboratory sample used to help the physician make a diagnosis.
4. **(B)** Defecation means the act of having a bowel movement or removing solid waste materials from the body.
5. **(A)** Sterile means that an object is completely free of all microorganisms. Steam under pressure (autoclave) will give complete sterilization.
6. **(C)** Carbon dioxide stimulates the respiratory center in the brain (medulla oblongata).
7. **(C)** Protein substance in the urine is called albuminuria. It results from the failure of the kidneys to filter.
8. **(B)** Protein is the body's vital building material that makes up the basic structure of all cells.
9. **(C)** The gallbladder stores and concentrates bile, which is used to break down fats into droplets and aids in the absorption of fatty acids and glyceral. Therefore, fats are restricted when there are diseases of the gallbladder.
10. **(B)** Water-soluble vitamins include vitamin C and vitamin B complex.
11. **(A)** Iron and calcium are the minerals most often deficient in the American diet.
12. **(C)** Tetany, which is due to lack of calcium, may be corrected by increasing milk or milk products, which are rich in calcium salts. Drugs containing high amounts of calcium may be given intravenously in emergencies.
13. **(D)** Constriction of the blood vessels prevents loss of heat from the blood through the skin.
14. **(A)** Milk contains only about 0.1 milligram of iron per cup. The recommended daily amount is 15–18 milligrams.
15. **(B)** Food proteins supply our bodies with nitrogen to replace that lost in urine, feces. and perspiration.
16. **(D)** The electrical charge results when a neutral atom or group of atoms loses or gains one or more electrons during chemical reactions.
17. **(B)** The cell is the unit of structure and function of all living things. The simplest organisms consist of one cell only.
18. **(D)** Osmosis is the diffusion of water through a semipermeable membrane from a region of greater concentration of water to a region of lesser concentration.
19. **(B)** From the word *cardiology,* meaning the study of the heart's physiology and pathology.
20. **(C)** Greenstick fractures are incomplete fractures with a longitudinal split of the shaft. They usually occur in long bones of children.
21. **(A)** Environmental factors are the relationships of living things to their surroundings.
22. **(C)** The fluid-like residue of digestion found in the colon contains valuable water, which is absorbed into the blood stream.
23. **(D)** After ovulation the egg travels into the fallopian tube. If sperms are present, the union of the sperm and the egg (fertilization) takes place in the fallopian tube.
24. **(D)** Photosynthesis is the process by which certain living plant cells combine carbon dioxide and water, in the presence of chlorophyll and light energy, to form carbohydrates and release oxygen as a waste product.
25. **(B)** The atmosphere is composed of about 78 percent nitrogen.
26. **(B)** Enzymes are protein substances that act as biochemical catalysts. They affect the rate at which a specific reaction occurs.
27. **(A)** Essential amino acids are those that cannot be manufactured by the body and, therefore, must be included in the daily diet.
28. **(C)** The barometer is an instrument used to measure air pressure. It is used in forecasting weather.

29. **(B)** An elevation of body temperature above normal is referred to as fever or pyrexia.

30. **(D)** The otoscope is a lighted instrument used to examine the ear canal, eustachian tube, eardrum, and the middle ear.

TEST 3: HEALTH AND SCIENCE

30 QUESTIONS • TIME—25 MINUTES

Directions: For each question in this test, choose the answer that you consider correct. Blacken the appropriate space on your answer sheet.

1. The body's continual response to changes in the external and internal environment is called

   (A) homeostasis
   (B) diffusion
   (C) osmosis
   (D) filtration

2. The ability of a cell to reproduce is called

   (A) osmosis
   (B) crenation
   (C) lysis
   (D) mitosis

3. The immunity that occurs when a person is given a substance containing antibodies or antitoxins is called

   (A) active
   (B) autoimmune
   (C) passive
   (D) permanent

4. The part of the cell necessary for reproduction is the

   (A) cytoplasm
   (B) nucleus
   (C) protoplasm
   (D) cytoplasmic membrane

5. The hormone that regulates the metabolic rate of the body cells is

   (A) oxytocin
   (B) aldosterone
   (C) thyroxin
   (D) cortisone

6. The sudoriferous glands secrete

   (A) sebum
   (B) perspiration
   (C) hormones
   (D) synovial fluid

7. Tanning of the skin is due to

   (A) keratin
   (B) sebum
   (C) sweat
   (D) melanin

8. The ovaries produce the hormones

   (A) estrogen and testosterone
   (B) progesterone and testosterone
   (C) estrogen and progesterone
   (D) progesterone and prolactin

9. The tissue that forms a protective covering for the body and lines the intestinal and respiratory tract is called the

   (A) periosteum
   (B) pericardium
   (C) epithelium
   (D) connective tissue

10. The hip joint is an example of a

    (A) ball and socket joint
    (B) hinge joint
    (C) pivot joint
    (D) saddle joint

11. The endocrine gland that prepares the body for the "fight or flight" response is the

    (A) adrenal cortex
    (B) adrenal medulla
    (C) pituitary
    (D) thyroid

12. Tears drain into the nose through the

    (A) ciliary body
    (B) lacrimal gland
    (C) eustachian tube
    (D) nasolacrimal duct

13. Respiration and heart rate are controlled by the

    (A) cerebellum
    (B) cerebrum
    (C) medulla oblongota
    (D) pons

14. The main function of the large intestine is to

    (A) absorb digested food
    (B) absorb water from waste materials
    (C) produce digestive enzymes
    (D) secrete digestive enzymes

15. The hormone produced by the adrenal glands is

    (A) progesterone
    (B) estrogen
    (C) testosterone
    (D) aldosterone

16. The sloughing off of the endometrium is called

    (A) menarche
    (B) menopause
    (C) menstruation
    (D) myometritis

17. The dorsal cavity has two subdivisions, namely

    (A) thoracic and abdominopelvic
    (B) cranial and spinal
    (C) thoracic and spinal
    (D) medial and lateral

18. The chamber of the heart that receives venous blood from body tissue is the

    (A) right atrium
    (B) left atrium
    (C) right ventricle
    (D) left ventricle

19. The major work of the heart is completed by the

    (A) right ventricle
    (B) left ventricle
    (C) right atrium
    (D) left atrium

20. The shape of the eyeball is maintained by the

    (A) aqueous humor
    (B) vitreous humor
    (C) eye muscles
    (D) eyelid

21. The inner lining of the heart is the

    (A) endocardium
    (B) myocardium
    (C) pericardium
    (D) pleura

22. The muscular structure that forms the floor of the pelvis is the

    (A) peritoneum
    (B) perineum
    (C) mons pubis
    (D) rectus abdominis

23. The large, round portion at the upper and lateral portion of the femur most often involved in hip fractures is the

    (A) acetabulum
    (B) acromiom
    (C) greater trochanter
    (D) tricuspid valve

24. One of the large muscles that is used in climbing stairs and that forms most of the buttocks is the

    (A) gluteus maximus
    (B) gluteus medius
    (C) vastus lateralis
    (D) vastus medialis

25. The basic unit of function of the kidney is the

    (A) medulla
    (B) hilus
    (C) nephron
    (D) cortex

26. Which of the following is abnormal for urine?

    (A) clear, amber liquid
    (B) nitrogenous waste products
    (C) slightly aromatic
    (D) high specific gravity

27. The hormone that regulates blood composition and blood volume by acting on the kidney is

    (A) antidiuretic (ADH)
    (B) aldosterone
    (C) parathormone
    (D) oxytocin

28. Composition of urine normally includes

    (A) creatinine, urea, water
    (B) creatinine, ammonia, sugar
    (C) nitrogen wastes, sugar, hormones
    (D) nitrogen wastes, water, pus cells

29. An injury to the left motor area of the cerebrum would cause paralysis of

    (A) the right side of the body
    (B) the left side of the body
    (C) both arms and legs
    (D) both arms

30. Electrolyte balance is maintained chiefly by the action of the

    (A) bladder
    (B) kidney
    (C) islets of Langerhans
    (D) gonads

TEST 3: HEALTH AND SCIENCE ANSWER KEY

1. **A**	11. **B**	21. **A**
2. **D**	12. **D**	22. **B**
3. **C**	13. **C**	23. **C**
4. **B**	14. **B**	24. **A**
5. **C**	15. **D**	25. **C**
6. **B**	16. **C**	26. **D**
7. **D**	17. **B**	27. **B**
8. **C**	18. **A**	28. **A**
9. **C**	19. **B**	29. **A**
10. **A**	20. **B**	30. **B**

TEST 3: HEALTH AND SCIENCE EXPLANATORY ANSWERS

1. **(A)** The body is constantly stabilizing and equalizing its environment to prevent any sudden or severe changes.
2. **(D)** The DNA molecules in the nucleus of a cell duplicate themselves and the cell divides, forming two cells.
3. **(C)** In acquiring passive immunity the body of the recipient plays an active part in response to an antigen.
4. **(B)** The functional unit is suspended near the center of the cell and has the property of division.
5. **(C)** Produced by the thyroid gland, thyroxin controls the rate at which glucose is burned and converts it to heat and energy.
6. **(B)** Sweat glands are distributed in the skin and produce perspiration, primarily water.
7. **(D)** Melanin, a brown pigment, increases when exposed to sun.
8. **(C)** Estrogen and progesterone promote development of female sex characteristics and regulate menstruation.
9. **(C)** Epithelial tissue has many forms—flat and irregular, square, long and narrow—that are arranged in single or many layers to form a protective covering and lining.
10. **(A)** The ball-shaped head of the femur fits into the concave socket of the hipbone and allows for a wide range of motion.
11. **(B)** Adrenaline is released from the adrenal medulla to prepare the body for emergency situations.
12. **(D)** A small opening into the nose at the inner corner of the eye allows the fluid to drain through.
13. **(C)** Many gray-matter areas that form the cranial nerves are located in the medulla oblongota and are involved in the control of vital activities.
14. **(B)** As peristalsis moves content along, water is absorbed through the walls into the circulation, and the remaining cellulose passes on to the rectum.
15. **(D)** Aldosterone is the hormone released from the adrenal cortex that helps regulate sodium and potassium balance.
16. **(C)** The shedding of the lining of the uterus occurs if the egg has not been fertilized by the sperm.
17. **(B)** Dorsal pertains to the back; the cranial and spinal cavities contain the brain and the spinal cord.
18. **(A)** Deoxygenated blood returns from the body tissues via the superior and inferior vena cava into the right atrium.
19. **(B)** The left ventricle has the major responsibility for pumping blood into the aorta to be dispersed throughout the body.
20. **(B)** The jellylike substance prevents the eyeball from collapsing inward.
21. **(A)** The endocardium is a smooth lining, which helps blood flow smoothly through the heart.
22. **(B)** The perineum is the external region between the vulva and anus in the female or between the scrotum and anus in the male and forms the pelvic floor.
23. **(C)** The greater trochanter is the ball-like head that articulates with the hipbone.
24. **(A)** The gluteus maximus is part of the hips and buttocks.
25. **(C)** Nephrons are responsible for the processes of filtration, absorption, and secretion.
26. **(D)** Normal urine has a low specific gravity.
27. **(B)** Aldosterone is released by the adrenal cortex in response to decreased blood volume, decreased blood sodium ions, or increased potassium ions.
28. **(A)** Water plus creatinine and urea, which are nitrogenous wastes, are normal substances in urine.
29. **(A)** The left motor control center in the brain controls the right side of the body because of the crossing of the nerve tracts within the brain.
30. **(B)** When the water intake is excessive, the kidneys excrete generous amounts of urine; if the water intake is lost, they produce less urine. The process is regulated by hormones.

UNIT XIII: READING COMPREHENSION

Please Review Unit IV, Pages 263–290, Before Completing This Section.

READING COMPREHENSION TESTS ANSWER SHEET

TEST 1

1. Ⓐ Ⓑ Ⓒ Ⓓ
2. Ⓐ Ⓑ Ⓒ Ⓓ
3. Ⓐ Ⓑ Ⓒ Ⓓ
4. Ⓐ Ⓑ Ⓒ Ⓓ
5. Ⓐ Ⓑ Ⓒ Ⓓ

TEST 2

1. Ⓐ Ⓑ Ⓒ Ⓓ
2. Ⓐ Ⓑ Ⓒ Ⓓ
3. Ⓐ Ⓑ Ⓒ Ⓓ
4. Ⓐ Ⓑ Ⓒ Ⓓ
5. Ⓐ Ⓑ Ⓒ Ⓓ
6. Ⓐ Ⓑ Ⓒ Ⓓ

TEST 3

1. Ⓐ Ⓑ Ⓒ Ⓓ
2. Ⓐ Ⓑ Ⓒ Ⓓ
3. Ⓐ Ⓑ Ⓒ Ⓓ
4. Ⓐ Ⓑ Ⓒ Ⓓ
5. Ⓐ Ⓑ Ⓒ Ⓓ
6. Ⓐ Ⓑ Ⓒ Ⓓ

TEST 4

1. Ⓐ Ⓑ Ⓒ Ⓓ
2. Ⓐ Ⓑ Ⓒ Ⓓ
3. Ⓐ Ⓑ Ⓒ Ⓓ
4. Ⓐ Ⓑ Ⓒ Ⓓ
5. Ⓐ Ⓑ Ⓒ Ⓓ

TEST 5

1. Ⓐ Ⓑ Ⓒ Ⓓ
2. Ⓐ Ⓑ Ⓒ Ⓓ
3. Ⓐ Ⓑ Ⓒ Ⓓ
4. Ⓐ Ⓑ Ⓒ Ⓓ
5. Ⓐ Ⓑ Ⓒ Ⓓ

READING COMPREHENSION TESTS

TEST 1: READING COMPREHENSION

5 QUESTIONS • TIME—8 MINUTES

Directions: Following the passage below, you will find a number of incomplete statements about the passage. Select the word or expression that most satisfactorily completes each statement. Blacken the corresponding space on your answer sheet.

How can we know that the birds we see in the South in the winter are the same ones that come north in the spring? John J. Audubon, a bird lover, wondered about this. Every year he watched a pair of little phoebes nesting in the same place. He wondered if they were the same birds and so decided to put tiny silver bands on their legs. The next spring back came the birds with the bands to build their nests on the walls of farm buildings in the neighborhood. The phoebe, it was learned, wintered wherever it was warm enough to find flies. In summer, phoebes could be seen from Georgia to Canada; in winter, anywhere from Georgia to Florida and Mexico. The phoebe was the first kind of bird to be banded, and Mr. Audubon was the first birdbander. Today there are thousands of birdbanders all over America, people who band all kinds of birds.

The government of the United States has a special birdbanding department that makes all the birdbands. The bands do not hurt the birds because they are made of aluminum and are very light. They come in different sizes for different-sized birds. Each band has a special number and the words, "Notify Fish and Wildlife Service, Washington, DC." Anyone who finds a dead bird with a band on one of its legs is asked to send the band to Washington with a note telling where and when the bird was found. In this way naturalists add to their knowledge of the habits and needs of birds.

1. The title below that best expresses the main theme or subject of this selection is

   (A) The Migration of Birds
   (B) The Work of John Audubon
   (C) The Habits and Needs of Birds
   (D) Studying Bird Life Through Birdbanding

2. According to the selection, Audubon proved his theory that

   (A) birds prefer a diet of flies
   (B) birds return to the same nesting place each spring
   (C) silver is the best material for bird-bands
   (D) phoebes are the most interesting birds to study

3. Audubon's purpose in banding the phoebes was to

   (A) satisfy his curiosity
   (B) notify the government
   (C) start a birdbanding department
   (D) gain fame as the first birdbander

4. The migration habits of phoebes depend upon

   (A) nesting places
   (B) the help of bird lovers
   (C) the available food supply
   (D) the number of young birds

5. Which statement is true according to the selection?

   (A) Residents of Georgia may expect to see phoebes all year long.
   (B) The weight of a band causes a bird considerable discomfort.
   (C) The government offers a reward for information about dead birds.
   (D) Phoebes are more plentiful in the East than any other kind of bird.

TEST 2: READING COMPREHENSION

6 QUESTIONS • TIME—10 MINUTES

Directions: Following the passage below, you will find a number of incomplete statements about the passage. Select the word or expression that most satisfactorily completes each statement. Blacken the corresponding space on your answer sheet.

It is important to understand just what we mean when we talk about stress, and theoretical definitions of stress abound. Probably the best definition was offered by the renowned stress researcher Hans Selye, who summarized stress as ". . . any bodily change produced as a response to a perceived demand being placed upon the individual." This definition highlights the notion that there are two important facets to stress: the psychological (or menial) and the physiological (or physical).

Stress can be typically negative events, called "distress," as well as the more positive happenings in life that nonetheless demand change and adjustment. After a demand is perceived, bodily or physical changes occur as a reaction. These biological responses typically include increased heart rate, respiration rate, blood pressure, and muscular tension, shallow (rather than deep) breathing, and the increased release of certain so-called stress hormones such as adrenaline and cortisol.

Such bodily changes occur for what is commonly known as the "fight-or-flight" response. The fight-or-flight response served a purpose ages ago, when acute, sudden stressors such as animal predators immediately threatened a person's existence. Successfully fighting off or fleeing from the threat greatly increased one's chance of survival. And, as with other creatures, our fight-or-flight stress reaction became "wired in" as a protective mechanism.

Stress continues to serve us today, as mild to moderate levels of stress can sharpen our alertness and motivate positive growth, spur the need to accept challenges, and promote change in our lives. Stress becomes a problem only when you consider the nature of some of our stressors. Unlike the saber-tooth tigers of long age, today's stressors tend to be more chronic in nature. Most people struggle with the demands of health problems, interpersonal difficulties, financial worries, and negative or critical self-imaging, to name just a few. These concerns have a propensity to stick around. When you begin to experience any one of them, your body reacts with predictable changes. However, because these stressors usually stay around and dominate parts of our existence for long stretches of time, the bodily changes that get "turned on," stay "turned on," which can cause or influence numerous undesirable consequences.

Chronic stress can contribute to such physical problems as migraine headaches, lower back pain, ulcers, digestive disorders. TMJ (temporomandibular joint) syndrome, suppressed immunity, and, of particular concern to people with diabetes, difficulty controlling blood sugar. There is even some evidence that cardiovascular disease, high blood pressure, and certain types of cancer can be adversely affected by stress. Chronic stress also appears to contribute to many psychological and behavioral disorders such as depression anxiety disorders, and low self-esteem.

Everyone attempts to cope with the stress in their lives, whether they do so consciously and deliberately or not. Unfortunately, many of the strategies people use to deal with stress actually produce additional sources of stress. Overeating, excessive alcohol consumption, cigarette smoking, and drug use are examples of stress management attempts gone awry.

Any effective strategy of stress management needs to do more than just distract you from that which is causing the stress. It needs to address both the physical and the psychological aspects of stress. To efficiently deal with stress, you must first get to know yourself and observe how stress tends to affect you, both physically and psychologically.

"Women and Diabetes: Strategies for Handling Stress"

1. According to Hans Selye, stress is stimulated by a(n)

   (A) environmental change
   (B) bodily change
   (C) perceived demand
   (D) physiological and psychological conflict

2. The physiological symptoms of stress are a result of

   (A) secretion of adrenalin and cortisol
   (B) suppression of adrenaline
   (C) accumulation of cortisol
   (D) absence of adrenaline and cortisol

3. The main problem presented by stress in Diabetics is the

   (A) blood sugar rises
   (B) blood pressure drops
   (C) immune system is suppressed
   (D) stomach develops ulcers

4. The theoretical basis for the effects of stress is based on the

   (A) interaction of the physiological and psychological self
   (B) interaction of the self with the environment
   (C) relationship between change and coping
   (D) relationship between change and growth

5. An effective method of coping with stress would be

   (A) focusing on the pleasure of eating
   (B) inducing relaxation by drinking alcoholic beverages
   (C) delaying stopping smoking
   (D) adapting to change

6. According to this passage

   (A) stress causes cancer
   (B) stress can be controlled
   (C) all stress is harmful
   (D) all stress is continuous

TEST 3: READING COMPREHENSION

6 QUESTIONS • TIME—10 MINUTES

Directions: Following the passage below, you will find a number of incomplete statements about the passage. Select the word or expression that most satisfactorily completes each statement. Blacken the corresponding space on your answer sheet.

Since 1910, more American women have died of heart disease than of any other cause. But for most of this century, physicians and researchers treated heart disease almost exclusively as a man's problem. When the American Heart Association held its first public conference for women in 1964, it focused on how women could help protect their *husbands'* hearts.

How could doctors and scientists overlook such a clear threat to women's health for so long?

For many years, heart-disease researchers concerned themselves primarily with *premature* heart attacks—heart attacks that strike down the young or middle-aged rather than the elderly. When women get heart disease, however, they tend to develop it 10 to 15 years later than men; thus, they are more likely to have heart attacks when they are past middle age.

For much of their lives, the sex hormone estrogen offers women substantial protection from heart disease. Only around age 55 does the rate of heart disease in women start to climb, both because estrogen levels drop after menopause and because other risk factors for heart disease become more common at the same age.

The age difference makes heart disease appear a more dramatic problem in men than in women; it's somehow more shocking when a heart attack hits a 50-year-old than when a 65-year-old is the victim. Indeed, the fact that men develop heart disease earlier than women means the disease may have a greater impact on their lives, and offers some justification for putting a greater emphasis on studying heart disease in men than in women. But until recently, researchers have done much more than that: They have systematically and almost completely excluded women from studies of all aspects of coronary heart disease.

One major heart-disease study did include women in virtually equal numbers with men, but the data were misinterpreted in a way that actually added to the confusion over women's risks. The Framingham Heart Study has been following more than 5000 men and women since 1948 to chart the causes and course of heart disease. Among other factors, the researchers identified people with chest pain, and assumed that they were suffering from angina, a symptom indicating that narrowed coronary arteries are supplying inadequate amounts of oxygen to the heart muscle.

Angina often precedes a heart attack. But in the mid-1950s, the Framingham researchers found that men with chest pain were much more likely than women with chest pain to have a heart attack within five years. They concluded that heart disease was simply not much of a threat to women.

There are two problem with that conclusion. First, many women with chest pain turn out not to have angina at all. A major study published in 1982 revealed that fully half of all women with chest pain who underwent coronary angiography—an X-ray procedure for visualizing the arteries of the heart—did not have blockages. (The same was true of only 17 percent of the men.) And second, in the 1950s most of Framingham's women were still too young to be at high risk for heart attack. A later analysis of the Framingham data showed that heart disease in women develops more gradually than in men. Women are more likely to experience angina for an extended period of time before suffering a heart attack.

Clinical trials—studies that test the effects of different treatments on a disease, rather than simply trying to understand the factors that lead to illness—have also tended to exclude women. Investigators have traditionally steered clear of testing any new treatments on women of childbearing age to avoid the confounding effects their hormonal cycles might have on test results, and to avoid unwittingly exposing a fetus by giving a drug to a woman who doesn't yet know she is pregnant. Many researchers have also excluded people over age 65, the age when women have the greatest heart-disease risk, out of concern that other illnesses in these older people would muddy the data. In clinical trials conducted over the past 30 years to evaluate treatments for heart attack, fewer than 20 percent of the total 151,000 subjects were women, according to a recent analysis in the Journal of the American Medical Association.

As a result, physicians have proceeded on the assumption that a treatment tested in men will work about equally well in women. Not necessarily. It is now clear, for instance, that the drug propranolol (*Inderal*), a beta-blocker commonly prescribed for high blood pressure and angina, is broken down far more slowly in women's bodies—an important consideration for dosage. Moreover, the potential of estrogen treatment to prevent heart disease in post-menopausal women is only now being tested in large clinical trials.

In 1985, the U.S. Public Health Service Task Force on Women's Health Issues ordered the National Institutes of Health to include more women in research, particularly research on heart disease. After several years of foot-dragging, the NIH established an office to ensure that women are appropriately represented in NIH-funded studies. Several large-scale clinical trials including women are now in the planning stage or underway. The clinical trial portion of the Women's Health Initiative—a $600 million, 14-year effort—will study the effects of a low-fat diet and hormonal therapy in preventing cardiovascular disease (as well as cancer and osteoporosis). It may be many years, however, before the decades of neglect are overcome.

"Heart Disease: Women at Risk"

1. The theory that estrogen protects women from heart disease is supported by the fact that
   (A) The rate of heart disease in women drops after age 55.
   (B) The rate of heart disease in women increases after age 55.
   (C) The incidence of heart disease in women is far less than in men.
   (D) Only post-menopausal women have heart disease.

2. Physicians and researchers have placed emphasis on heart disease in men more than women because
   (A) men develop heart disease earlier than women
   (B) more men die from heart disease than women
   (C) men are more prone to heart disease than women
   (D) men respond to treatment more readily than women

3. When comparing the occurrence of angina in men and women
   (A) angina often proceeds a heart attack in men
   (B) angina usually proceeds a heart attack in both men and women
   (C) the occurrence is more frequent in females
   (D) the occurrence is less frequent in males

4. The age when women are at greatest risk for heart disease is
   (A) 45–50
   (B) 50–55
   (C) 65–70
   (D) 70–75

5. It is important to conduct clinical research on both men and women because
   (A) preventative techniques are the same for both men and women
   (B) age differences in occurrence of heart disease indicate differences in causes
   (C) physiological differences lead to differences in responses to treatment
   (D) the impact of heart disease on an individual's life is the same for men and women

6. The focus of the NIH clinical trials for Women's Health Initiative is to study the
   (A) relationship between the aging process and the occurrence of heart disease
   (B) factors that lead to high risk for heart disease
   (C) female responses to drugs used to treat heart disease
   (D) effects of diet and hormonal therapy on prevention of heart disease

TEST 4: READING COMPREHENSION

5 QUESTIONS • TIME—8 MINUTES

Directions: Following the passage below, you will find a number of incomplete statements about the passage. Select the word or expression that most satisfactorily completes each statement. Blacken the corresponding space on your answer sheet.

Can creativity evolve with aging—maybe even flower with aging? If you belong to the "can't teach an old dog new tricks" school of thought, you may think that unless you have been an artist or writer or musician your whole life you are unlikely to be one in midlife—that increased creativity isn't compatible with growing old.

But research into fields as varied as neurology, behavioral science and art history says otherwise. So do the thousands of people who are finding that different types of creativity can accompany aging.

There is the artistic creativity of people like Bill Traylor, a folk art painter who did not pick up a paintbrush until he was 85 years old.

There is the exhilaration of the 81-year-old whose late-life burst of creativity led to her discovery of literature, a discovery she felt changed her life.

Then there is social creativity, a deftness with interpersonal relationships, that older people, the keepers of the culture, have traditionally offered.

The point is not that every older person can or should be a Picasso, but that aging precludes neither productivity nor creative energy. Moreover, creative capacity after age 65 is considerably more common than most people realize.

Creativity at older ages is not just a matter of anecdote; science has shown that the potential for intellectual growth with aging has biological underpinnings. Studies of the brain show that, in response to a more stimulating or challenging environment, brain cells sprout new extensions, improving their communication with other brain cells.

The same studies, along with behavioral research, indicate that brain cells respond to mental exercise just as muscle cells respond to physical exercise. Science, in short, supports the maxim "use it or lose it" when it comes to the aging brain.

There are several ways of categorizing the creative impulses of older persons:

- creativity that continues with aging;
- creativity that commences with aging;
- creativity that changes with aging;
- creativity in response to late-life loss.

There are famous examples of older people exuding creativity throughout their lives—Picasso experimenting with new styles of painting in his 90s, Verdi composing new operas in his 80s, George Bernard Shaw writing new plays in his 90s.

"Contemplating Creativity" by Dr. Gene Cohen
Reprinted with permission from AARP Bulletin, *April 1997*

1. According to this passage, the relationship between aging and creativity can be

   (A) direct
   (B) indirect
   (C) mutually exclusive
   (D) unpredictable

2. Bill Traylor is an example of which one of the following types of creativity?

   (A) composing music
   (B) social creativity
   (C) literature discovery
   (D) folk art painting

3. A theoretical basis for creativity at older ages is

   (A) intercommunication among brain cells expands in response to physical exercise
   (B) intercommunication among brain cells expands in response to stimulating environments
   (C) intellectual growth increases in the aging brain
   (D) intellectual growth decreases in the aging brain

4. According to this passage, one would expect to see more creativity in the aged when the person
   (A) is a bus driver
   (B) works with embroidery
   (C) is a teacher
   (D) is a bird-watcher

5. Which one of the following statements is true?
   (A) All aged people are creative
   (B) Only people who have been creative in younger life can be creative in older life.
   (C) The first sign of creativity may occur in older life.
   (D) Only one type of creativity is seen in aged people.

TEST 5: READING COMPREHENSION

5 QUESTIONS • TIME—9 MINUTES

Directions: Following the passage below, you will find a number of incomplete statements about the passage. Select the word or expression that most satisfactorily completes each statement. Blacken the corresponding space on your answer sheet.

A nearby flow of water is a very convenient place to dispose of waste materials, and people have been doing this for many years. If the right chemicals are dumped into the water, it can be beneficial. Lakes tend to follow a course from being deep, clear, nutrient-poor lakes to becoming shallow and more productive nutrient-rich lakes. This is the natural course of most lakes, and the addition of chemicals such as phosphates and nitrates can actually accelerate this process. To a certain extent, this is good, and it has been done intentionally in some cases: but when carried to extremes, it can Icad to a man-made natural disaster. The water produces so much algae that most other forms of life cannot exist, and the lake chokes to death. In most cases, factories and sewage drains have carried this addition of chemicals too far.

Another consequence of dumping waste material into waterways, especially lakes, occurs when the waste contains metals, such as copper. Some metals literally cover the lake bottom and kill off all the bottom-dwelling organisms. Since many of these organisms are responsible for the decomposition of organic material on the bottom, the removal of these animals results in a great deal of the organic material remaining undecomposed, and this decreases the nutrient content of the environment.

The dumping of waste materials from combustion into the air is quite obvious every time you look at the skyline of any major industrial area: Dumping poisonous materials into the environment has resulted in the destruction of many of our oxygen-producing plants and has driven many animals from our immediate environment. Another result that strikes perhaps closer to home is the increase in lung disease attributed to air pollution. Moreover, the propellants from aerosol cans cause problems by deteriorating the ozone layer of the atmosphere. This depletion allows greater amounts of ultraviolet radiation to reach the surface of the earth. This higher level of radiation reputedly causes an increase in skin cancer.

Both air and water pollution are a retaliation by nature to man's abuse. We assume that the dumping of wastes into the environment is a one-way process, and we do not count on any repercussions. But the cost of dumping garbage into the environment is slowly coming back to haunt us. Whether it be by the return of mercury and DDT to us in our food, or the destruction of shields in the atmosphere that protect us from being burned by the sun's radiation, we will pay for our assaults on the environment.

1. The title that best expresses the main idea of this section is
   (A) Save Our Lakes
   (B) Man's Responsibility Toward Nature
   (C) Air Pollution
   (D) How Pollution Causes Cancer

2. According to this passage, one of the negative results of dumping waste chemicals into lakes is the

   (A) increased growth of algae, which kills other organisms
   (B) discoloration of water
   (C) limitation of recreational activities
   (D) increased temperature in the water

3. Two causes of air pollution are

   (A) smoke and copper
   (B) aerosol cans and recycling of waste materials
   (C) decomposition of organisms and deoxygenation of plants
   (D) dumping of waste materials and use of aerosol cans

4. The author's attitude toward environmental protection is

   (A) complacency
   (B) pro-conservation
   (C) indifference
   (D) apathetic

5. The author's reference to the driving of animals from our immediate environment implies

   (A) migration
   (B) extinction
   (C) destruction
   (D) poaching

READING COMPREHENSION TESTS ANSWER KEY

TEST 1

1. **D**
2. **B**
3. **A**
4. **C**
5. **A**

TEST 2

1. **C**
2. **A**
3. **A**
4. **A**
5. **D**
6. **B**

TEST 3

1. **B**
2. **A**
3. **A**
4. **C**
5. **C**
6. **D**

TEST 4

1. **A**
2. **D**
3. **B**
4. **C**
5. **C**

TEST 5

1. **B**
2. **A**
3. **D**
4. **B**
5. **A**

NOTES

NOTES

NOTES

NOTES

NOTES

NOTES

NOTES